Discovering
Optimal

JOSEPH GIBBONS

FOREWORD BY KARISSA KOUCHIS

Discovering Optimal

SHIFT YOUR NARRATIVE,
TRANSFORM YOUR HABITS,
BOOST YOUR ENERGY

Figure.1
Vancouver / Toronto / Berkeley

Cataloguing data is available from Library and Archives Canada
ISBN 978-1-77327-211-5 (hbk.)
ISBN 978-1-77327-212-2 (ebook)
ISBN 978-1-77327-213-9 (pdf)

Design by Naomi MacDougall
Author photograph by Kendra Ruth Photography

Editing by Steve Cameron
Copy editing by Jane Broderick
Proofreading by Marnie Lamb
Indexing by Stephen Ullstrom
Jacket artwork *Along the Way* by Rachel Albano, www.rachelalbano.com

Images of *Sinai Health Magazine* on p. 89 are reprinted with permission.

Printed and bound in Canada by Friesens

Figure 1 Publishing Inc.
Vancouver BC Canada
www.figure1publishing.com

Figure 1 Publishing works in the traditional, unceded territory of the xʷməθkʷəy̓əm (Musqueam), Sḵwx̱wú7mesh (Squamish), and səlilwətaɬ (Tsleil-Waututh) peoples.

FOR LAUREN, JAKOBY, AND ELIJAH.

Words on a page could never properly express the immense love and endless gratitude I have for you all. Lauren, you are the love of my life—this book would not be possible without your sacrifice, grace, and loving tenderness. Jakoby and Elijah, you are my greatest source of inspiration and joy—your humor, creativity, and boundless enthusiasm motivate me to approach life with levity and curiosity.

Contents

Foreword

IF YOU'RE LUCKY, at some point in your life's journey you'll be gifted with an opportunity to enhance your health or completely transform it—either by pure desire or by way of desperation. The great news? With that very opportunity comes the potential for a new kind of life. A life of vibrancy, healing, undeniable passion, honor, self-trust, and self-respect. Since you're reading this, there's a chance you're at this lucky turning point in your life. And if you are, know that it's not happening by accident. There's an incomprehensible intelligence—far beyond what the human mind can understand—that plays its part in shaping the challenges that lie before us. And contained within the sacred core of our challenges can be a lesson, and fertile ground for transformation.

You hold in your hands a book that has the capacity to help you radically awaken to the healthiest version of your physical, mental, emotional, and spiritual self. *Discovering Optimal* is an instruction manual for accessing a kind of health and well-being that is rarely discussed or taught in our society and culture at large. This book is truly a gift to our planet; it's a practical wake-up call about what it takes to transform our habitual patterns and behaviors so we can live steeped in joy, passion, and purpose with energy and health far beyond what we often think is possible.

As a civilization we've fallen asleep—running on autopilot unfazed by our less-than-optimal health and less-than-ideal happiness. The scary thing is this has become the new normal. People assume restless sleep, poor digestion, brain fog, anxiety, depression, low energy, low sex drive, moodiness, and even general sadness are simply normal. This couldn't be farther from the truth of how nature intended our vessels to be used.

We've been gifted the most incredible machine ever created—the human body. And it is our responsibility to optimally care for it so it can thrive (and therefore you can too). Do you remember what thriving looks and feels like? Under the stacking layers of exhaustion, stress, sickness, and disease it can be quite hard to reassociate to those early dreams that you created when you had all the health and energy you could ever desire. Reawakening these desires is important, and this book is part of your journey to getting there, I promise.

Do you remember what thriving looks and feels like?

The beautiful truth is the version of life you want, wants you back. But the way we've programmed ourselves to operate—and some of the beliefs we perpetuate—is preventing what we want from coming to us. Our role, as this book so eloquently outlines, is to identify our personal blocks and, with love, transmute them, open them, and break them down so that we can live our lives with the purpose, clarity, and energy that's inherent to our nature.

I could not be more thrilled that my dear friend Joseph has finally brought his life experience, learnings, and wisdom to the world in this way. I've had the pleasure of developing a meaningful friendship with Joseph through my work with Tony Robbins and have observed many years of his dedication and complete commitment to what he teaches. In these pages Joseph will lovingly guide you through the process of uncovering what no longer serves you, identifying your unique patterns and habits that restrict you, and highlighting the simple (yet sometimes difficult) choices you can make every day to honor your body, and your life—all to help you live out your purpose on this planet.

Please keep in mind, to get the full benefit from this book it will take radical responsibility. When it comes to our health and life there is no one to blame if you aren't living optimally (not even yourself!). However, the phrase "I own it. I will transform it." may be a supportive tool in your evolution. The truth is that nothing outside of us has ever had the power to shape our reality, even if we have let it be so in the past. So, it is officially time to take your power back, to put the responsibility for your wellness into your hands, and to ride the empowering wave of potential into the life that awaits you. With this book, and with Joseph as your guide, you will without a doubt ride that wave to the shore of optimal living.

The teachings, habits, and daily practices shared in this book have shaped and changed my life. It is an honor to be an ambassador for these teachings and for my dear friend Joseph, who is deeply congruent with his world and mission. Buckle up, your life is about to flip upside down for the better. Embrace it all.

KARISSA KOUCHIS
Speaker, Host, Self-Discovery Advocate
National Speaker for Tony Robbins

Introduction

YOU DON'T HAVE to stumble your way through life any longer.

I'm willing to bet that many of you reading this are tired from morning to night, that you "require" caffeine to start your day, and that you regularly struggle to get deep, restful sleep. Your endless to-do list and consistent stress have depleted you to the point of utter exhaustion. You're living below your capacity. And in some cases well below it.

The concept of waking up refreshed, having sustainable energy all day, and falling asleep easily might be a truly foreign concept to you, but it doesn't have to be. There's another path you can take, one that's both universal and specific. *Discovering Optimal* is designed to help you determine your unique blueprint for optimal health and wellness.

After working with thousands of people in workshops, lectures, seminars, conferences, and retreats, I've clearly realized that everybody wants some version of the same thing—they want *everything*! They want to wake up feeling rested; they want to have more daily energy; they want more time with their loved ones; they want to be stronger, more flexible, less stressed, and generally more satisfied with their life.

Here's the good news. If you have the willpower and are willing to do what's necessary to gain momentum and then sustain it, you'll discover that a brighter life exists for you. Joy and fulfillment are out there, and you deserve it!

Everything starts with the choices we make. Our choices are often rooted in a set of habitual practices—some good and others bad—that have been established over decades. To break free from undesirable habits, you need the courage to face your current behavioral blueprint and the discipline to implement the behavioral changes that are necessary to alter it.

It's not easy. In fact, it's downright difficult. But life hacks and fad diets aren't enough to fundamentally recharge your life.

As you will read, my journey to optimal health and wellness was anything but linear. Sometimes my lack of energy was due to external circumstances, and other times I was my own worst enemy. In the pursuit of my optimal life, my entire thirties were spent obsessively trying to discover the "golden formula" for boundless energy, consistent happiness, and youthful enthusiasm. The truth is there's no formula in existence that doesn't require deep introspection to understand, accept, and sometimes change the way you think of yourself and the world around you. This journey has forced me to face and challenge the paradigm and blueprint I'd been following for decades. In the process I had to dig deep and uproot long-held beliefs and discard anything that wasn't serving my life's missions.

Discovering Optimal will guide you through an introspective process that will reveal your unique health needs, recalibrate your internal physiology, realign your health and behavioral priorities, recharge your mind, and help with the implementation of strategies to revitalize your well-being.

Everything starts
with the choices we make.

WE ALL HAVE 168 hours in a week—and for many of us this never seems enough. How are we supposed to juggle work, sleep, family, socializing, and hobbies, and still find the time to eat right, exercise, and de-stress? It starts with the foundation.

Building a solid house requires a sturdy foundation—one that can handle a lot of pressure. The same is true of you. Your foundation must be made robust by the energy that's required to live your life. When you're tired, burnt out, and stressed, every task is a challenge. "Fatigue," former Green Bay Packers coach Vince Lombardi famously said, "makes cowards of us all."

When you're tired, everything seems more difficult. When you're energized, those tasks don't seem quite as challenging. It's no wonder caffeine is the most widely used psychostimulant in the world.[1]

If you're reading this book because you want consistent and sustained energy, then it must be derived from your own physiology. This may require a shift in your psychology and your habits. You must curate a life that results in more energy, not less.

Reflect for a minute on the children in your life (or in your neighborhood). Think about the ones who aren't glued to a screen and actually get outside and play. They are creative, funny, and have boundless energy and enthusiasm. Have you ever stopped to think about why this is? No? Then think about it now. Go ahead . . . I'll wait . . .

One of the reasons why children are energetic is that their bodies are performing closer to their intended design. Their physiology hasn't been subjected to decades of too much sitting, too little sleep, excessive stress, poor dietary and lifestyle choices, and managing an unmanageable to-do list.

The problem with this picture of energetic children is that, if they aren't careful, they're going to end up like most adults today: sick, tired, and sluggish. What a shame.

Our twenty-first-century world doesn't value rest and regeneration. It values irrational levels of productivity, endless to-do lists, and demanding schedules. In short, we've begun to value breadth rather than depth. And one of the tools we use to keep treading water in our modern-day world of more, more, more is stimulants.

Coffee, energy drinks, and soda can give you the burst you need to get through lengthy to-do lists and long days. But, unfortunately, the more you chase that euphoric, energetic feeling with those stimulants, the farther away you get from what we all desire: consistent energy! We tax our body all day and all night, inhibiting the natural circadian flow of hormones and enzymes that are designed to keep you stimulated and alert when required and relaxed and tired when it's appropriate.

The strategies outlined in this book are designed to work with you in the development of an optimal way of approaching your health and wellness. It all begins with increasing your energy level. Once we've done that, the rest is easy (or at least easier than it would otherwise be).

To achieve what you desire most, you must go beyond goal-setting. Your inner dialogue must change from "I want" to "I will," from "I'll try" to "I'll do," and from tomorrow to today. So, then, let's do it. *Today.*

In Part I of the book I'll share firsthand accounts of what's at stake if you don't manage your time and energy properly. I'll also help you to identify the obstacles that are impeding your ability to achieve more energy, better immunity, increased happiness, and deeper fulfillment in life. Identifying the obstacle isn't always easy; it may take some deep introspection if the repeated behavioral patterns stem from your subconscious.

Once your obstacles are determined, Part II will help you to uncover the "root" of your issue. For some, the root may be easy to determine; for others, it may be very difficult. If you have repeated and unwanted behavioral tendencies, then you haven't exposed the origin of your issue, which is why it has continually resurfaced in your life.

In Part III you'll learn how to optimize your energy, immune system, happiness, and purpose in life. You'll discover strategies that are scientifically proven to enhance your overall well-being and outlook.

Finally, in Part IV you'll choose the techniques and strategies that best fit your lifestyle. You'll curate an optimization plan that allows you to grow and evolve daily. Systematic increases in well-being help to ensure long-term and sustained success.

It May Get Worse before It Gets Better

Every time my wife and I do a deep clean or a purge of our house, we get to a point where the house is a disaster. There are clothes, boxes, and stuff everywhere. We inevitably ask why we decided to embark on this journey. Why today?

Continuing to shove items into closets and under beds seems, at that moment, the best choice. However, to achieve a clean and organized house we know that we must wade through the mess to reach our goal. The same is going to be true for you. The longer you've put off taking care of yourself—the longer it's been since you felt energetic and fully present— the more "clutter" you'll have accumulated. Meaning it's likely going to get worse before it gets better.

If that scares you, you can easily close this book and retreat to the same "comfortable" behaviors that led you here. But one thing I can guarantee: putting it off any longer will result in more internal clutter and disarray. The further delay could result in the development of a chronic condition or disease that doesn't allow for a full restoration. The time to start the restoration process was yesterday, but we'll settle for today.

Don't get down on yourself for not doing something sooner. Be proud of yourself for deciding to do something today. No one is perfect. You're

CAFFEINE AND YOU

We all love the burst of energy that caffeine provides. But that jolt of energy is due to an exogenous (from outside the body) substance and isn't sustainable. Over time it slowly changes your brain chemistry to the point where you require more and more caffeine to induce that "energetic" feeling.[2]

The physiology behind this is simple. In your brain you have adenosine receptors, and as adenosine builds up in your brain it binds to the receptors and induces sleepiness. This is great at bedtime but not as desirable during the day. When you feel a lull of energy and opt for caffeine in any form, the caffeine (which has a molecular shape similar to adenosine) binds to the brain's adenosine receptors and negates its ability to induce sleepiness. Bam! Energy! But our body doesn't give up its natural rhythms so easily. To combat the consistent buildup of adenosine, the brain makes more adenosine receptors.

So, if you regularly drink caffeine, you need even more to fill those new receptors, and eventually the cycle may continue to the point where you no longer feel any perky effects of caffeine.

Further, if you consume caffeine too late in the day it will cause sleep disturbances,[3] and, when combined with a stressful lifestyle, caffeine can negatively impact your hormone-releasing adrenal glands (which help regulate your immune system and your stress response), causing fatigue in that organ and a lowering of overall function.[4]

It should be noted that coffee isn't necessarily a bad thing. In fact, for people who consume it in moderation—less than 400 mg of caffeine per day[5]—there are a lot of potential health benefits, such as the high amount of antioxidants,[6] lower incidence of type 2 diabetes and cardiovascular disease,[7] and for my slightly constipated friends . . . it gets things moving.[8]

The caffeine content of drinks (coffee, soda, tea, etc.) varies dramatically. You might have as little as 2 mg in a cup of decaffeinated coffee[9] and as much as 475 mg in an extra-large (Venti), blonde roast Starbucks coffee.[10] Thankfully, determining the caffeine content of your favorite drinks is easier than ever today because of the internet.

going to face setbacks. But be sure to celebrate the small wins, because, as you'll learn, you have to fight hard for each one of them. **So take a moment and celebrate your commitment to change.**

MY MISSION

Optimal health and happiness for me and my family—that's my most important life mission. While I innately understand that this will always be a moving target—one that requires patience, planning, anticipation, and the ability to continually adapt—because of the work I've done to acknowledge, understand, and address those behaviors, I now know the steps that are required to rid my life of unhelpful habits. As a result, I possess a deep understanding of what's necessary to keep us happy, healthy, and feeling our best selves.

My second mission is to help as many people as possible to enhance their overall vitality and wellness. That's why I've written this book.

What's your mission?

If you don't know the answer to this question, that's okay. However, I want you to start brainstorming ideas. Later in the book there's an activity designed to help you articulate your mission so that your subconscious brain doesn't flounder or become confused about its objective.

My missions serve as a guiding force in my life. Whenever I feel things drifting off course, I'm reminded of what my ultimate missions are and I quickly return home. I want the same for you.

PART I

Identifying the Obstacles

"Knowing yourself is the beginning of all wisdom."
—ARISTOTLE

W E ALL EXPERIENCE obstacles daily. For some, however, the obstacles have a significant impact on their ability to live with flow. The consistent compounding of stress on the body and mind with toxins, distractions, malnutrition, and lack of recovery, among other things, means that your physiology is always playing catch-up, never able to flow with ease.

It can be challenging to follow the recommended health advice, especially since it can be confusing to someone unfamiliar with this field of study. With the explosion in online health coaches and trainers, how are you to vet the advice you're bombarded with? Especially when the advice given is conflicting and contrary to what you've learned.

Self-education and the discovery of resources and people you trust is a positive step toward eliminating the confusion. In addition to using trusted resources, you must learn to master the language of your body. Each day, your body (and mind) provides clues as to what it needs more or less of. *Discovering Optimal* will help you to understand how to listen and decipher the language. To begin, you must become clear about the obstacles that have been impeding your ability to live optimally.

CHAPTER 1

The Painful Way I
Came to Find My Path

*"Take the opportunity to learn from your mistakes: find the cause
of your problem and eliminate it. Don't try to be perfect; just be an
excellent example of being human."* —TONY ROBBINS

BEFORE WE BEGIN, let me say that there's no magic elixir, secret diet, or new gym trend that will solve your problems. As I said in the Introduction, you can't achieve optimum wellness, happiness, and vitality without doing the uncomfortable work of looking within and challenging the preconceived notions you have about the way you live and function.

Take me, for example. While I've always pursued optimal health and wellness, I haven't always been successful at it. My pursuit sometimes yielded fantastic results and other times fell completely flat. This would often lead me to scratch my head and wonder why my health and energy fluctuated so much. With every bad day I'd obsessively try to find the answer as to why my energy was subpar or why I felt anxious and sick. I'd research voraciously and become consumed with finding the solution to my problem.

As time rolled on, and my health continued to deteriorate, I hurled myself into books, articles, and documentaries on nutrition, exercise, sleep, meditation, faith, supplements, alternative medicine, and on and on and on. It was through this process that I experienced some of my darkest days. I became confused as to how I could be doing so many of the positive things I was learning but still see a rapid decline in my overall wellness. So, in essence, I began writing this book for two reasons: desperation and hope.

I had become desperate. I'd been running my body, mind, and soul into the ground for years. I continued to draw from what I believed was an endless well of energy. I was grossly overworked, chronically under-slept, and helplessly unhappy. I took for granted my mind and body. I got up every morning and told it to grind again—no breaks, no rest, no complaining.

I failed to listen to my cues. My body was weeping and desperately needed me to pull back, rest, and recover. But instead, I punished it day after day until the inevitable happened. It broke.

You see, I grew up thinking that "doing it on your own" was a manly thing. It represented pride, and pride was good, right? When faced with a challenge or conflict, the voice in my head would say: I can do it alone—doing it alone builds character and it won't burden anyone else. No one needs to know what I'm going through; I'll just keep gritting my teeth and grinding on until I overcome this, or at least until whatever challenge I'm faced with passes—be it an excessive amount of work, a breakup, an illness, or even the loss of a loved one. I can do it alone. That became my motto in life.

This life approach worked well for the most part (at least to the outside observer). It helped me to get through graduate school, land my dream job, and marry my amazing wife. And, looking back at my history, there isn't much that I'd change, because the challenge of those things shaped who I am today. However, just as I've learned from the mistakes of people before me, you can learn from mine, and in the process save yourself a lot of unnecessary headache and heartache.

I desperately researched everything I could on food, supplements, spiritual practices, the subconscious mind, meditation, energy, sleep, nature, and Eastern medicine. My stubborn brain convinced me yet again that the solution was out there, just begging to be discovered. If I could tailor the perfect cocktail of nutrition, supplements, exercise, and what have you, then I wouldn't have to face the real problem: that my mind and body weren't just tired; they were utterly exhausted and incapable of rising to the next task I demanded of them. My way of life had been threat-ened by the collapse of my mental and physical health. So I prepared for that threat as earnestly as I could.

I recruited an army of health providers to help with this. At the head of my army was my naturopath, with whom I would consult several hours a week. Yet, no matter what I did, the enemy continued to advance. When this happened, I tweaked my strategy and pushed forward yet again, and again, and again. **I did this until I wasn't just exhausted; I was broken**.

BROKEN

If you've experienced a mental or physical breakdown yourself, then you know the despair, the exhaustion, and the immense stress associated with it. If that's you, and you're still trying to claw your way back to some semblance of positive health, you can save a large amount of time by learning the techniques that have worked for me (and for the many others who came before me). However, if you're currently experiencing a breakdown, please seek professional help to begin your healing process. To complement your professional guidance, begin to implement the strategies in this book that resonate with your lifestyle, goals, and abilities. And if you haven't broken, let's aim to keep it that way!

Given the unreasonable demands our modern world places on us, it's obvious that there will be many, many people dealing with the ramifications of burnout and persistent exhaustion. The scariest part of breaking down for me was not knowing the repercussions. If your body or mind has reached its limit, you've now made yourself susceptible to your familial gene pool. As you'll soon see, my third breakdown led to a mental health issue for which there's no known cure—and is one of the reasons why I chose to learn as much as I have on health, wellness, energy, and vitality.

Whether you're currently being overtaxed in the physical, mental, or emotional realms, the outcome is the same: detrimental health and the potential for chronic conditions or disease. Please read about my breakdowns, take them as a cautionary tale, then learn (and implement!) the strategies I've used to achieve optimal health and vitality for myself.

April 15th, 2010

It was a Thursday afternoon. I stood in front of my Programming for Diverse Populations class at Algonquin College in Ottawa, Ontario, ready to give my final lecture of the week. Suddenly, as I began to speak, it felt as if someone flicked off a light switch in my head. That may sound confusing, but it's the only way I can describe what it felt like. I opened my mouth to address the class, but there was just one problem: nothing I said was coherent—I'd lost the ability to talk. Noise came out, but I couldn't form words properly. After a few moments of gibberish, I commanded my mouth to speak the words in my head, but it refused. Standing there, dazed and confused, I made several more attempts to autocorrect this odd problem and speak a coherent sentence. **What on earth was happening to me?**

After what seemed like an eternity in front of my students, I got just enough words out to tell them that class was canceled. I apologized, walked out of the college, and headed straight home.

For context, the eight months preceding my inability to speak in front of my class, I worked in the exercise physiology lab at the University of Ottawa 26 hours per week, started my teaching career at Algonquin College, where I taught eight courses, and had a personal training business that I ran out of a local gym. I worked seven days per week and averaged less than four hours of sleep per night. On top of all that, my girlfriend of six years had broken up with me. She provided no explanation and showed no empathy. She simply disappeared from my life one day, leaving me confused and in despair.

How did I deal with that? I did what came naturally: I dove headfirst into my work and ignored every other dimension of health. My physical, nutritional, social, and mental health all suffered. Balance ceased to exist. Around the six-month mark, my extreme lack of self-care began to manifest in bizarre physical issues. Out of nowhere, all of the acne that I'd had as a teenager came roaring back, I started to get small white flashes in the corners of my eyes, and one of my testicles began to consistently throb. (That sentence was more awkward for me to write than it was for you to read, I promise.)

So what did I do? I got medication for the acne, an eye exam for the spots, and a testicular exam for the throbbing. Not once did my overworked brain consider the fact that my body was tapped out of resources due to the lack of compassion I was showing it. Surely there had to be a way to continue grinding my way through work while finding a path to physical recovery and the resolution of my newfound ailments.

Thankfully, the sudden mental vacancy I experienced in front of my students happened toward the end of the semester and I made it through my contracts at both the college and the university. Then I had only to focus on my training business—and I slowly began to recover. If this had happened mid-semester, I surely would have tried to "man up" and the consequences would have been much worse.

Does any of this sound familiar to you? Do you avoid dealing with difficult-to-manage areas of your life by overindulging in one space in order to have some semblance of control?

It isn't uncommon, and don't blame yourself if this pattern of behavior describes your tendencies. When reflecting on your own decisions, try to stay clear of judgment. There's a host of internal and external reasons why someone acts the way they do. We aren't here to critique our past. We're here to acknowledge our past and understand and accept that parts of our blueprint serve us well while others don't. Simple as that.

November 11th, 2016

To make a long story short, there were a few things at play here. First, my hopes of surprising my girlfriend, Lauren, by whisking her away for a romantic weekend so I could propose to her were dashed by a music gig she had and was unable to cancel. Second, it was Remembrance Day (Veterans Day to my American friends). My mother, whom I loved dearly, had died seven months before and, in typical fashion, I'd done everything in my power since her death not to grieve. You see, back then I didn't cry, I didn't share my emotions, and I wouldn't tell the truth about how I was doing; instead, I'd shrug my shoulders, say I was fine, and carry on.

However, watching the tributes to the fallen soldiers, and the emotion behind them, caused a guttural reaction of sorrow in me. The reality of my mother's death and all the emotions I'd pushed deep inside rose to the surface in a sea of confusion and tears. So how did I decide to deal with this? I concluded that the best course of action would be to have some drinks, hang out with friends, watch my beautiful girlfriend sing, and wake up the next day as if I'd never had an emotional breakdown—one that was 21 months in the making (since hearing of my mother's stage 4 cancer diagnosis on February 13th, 2015).

With Lauren's gig now over, I was drunker than I'd been in years, and we headed home (after a quick stop to fill my stomach with multiple Big Macs—yes, multiple). I knew that the next day I'd feel terrible, but at least it would just be a hangover, something that would pass. I could then push my emotions back where they belonged, stuffed deep inside (probably beside that piece of gum my parents had convinced me would stay in my stomach for years).

Yes, I was hung over the next morning, very hung over in fact. But this time was different. My jaw felt like I'd gone 12 rounds with Mike Tyson. I ground my teeth so badly while sleeping that any movement of my jaw caused extreme pain. Lauren lovingly coddled me with comfort food and laughter; she assured me that I'd feel better the next day. She was right, sort of. Although the headache and urge to vomit were gone, the jaw pain wasn't.

Over the next two weeks I spent my days consciously avoiding what had taken place on November 11th—the fact that my body and mind were finally processing my mom's death. However, with the emotional flood-gates now open, my body went through a grieving purge every time I slept, since that was the only time I'd let my guard down. I was tormented in my sleep and woke up each morning as if all the great boxing heavyweights of the past had joined Tyson for a few jabs and uppercuts.

Finally, I took Lauren's advice and saw a psychologist. For many, going to a psychologist might be an easy thing, but for me it was very difficult. A few years earlier I had seen a psychologist for just one visit. I went to him because I lost my best friend to suicide in June of 2013. I was tormented to the point of sleeplessness by how I could have saved Andrew. I researched hard and finally found someone I thought I'd feel comfortable sharing my pain with. After I explained to him what had happened and how Andrew had died, he said to me, "There's a special place in hell for people who commit suicide." *What*?! These are the words of a trained professional? I quickly left, never to return. That's it, I thought: this confirms that deal-ing with things on your own, quietly, is the best method. This experience kept me from talking to anyone about his death for years.

Snap back to 2016, and I knew that not all psychologists were like the one I saw to help me grieve for Andrew. However, I still feared going. What would I have to say and how would it make me feel? To protect myself, I initially treated my sessions like research, with a pen and pad, ready to jot down the steps needed to make these bad feelings go away. I went in looking for the secret formula for making it all better.

"I'll follow your script to the letter if it will make the pain go away," I told the psychologist. But, as I came to realize, emotional health, grieving, and the heartache of loss don't work like this. She provided no secret formula, though she did help me to process my grief by slowly opening the emotional vault that I'd worked so hard to seal shut.

Think about a time when you had emotions bubble to the surface. Did you instinctually cram them back down? Did you have your own version of Keep Calm and Carry On the way I did?

Again, this kind of thinking is all too abundant in our society. As we go forward through this book, I'll occasionally share reflective exercises that will help you to snap out of this limited and self-harming mindset and instead focus on how to better serve yourself in times of immense need.

February 5th, 2017

Not quite three months out from my emotional breakdown over my mother's death, and about two months into my one-hour weekly sessions with my psychologist, I had the strangest and most worrisome breakdown of my life.

What was most alarming was that this breakdown took place during one of the happiest and most productive times of my life. I was engaged, I had a smooth start to a very busy semester at work, and I was getting a lot of great research done for a side business that I wanted to get off the ground. Life was good. I had largely given up caffeine and alcohol. I was exercising daily and eating well. My schedule was incredibly full, but I enjoyed it. I needed every day to be a productive one, so I planned my life to maximize my energy levels—that was the only way I'd succeed with any form of sanity.

And the plan was working!

January was great. In fact, my energy was so good that during a stretch of 12 straight working days I had just as much energy at the end of the day as at the beginning. That stretch even included a two-day personal training workshop and certification exam where I spent 14 hours each day teaching and testing candidates. Surely I should have been exhausted by the end of those days. But I wasn't. I felt great! Even though my life was grossly imbalanced in favor of work, I was happy, productive, and enjoying life; the planning of a healthy lifestyle to combat the rigors of a heavy schedule was paying off!

After that workshop I headed into another week of work, which brings us to Friday, February 3rd, two days before my breakdown. As usual, I got up at 5:30 a.m. to teach an 8 a.m. class. I worked all day, then went to my weekly ball hockey game from 6:30 to 9 p.m. From there I headed to downtown Toronto to watch Lauren and her band play. They finished at 1 a.m. and we got home about 3 a.m. (a nearly 24-hour day of continual mental and physical output—an all-too-often occurrence for me).

The next morning I got up early (rest is for the weak and unmotivated, right?) to take in back-to-back lectures on gut health at a local health-food store. Then on Sunday, February 5th, we headed off to meet Lauren's friends for brunch; this may seem insignificant, but since these people were new to me there was an elevated energy output required (as Brené Brown describes it, an "F'ing first time,"[1] which I'll expand on in Chapter 2, page 32). After brunch we went to a coffee shop to do a little work—then *bam!* Something hit me. All of a sudden, my head felt "off"—a little dizzy and a little disengaged. So we packed up and headed home. Nothing that a good night's sleep couldn't solve. Or so I thought.

The next morning the sensation was still there, and it had magnified. It was now much worse. I felt as if I was in a dream state, neither fully awake nor fully asleep. When in conversation with anyone, I felt completely disengaged. It was as if I was watching myself from the outside, robotically going through conversations with coworkers, students, and even family. I felt numb and apathetic toward everything.

Every conversation I engaged in felt like trying to solve a complex math equation (and I'm terrible at math). To get the desired outcome, which in those cases was a routine exchange of words (a simple conversation), I had to intently focus on every word coming from the speaker's mouth. I had lost the ability to passively listen to the words of the speaker and provide a coherent response. It was as if the neuron highway in my brain had a massive, 100-vehicle pileup. I could eventually get past the wreckage, but it took time—a lot of time.

When the symptoms were at their worst it felt as if the words coming from someone's mouth entered my brain one by one. Instead of hopping into a supercharged race car to go from their mouth to my brain, they opted for a slow and stubborn donkey. Each conversation left me feeling exhausted.

I avoided people as much as I could. And when I knew a conversation with someone had to take place, I pumped myself up for it. Even the briefest of conversations took all my mental energy. It would leave me frustrated and exhausted. I felt like my bedside lamp. Yes, my lamp. You see, the lamp beside my bed has 20 different light settings. If the brightest setting, at 20, represents being fully present—vibrant and energetic—then the events of February 5th brought me from a 20 to a 10 immediately; the light had become dimmer. With each passing day and with each conversation the light got a bit dimmer. My focus, attention, comprehension, and motivation were decreasing. It was as if the light in my brain was going out. Every day I feared what would happen if the light dropped to zero.

My sensations continued to get progressively worse. The light in my head was nearly off completely. I felt like a robot, devoid of emotion. Fearing the worst, I worked diligently to determine the cause. Was it purely mental, purely physical, or both? I went to multiple medical doctors. None of the experts had seen my symptoms before. A lot of caution was taken and multiple tests were conducted. I had an MRI, a 24-hour sleep-deprived electroencephalogram (EEG), five rounds of blood work, appointments with medical doctors, including endocrinologists, and several psychology visits, and nothing came back conclusive.

It wasn't until a year or so later that I was properly diagnosed. I had overworked my brain to the point of developing a depersonalization/derealization disorder, one that I live with to this day. Essentially my brain was doing a hard reboot to protect itself from my go, go, go lifestyle. My brain went into survival mode—it had shut down to protect itself.

YOU MIGHT BE asking yourself how I made it through those seven years without having even more breakdowns. It was as if I was walking a tightrope: if I didn't eat near perfectly, engage in the appropriate amount of exercise, and get adequate sleep (not optimal sleep, just adequate sleep to barely avoid breaking down), I'd begin to sway uncontrollably. My balance waivered for those seven years.

I learned the hard way that our bodies are not endless wells of energy that we can draw from whenever we want and expect no repercussions. There's always a price—and I've paid that price many times.

To feel as energetic and happy as the children in your life, you must manage your energy just as you would your finances. Failure to do so leaves you with progressively fewer and fewer resources, which results in less energy, joy, and vitality. And if you continue to take more than you replace, you'll force your brain and body to make sacrifices just to survive. In doing so, you're left vulnerable to diseases and infections that could ultimately kill you.

Even though this diagnosis has no cure, later in the book I'll explain how it's shaped my life for the better, how I use my depersonalization to my advantage. But before I was able to view this condition as a blessing, I worried incessantly about it. I thought to myself: it's now or never—without an immediate and holistic intervention I may never fully recover.

I finally surrendered to the reality that my current and future health required a deep and sustainable reboot—particularly with the long-held beliefs and tendencies of my subconscious brain. The decisions I'd made to that point had led to where I was, so a proper recovery strategy required that I recalibrate my physiology, retool my self-care strategies, engage and accept my spiritual self, and readjust the expectations I had of myself.

These weren't easy things to implement and I certainly stumbled along the way. Here's hoping you're starting from a baseline that's not as severe as mine was. But no matter where you're starting from on your journey to discovering your optimal self, you can trust the fact that people all over the world have come from similar backgrounds and experiences as you—and have taken similar steps and actions to recharge their life. You can do it!

I Walk down the Street

The breakdowns I've had, and the stumbles between those breakdowns, aren't what define me. While I'm eternally grateful that I have people around me who can help me get back on my feet, if I don't learn from my faults I'm destined to repeat them. One of my favorite poems is by Portia Nelson. It's titled "There Is a Hole in My Sidewalk: The Romance of Self-Discovery."[2] Without providing you with context as to how it's helped me, I want you to read it and decipher the message for yourself.

CHAPTER I
I walk down the street.
There is a deep hole in the sidewalk.
I fall in.
I am lost . . . I am helpless.
It isn't my fault.
It takes forever to find a way out.

CHAPTER II

I walk down the same street.
There is a deep hole in the sidewalk.
I pretend I don't see it.
I fall in again.
I can't believe I am in the same place.
But, it isn't my fault.
It still takes a long time to get out.

CHAPTER III

I walk down the same street.
There is a deep hole in the sidewalk.
I see it is there.
I still fall in . . . it's a habit . . . but,
My eyes are open.
I know where I am.
It is my fault.
I get out immediately.

CHAPTER IV

I walk down the same street.
There is a deep hole in the sidewalk.
I walk around it.

CHAPTER V

I walk down another street.

CHAPTER 2

Hard Truths

"Insanity is doing the same thing, over and over again, and expecting different results."—ALBERT EINSTEIN

I'VE DEDICATED MY life to finding ways to enhance my mental, physical, spiritual, and emotional being. I use that knowledge to improve my life—and I package that content to help my college and university students realize their full potential. Life has brought me to my knees on several occasions. After each knockdown I learned new skills and continued to refill my arsenal. With decades of schooling, research, and experience, I always knew that the achievement of my goals (optimal mind, body, spirit, and vitality) was very close, but there was always something holding me back. Once that something was discovered, my labor paid off in spades.

The missing component to my struggle was so simple that I'm sometimes hard on myself for not listening to my mom all those years ago. But then I quickly realize that if I'd listened to her I wouldn't have accrued the experience and information I use daily to help other people find their path to optimal health and wellness. **The missing link for me was rest.**

I obsessively worked on every other dimension of health while neglecting the warning signs that my body and mind needed to recharge and revitalize. Once life (and my wife) forced my hand and demanded that I rest, I made it my full-time job to do just that. And for months I rested.

For most of my life I viewed "rest" as unproductive time. So, at first, resting was very uncomfortable because it felt foreign to me. I had subconsciously trained my brain to associate "productivity" with tangible accomplishment, not with rest. But as time went on something incredible happened. By resting, I found that the other strategies I'd adopted from all my time researching and adapting my routines were finally beginning

I understand that many of you reading this may not be in a position to completely rest. That's why, throughout this book, I outline strategies for you to incorporate into your life so you don't get to where I was, where nothing except absolute rest would help. I'm fortunate to have summers off from teaching and to have a partner to help raise our children. I'm forever grateful for these things.

to pay off. My energy, mental clarity, vigor, vitality, and enthusiasm for life had skyrocketed. By resting, I flourished.

Considering how close I was (without even knowing it) to optimal health and wellness, I'm reminded of the story "Three Feet from Gold" included by Napoleon Hill in his famous book *Think and Grow Rich.*[1] It's the story of a man who was determined to cash in on the Colorado gold rush. He bought the necessary equipment and began mining. He was successful at first, but when the gold stopped coming he decided to quit and sell his equipment. He sold it all to a "junk man" for just a few hundred dollars. The resourceful junk man knew he couldn't do it alone, so he hired a mining engineer, who did some calculating for him. The engineer determined that the previous miners were off course by a mere three feet! This meant that if they had recalculated their mining direction or hired someone to help them determine where the gold vein was, they would have amassed a huge fortune. Instead, the gold went to the resourceful junk man.

The moral of the story for me is twofold:

1. Your goals, health, and ideal life might be closer than you realize.

2. When you encounter a roadblock to your goals, use your resourcefulness to find someone who can help you to navigate through it.

Commitment over Convenience

For most people, their current health is a direct reflection of the decisions they've made in the preceding days, weeks, months, and years. Now, of course, there are some people who will, unfortunately, develop certain physical diseases or mental health issues through no fault of their own;

they make great choices but fall victim to their genetics. That doesn't represent most people. Most people, knowingly or unknowingly, make decisions every day that bring them either toward or away from health and vitality. If you think that what happens in your life is a complete fluke, then you're going to end up a victim of ignorance.

It's apparent that far too many people die early from the choices they've made.[2] Some people are aware of their poor choices, while others are not. Consider the boiling frog fable. The premise is that if a frog is put into a pot of boiling water, it will immediately jump out. Conversely, if you put a frog in tepid water, then gradually increase the temperature, it won't perceive any danger and therefore will boil to death. The frog won't know that death is imminent until it's too late. This is true of people who are oblivious of the poor dietary and lifestyle choices they're making: **they're slowly boiling themselves to death**.

To avoid this, you're going to have to take responsibility for your life to ensure that you have the best possible chance of living with optimal health and vitality.

When trying to teach my clients or my students about behavioral change, I use the analogy of a person and a cliff. With each poor decision, be it the choice to continue smoking, drink too much, take drugs, not get enough sleep, or improperly deal with emotions, among a host of other bad decisions, you're taking steps toward the cliff's edge, toward the drop. That drop could mean cancer, heart disease, diabetes, depression, anxiety, and even death. How much your body (and mind) can handle before it can handle no more is dependent on numerous factors (genetics, comorbidities, access to care, and your nutrition, among others), but two things are certain: No one is immune, and everyone has their tipping point; this is the point of toxic exposure, where you've now opened yourself up to the repercussions of your choices.

Identifying Your Behaviors and Habits

"Knowing others is intelligence; knowing yourself is true wisdom. Mastering others is strength; mastering yourself is true power."—LAO TZU

Remember the feeling—this is perhaps the best teaching tool I can provide. If you're really motivated to learn how your behaviors and habits influence

CRISIS: DANGER OR OPPORTUNITY?

"Among other things, crisis represents opportunities to grow in wisdom. When you approach each crisis with this attitude you will pluck the opportunity out of each situation and benefit from it."–BOB PROCTOR

In life we all encounter challenging times. With each encounter we're given a choice: to dwell on what has taken place and live in the negative, or to find some good in what has happened and therefore move forward in a positive way. This doesn't mean that challenging times won't require time to grieve; but once the grieving has subsided, if you don't move out of the negative state, more of your life will be taken away from you.

You might be uncomfortable with where you are—perhaps you're very uncomfortable. But that just means it's the perfect time to make a change. In Chinese the word "crisis" has two symbols: one represents a time for danger and the other a time for opportunity. **You get to choose.**

Some people will see every challenge and crisis as a threat and therefore respond from a place of fear, desperation, and worry. Others will objectively acknowledge the crisis, then search for meaning, direction, and an opportunity to grow from it. If you're honest with yourself, which category do you fall into when crisis arrives?

your outcomes, energy, performance, and happiness, to name a few areas, then learning to recollect *how* you feel is crucial in the recovery and rejuvenation process. So, when you feel tired, happy, sad, angry, excited (or any distinct and elevated emotion) take a moment to reflect on the minutes, hours, or days preceding that moment. What was happening (or did happen) that might have contributed to your emotional or physical state?

It might not be one thing but many. And learning to pause and reflect meaningfully on your emotional and physical state as it relates to your behaviors and habits will enable you to uncover those things that are not serving you well on your path to optimal living. You'll begin to gain insight into what your body and mind need more or less of.

For example, if you drink alcohol, then you've likely had a hangover or two in your life. This is a perfect example of cause and effect. For most, it's very clear that when they consume too much alcohol it typically leads to exhaustion, brain fog, and headaches the next day.

The key is finding all the behaviors (food choices, amount of physical activity, sleep quality, etc.) and scenarios (work-related stress, people who bring you joy or anxiety, etc.) in your life that elicit responses from your body and mind that are both positive and negative. In time you'll learn to reduce the negative behaviors, properly prepare for stressful scenarios, and subsequently introduce more of the positive behaviors and people into your life.

While the link between alcohol and hangovers is very clear, the links between how you feel and other behaviors (poor diet, increased stress, limited deep sleep, and emotional distress, to name a few) are typically less understood. There isn't a formula that works for everyone, because our needs in the physical, nutritional, emotional, and spiritual realms are unique. Finding the right balance for you starts with discovering what does and doesn't work.

Sometimes there may be behaviors that you know will lead to an outcome that isn't desirable, yet in weighing the pros and cons you make the choice to continue that behavior anyway—and that's okay; the problem arises when you make too many of those poor choices, which compound and cause your health to continuously suffer.

The body is a very resilient entity, capable of cleaning up most of the mess you leave it with each day. But everyone and everything has its limits. Consistently pushing the boundaries means that your body is overworking. And what happens when we overwork? Eventually we crash.

Physiologically, when demand regularly exceeds capability, what's left is a pileup of waste and congestion in your hard-working organs.

Here are a few examples of what physiological "excess" can lead to within our bodies over time:

- Too much sugar = type 2 diabetes[3]
- Too much alcohol = cirrhosis of the liver[4]
- Smoking = lung cancer[5]
- Too much saturated fat = heart disease[6]

There are thousands of other links between what you chronically over-consume, or under-consume, and the health risks that come with those behaviors. And negative physiological outcomes are accelerated when combined with stress. In fact, it has been estimated that 60 to 80 percent of doctor's visits are attributed to stress-related ailments and complaints.[7] But, unfortunately, it has been found that only 3 percent of "visits included stress management counseling by primary care physicians."[8]

The way that stress permeates our mental and physical self demonstrates that nothing we do operates in a vacuum. You can't be broken in one area and not expect repercussions in another.

Helping people to recognize the barriers that impede the progress of their health and wellness isn't always easy. We all have daily habits and routines we'd like to see improved. Some of the biggest contributors to a person's discomfort and unhappiness are very apparent, while others are hidden and unknown to the individual. Have a look at the list of categories and determine where you reside due to your habits.

1. You have unhealthy habits that are distinct and obvious.

    Some individuals who reside in this category may be motivated to change their habits but each attempt is followed by failure and the eventual return to the negative behavior. Unfortunately, lack of success isn't always attributed to an absence of willpower or motivation. Many people in this category are extremely motivated yet the behavior continues to find its way back into their life.

    Imagine that bad habits are like weeds in a garden. A motivated person who's failing to achieve sustained success is likely ripping the weeds from the ground only to find that they keep "miraculously" popping up again. Motivation can take a person only so far. The reason why the weeds keep popping up is that the root problem hasn't been uncovered—in other words, people in this predicament haven't dug deep enough.

2. You have unhealthy habits but due to a lack of knowledge in the area, combined with "clever" marketing, you believe you're making a healthy choice.

    Big corporations employ an arsenal of tactics designed to make you look one way when the truth lies in another direction. It is corporate misdirection used to disguise the truth. The deception most often happens with our food. Much of what's advertised as wholesome and nourishing is filled with unhealthy, cheap, synthetic ingredients that pull you farther away from your desired destination of optimal health.

That's not to say all food advertised as wholesome and nutritious is junk pretending to be healthy, but buyer beware!

As an example, I grew up believing that having a muffin for breakfast was a smart choice, as many muffins are made with nuts and fruits. It seemed logical: muffin equals healthy. That was programmed into me and many others through a general lack of knowledge about nutrition, combined with commercials and clever packaging that highlighted what the food companies want you to notice: things like whole grains, fruits, and nuts. Even a 1988 L.A. Times article titled "Muffin Madness: Health Conscious Snackers Stir up New Yen for Old Favorite"[9] highlights the dichotomy of consumer perceptions (muffins are healthy) and nutritionists' understanding (muffins are unhealthy). And still, in 2023, you can find people assuming that muffins are healthy when we know, as UCLA nutrition professor Rosalyn Alsin-Slater told the L.A. Times in 1988, "Muffins are not a health food."[10]

If your bad habits are in this category, education is going to be your first tool. You don't know what you don't know, so where do you start? I'd suggest that you challenge your assumptions and objectively look at yourself from the outside, trying to notice clues to your habits that may require attention. You could take it a step farther: ask someone in your household if they know where your "muffins" exist—the blind spots that are keeping you from moving the health needle closer to optimal.

Throughout this book I provide some thinking for you on several health-related items that might help you to begin to challenge your assumptions and educate yourself.

3. Your bad habits are dressed in sheep's clothing.

If you reside in this category, it will take a little more sleuthing to root out the reason why you're not living in an optimal state. From the outside, your habits and routines appear generally healthy. However, if, like me, you're truly blind to the reasons why you can't quite achieve what it is you desire, you'll have to go deeper than those living with habits in the previous two categories.

For people in this category, there's a wolf lurking, ready to steal your happiness and joy. If you're anything like me, you can feel it. It will take a concerted effort and an open mind for people in this state to uncover the underlying habit stopping them from living optimally.

It may be that you need to reboot your mental and physical state in a radical way, just as I did. But if your missing link is uncovered and you put in the work to reset your habits, then those other positive health habits will finally be able to properly flourish, just as mine did.

Some people can listen to their mind and body and determine whether they've had too much of something. These people are able to then use their resolve and willpower to stop without issue. Others—or should I say most people?—struggle in certain areas to fight the temptation of one more TV show, one more drink, one more snack, or one more coffee. You know yourself very well, but this doesn't mean you won't lie to yourself from time to time.

People will do whatever they can to justify negative behaviors, because it's what they want in that moment. The occasional overindulgence may be fine, but you're here reading this book for a reason. You're looking for answers to why you're consistently tired, why you struggle to jump out of bed in the morning, why consistent happiness feels foreign to you, and why you don't feel truly fulfilled. You're ready to make a change and create a life system that correlates with the vision of yourself that makes you proud.

 ## Identifying Your Habitual Behaviors

The purpose of this exercise is to help you identify the habits and behaviors that are robbing you of the energy and vitality you crave. But the only way this will really work is if you're honest about yourself and you fully commit to this journey. There's a reason why you haven't done something about your behaviors yet (or if you have, there's a reason why your actions haven't stuck), and it's because doing something to change is harder than staying the course.

And if you've made efforts but haven't succeeded, that's a similar problem. Motivation isn't enough. The hard work of uncovering the root is where you need to focus your energy. The exercises that follow are the first of many in this book that will get you critically thinking about the choices you make. It's time to be courageous, let your guard down, and look at yourself objectively. What do you see? More importantly, what are you going to do about it?

In the table, circle all the unhealthy behaviors you engage in—the things you consume too much of (I never said this was going to be easy). Remember, not all of these are inherently bad, but, if not properly managed, that overconsumption or persistent indulgence can lead to an addiction. And if there's something else you think of, put it in one of the empty boxes.

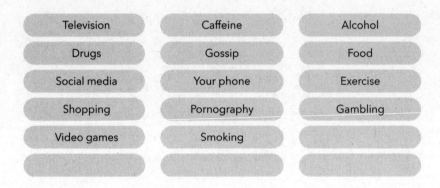

In relation to those things you've circled, ask yourself the following questions:

1. When you're finished with your overindulgence, how do you feel? Are you satisfied, upset, disappointed, content?

2. Can you live without it?   Yes / No

   If you answered No, explain why you can't live without it.

3. Project forward six months. Imagine you've abstained (or at least not overindulged); how does that make you feel?

By now you likely know whether you can develop a healthy relationship with your behaviors or if abstinence is the healthier route. Of course, there are certain things that can't be completely removed from your life. For example, if you have an unhealthy relationship with food, you can't just eliminate it; you must discover a new, healthier way for it to exist in your life. This is one of the reasons why eating disorders are some of the hardest disorders to treat.[11]

For those who can't realistically eliminate those habitual things that may lead to an addiction or disorder, it might be time to set up clearly defined boundaries and then enlist the help of family or friends to help you stay accountable. If your behavior is connected to a mental health condition, I urge you to contact a trained professional and begin healing as soon as possible.

"Identify your problems but give your time and energy to solutions."

—ANONYMOUS

The following table shows some of the issues I've struggled with and the solutions that I determined worked best for me (remember, just because it worked for me doesn't mean it's the best solution for you). Write your name in the blank spaces and then get critical about your issues and creative about your solutions.

Joseph's Issue	Joseph's Solution
Caffeine started to cause increased anxiety	Exercise first thing in the morning to get a more natural and sustainable influx of energy
Started each day in a reactive state (due to my kids dictating what time I got up)	Set my alarm for 90 minutes before my kids typically wake, and get up on my own terms
Watching "just one more show" and staying up late, which led to fatigue the next day	Purchased a TV power bar that automatically turns it off at 9 p.m.
Anxiety was increased when I had to rush	Prepare everything the night before

_____ Issue	_____ Solution

WHAT DO YOU (REALLY) NEED?

I'm an advocate of listening to your body. However, since our body gets used to routines, it grows to expect them. Just because a smoker craves a cigarette it doesn't mean their body needs it. Just because an alcoholic craves alcohol it doesn't mean they need it. The key is doing your research and/or finding trusted healthcare professionals and alternative health practitioners to help you determine what your body truly requires for you to live optimally.

I know I'm not the only person who's been told "breakfast is the most important meal of the day" at least a hundred times in their life. For decades I made sure I ate first thing in the morning. Due to the consistent regularity, my body was programmed to eat as soon as my eyes opened. Although my body was conditioned to crave calories at the beginning of the day, was this routine truly serving me? Yes and no. At certain stages in my life it certainly was, but at other times it may not have been.

Listening to your body is too broad a statement—it rings true in some cases but not in others. This is why education is your most powerful tool: it will help you determine, objectively, the habits you should alter.

F'ing First Time (FFT)

Researcher and author Brené Brown opened my eyes to the energy-draining and mentally taxing effects of doing something new for the first time.[12] Once I learned this, I became acutely aware of FFTs and the reason for my lack of energy the day after the event, task, meeting, or skill acquisition.

Not all FFTs are created equal. Some are very complex and time-consuming while others are short and relatively easy. The worst thing you can do for your energy and mental well-being is to batch FFTs together. For instance, if you're starting a new job where there's a steep learning curve, it probably isn't the best time to begin guitar lessons, learn a new language, or take on a home renovation.

As a family, we had one of our worst bouts of FFT batching when we moved to a new town. It was early September and the FFTs included me starting a new semester, Lauren beginning a new career, my elderly father moving in with us, the kids starting preschool (lots of tears in the first few weeks of drop-offs), starting home renovations, and meeting dozens of new people.

Learning about FFTs helped a lot. It helped to explain my exhaustion and showed that even small FFTs can seem daunting and draining when they're inserted into an unusually busy period in your life. We now actively anticipate FFTs—and if they're on the bigger side of the spectrum I make sure to incorporate the necessary rest following them.

For the record, FFTs are good! They help you to push the boundaries of your comfort zone, they help you to grow, and they help you to evolve. But, as with excessive exercise and emotional output, if you push too hard you'll move past the ability to quickly recover and will therefore suffer the consequences (exhaustion, burnout, and potential disease development).

It's time to be courageous, let your guard down, and look at yourself objectively.

CHAPTER 3

Burnout

*"Most people work hard and spend their health
trying to achieve wealth. Then they retire and spend
their wealth trying to get back their health."*

—DALAI LAMA

IT SEEMS THAT we've become addicted to work. In fact, many of us wear our overworking lifestyle like a badge of honor, equating it with success.

We've been taught that working hard is noble—that the more work you do, the more noble you become. Also, if you're required to work long hours, it's perceived that you possess characteristics that are in demand by employers. This is likely the reason why people like to tell you how hard they work—it proves that they aren't lazy and they're in demand. But as a society we're focusing on the wrong metrics to measure success and are attempting to achieve success from a severely disadvantaged position.

If we revisit our blueprint, dig deep into our ideological roadblocks, and learn to accept who we are and what we need, we can tap that potential inside us to achieve the things we deem important while inherently knowing when we reach our limits—and the dangers we face if we go over them.

Your Capacity for Work

Energy is simply the capacity to do. Some of us can do less than the average person, others more. However, we all have the *capacity* to do *more*. That might seem like an odd comment coming from someone who just told you about three breakdowns in the span of seven years, the last of which left him with an irreversible disorder. How can I be telling you that you have the capacity to do more? It's because of experience and education.

There's a general formula you must follow to progressively become stronger, smarter, and more capable. Whether your desires are mental or physical, you must employ recovery strategies that are in balance with the amount of work you're putting in. In addition, you must be acutely aware of when your mind or body is close to its breaking point and have the *will* and *fortitude* to pull away in order to prevent burnout and exhaustion.

The most difficult reality you might face is that just because someone else can, it doesn't mean that you can—at least not yet. Just because someone else can work 60 hours a week and manage with six hours of sleep per night it doesn't mean that you can. Just because someone else can safely exercise at a high intensity seven days per week it doesn't mean that you can. Self-awareness, self-restraint, and the desire to follow a healthy road map to success are paramount for the achievement of consistent growth.

Remember, you are your greatest experiment. If you have a curious mind and a desire for self-improvement, you'll tinker all your life in the pursuit of more energy, more capacity, more strength (mental, emotional, spiritual, physical), and more happiness and fulfillment. But be wise and learn to speak the language of your body (and mind)—a skill I'll help you learn in Part II.

What we know is that pushing a dimension of health too far will lead to excessive stress on the body or mind, and that's not good. Too much rest will lead to atrophy, and that's not good. So what's the correct amount of stress and the proper recovery that will lead to improvements? Well, when it comes to bolstering our physical, emotional, mental, and spiritual energy tanks, there's no universal formula that will work for everyone.

If you were to put me through a day in the life of a mixed martial arts fighter, a Fortune 500 CEO, or a stock trader, to name a few different professions, I'd likely end up exhausted. I simply wouldn't have the energy reserves, the muscular ability, the psychological strength, or the constant high-level attention span to endure what those professionals go through daily. I'd be able to do those jobs no more than I'd be able to be a line cook in a busy diner or an early childhood educator teaching a class of kindergartners.

Sure, I'd be coming to these endeavors as a fish out of water, but so are we all when we have our first forays in our professional lives. No one is born ready to take on the demands of their work and life; we become good at what we do by systematically adding more and more work incrementally so our body can continually recover and come back stronger.

Put another way, if you're the type of person who holds onto and suppresses your emotions, letting them all out at once will likely make you feel exhausted for days. Like a person who doesn't exercise much, if you haven't flexed your emotional muscles for a while, it won't take long to exhaust them. In all aspects of life, we must be conscious of our energy output and renewal. Essentially this means that you systematically plan your outputs and your recovery—and over time you'll have the capacity to give more energy to your pursuits because your tank is more robust.

" 'I'm too busy' just means 'I can't say no to the unimportant.'" —ROBIN SHARMA

Predicting Burnout

Our shift to overwork has not served us well. Currently there is no set of universal criteria for predicting if someone is heading toward a work-related burnout. However, according to researchers, there may be some predisposing factors that you should be aware of:[1]

- Extremely high expectations of oneself
- Extremely high expectations of one's work
- Poor stress tolerance
- Poor coping skills
- Lack of self-direction
- Socially strained work environment
- Vaguely defined job duties

Does any of that sound like you? The first two points sound like good virtues to have, don't they? Aren't we supposed to have high expectations of ourselves and our work?

I'd argue that we can, and we should, always put our best foot forward, so long as it doesn't lead to perfectionism and overwork. This distinction between being able to work within one's expectations and being aware of the pitfalls of how we operate is essential. If you're a perfectionist, this is something you'll want to address as you consider your capacity.

The Mayo Clinic proposes a series of questions that may help you to evaluate your work-related coping:[2]

1. Has your work made you cynical or critical?

2. Do you find you have to drag yourself to work and it's hard to get the day started when you get there?

3. Do your colleagues, customers, or employers annoy you?

4. Has your patience worn thin at work?

5. Do you suffer from low energy levels at work?

6. Do you find work disappointing?

7. Do you use food, drugs, or alcohol to feel better or to numb unpleasant feelings?

8. Have you noticed changes in your sleeping patterns or appetite?

9. Do you suffer from "unexplained" headaches, backaches, or other physiological ailments?

We all likely experience some of these things in the ebb and flow of our workweek, but if you are experiencing many of them simultaneously and often, that should be a red flag that you are overworked or are working hard at something that is unfulfilling. Either way, something needs to change for you. According to the authors of *Biohacker's Handbook*, biohackers have a manifesto as it relates to their work:[3]

1. Your work should be genuinely enjoyable and meaningful to you.

2. Aim for self-directed freedom at work—for example, regarding working hours.

3. Seek a positive and supportive atmosphere and a pleasant work environment.

4. Don't live to work; work to enrich your life.

5. Quality over quantity; impact over efficiency.

6. Allow yourself enough time for rest and recovery.

7. Take regular breaks and use them to get up and move.

8. One half of your working time should be about producing an output while the other half should be spent on input (making connections and learning new things).

9. Research and select the best tools for repetitive tasks.

10. Pay attention to posture, ergonomics, and working positions.

What is a biohacker? It's essentially an individual who aims to enhance or optimize their biology. They research, and use their findings to adjust their sleep, nutrition, supplements, exercise routine, brain health, and so on in a way that results in optimal performance in each of these areas.

Not everyone, at all moments in time, can genuinely enjoy the job they do that puts money in the bank and food on the table. And it goes without saying that many people struggle to make ends meet in jobs they don't enjoy. This is a travesty. For anyone in this situation, my advice is to find ways to achieve small wins at work that provide meaning for you and help to make your day fulfilling; also, I strongly encourage you to carve out time for yourself, outside of work, doing something that really gives you joy.

If you're lucky enough to have the freedom to implement some of the suggestions on this list, then I encourage you to review it every couple of months to see if there are elements of the manifesto that you can implement, or re-implement. Continually checking in with yourself is another important aspect of avoiding overwork.

"The Burn Is So Seductive"

Consider the following diagram, which was inspired by Neil Pasricha, author of *The Happiness Equation*.[4]

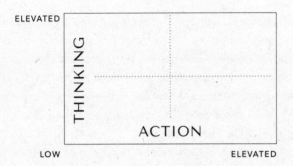

In a very simple way, he demonstrates to the reader the various states we find ourselves in. We're always thinking about something and we're always engaging in an action. Even when we're sleeping, we're engaging in an action (but this is at the low end of the spectrum). When I saw a similar illustration in his book, it highlighted what I already knew, but for some reason it really stood out and reminded me that I'd made that top right corner my home since I was a child. And when I wasn't burning at an elevated rate in this category, I was still either in the elevated-thinking (low-action) or elevated-action (low-thinking) quadrant.

DEATH BY OVERWORK

An extreme example of our energy renewal not matching our demands is when people literally overwork themselves to death. *Karoshi* is a Japanese term that translates as "death by overwork."

In the early 1950s, the Japanese prime minister, Yoshida Shigeru, decided that rebuilding Japan's economy was the top priority.[5] He had major corporations offer lifelong job security to their employees (often referred to as "salarymen") in exchange for their loyalty. It worked—the economy became stronger and stronger. The downside was that employee "loyalty" often meant working extremely long hours, which started to cause physical and mental health problems among Japanese citizens.[6, 7]

Cases of karoshi have risen since the first case was reported in 1969.[8] The typical cause of death in karoshi cases is heart attack or stroke.[9] It has become so bad in Japan that in 2018 there was a "No More Karoshi" protest in Tokyo.

Don't get me wrong. I've visited the low-thinking and low-action quadrant before, and I can remember just about every time I ventured into that strange land. The most vivid recollection of a trip into this quadrant happened on a camping holiday when my wife and I first started dating. We are both doers and thinkers, which are fantastic qualities when you need to get things accomplished but dangerous when you don't have a partner who provides the yin to your yang. That said, on this particular trip I remember the exact moment when I ventured into that quadrant, and IT. WAS. GLORIOUS. I can still remember the contentment that came over my whole body. It was a sense of peace that enveloped my entire being.

Lauren was sitting in a camping chair reading a book while I gathered kindling from the woods. As I walked through the forest picking up dry and brittle sticks from the forest floor, it hit me. My brain, and the incumbent thoughts that fill it, had suddenly slowed. If the pace of my thought pattern was typically represented by a sports car on a busy highway, then in that moment I got off at the nearest exit, left the car, climbed into a horse-drawn buggy, and was being toured through the most glorious countryside while slowly sipping wine. What a feeling.

At the time, I didn't know the physiological reason for the slowing of my elevated-thinking brain. I now know that I hit what some people call flow. My body, brain, soul, and spirit were all in the moment, living in harmony with one another. From a physiological standpoint, my usually ramped-up beta brain waves had crossed over into alpha waves. I hadn't discovered meditation and mindfulness at that point in my life, so the only times I had ever crossed into this brain-wave frequency were when I was drifting off to sleep, when I was waking up in the morning, or—in fleeting moments during the day—when I was daydreaming.

This moment in the woods wasn't fleeting; I leaned into it and enjoyed every moment of its presence. I cherished the crunching of the leaves and twigs beneath my feet, the soft whistling of the trees, the sensation of the firewood in my hands, and the beauty of the forest that surrounded me. Once I had gathered enough wood, I slowly walked over to the firepit and did the most primitive thing a human can do: I built a fire. I was still enjoying the glow of my zen-like pace. It felt so good that I held onto it for as long as I could.

Eventually I crossed back into a beta state, but not back into my usual high-frequency and high-cycles-per-second state. It was a much calmer state. I wasn't in my sports car on the highway, and I wasn't in a horse-drawn carriage. I was in a comfy SUV, driving at a relaxed pace on a beautiful country road.

Just as I can tell you the exact moment in the forest when I ditched the sports car, I can tell you the exact moment when I hopped back in. When our camping holiday was over, we headed back to the city—not just any city but Toronto, the largest city in Canada. We sat at a red light, still basking in the glow of our relaxing holiday. The light turned green and we proceeded to go forward when out of nowhere another driver cut us off, honked, and gave us the middle finger. Just a moment later I looked out my window and saw a guy stumble out of a bar and puke. Yup, my brain-wave frequency went back to its home, back to its comfortable high-frequency domain. I immediately felt my shoulders tense up and my respiration quicken. Well, it was fun while it lasted.

According to Pasricha, "Happy people alternate between boxes. They flip-flop. They swirl. They jump. They know where they are and they know how to create space."[10] So the question for you is, How do you create space? If you're reading this book, I'll bet you're really good at occupying all of the quadrants except the bottom left. Let's change that. Let's find your recharge station and make it a little more accessible and inviting. It's time to get out your metaphorical throw pillows and cozy blankets. We need to change your thoughts around what it means to visit this space from time to time.

To do so you must think of places and activities that cause a significant reduction in thinking and action. For overachievers this can be difficult, since productivity is like a drug for them. They believe that more will make them feel better. More, more, more. More action, more thinking, more earning, more likes, more shares, more friends, more stuff. The list never ends! But like all the overachievers who'd come before me and had found a way back to the lower left quadrant, I needed to begin associating the word "productivity" with something other than work and the checking of items on the constantly repopulating to-do list.

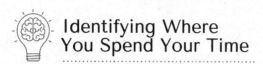 Identifying Where You Spend Your Time

Populate all four quadrants with the habits, behaviors, and/or activities that fill your life. It's important to note that no quadrant is inherently bad. But if you notice that the activities in your life are weighted to any particular quadrant, this will eventually lead to the exposing of that quadrant's flaws. For instance, if your habits and activities have you spending excessive amounts of time in the elevated-thinking and elevated-action quadrant, you're putting yourself at risk of burnout. Too much time in low thinking and low action may result in a breakdown of your relationships, issues with your employer, apathy, or loss of motivation. You can read an example of my activities and then list your own.

	Elevated Thinking & Low Action	Elevated Thinking & Elevated Action
T H I N K I N G	Researching Writing Reading	Teaching Attempting projects or tasks that are new to me (e.g., building a shed for the first time)
	Low Thinking & Low Action	**Low Thinking & Elevated Action**
	Watching movies/TV Group meditation Sauna time Praying Sleeping	Sports (other than golf . . .) Exercise

A C T I O N

"The richest, happiest and most
productive lives are characterized by
the ability to fully engage in the
challenge at hand, but also to disengage
periodically and seek renewal."

—JIM LOEHR AND TONY SCHWARTZ,
CO-AUTHORS OF *THE POWER OF FULL ENGAGEMENT*[11]

	Elevated Thinking & Low Action	Elevated Thinking & Elevated Action
T H I N K I N G		
	Low Thinking & Low Action	Low Thinking & Elevated Action

A C T I O N

Closer to Home

When my wife and I first began dating, something we bonded over was our passion for and dedication to our careers. It became our sheep in wolf's clothing. Lauren is a singer/songwriter. She has overworked herself in much the way I have. On New Year's Day in 2018 she went for a walk and penned the following to illustrate her tendency:

> caught up in the hustle
>   never slowing down
> who am I without worry
>   and the carving of new ground
>
> there's a pressure in the silence
>   a discomfort that I fear
> without a task or purpose
>   who I am is far from clear
>
> slow down, halt the demons
>   all the voices screaming
> should I go on to build a future
>   or stay the beaten path instead
>
> when I'm lost and lonely
>   the work will mask the pain
> a cycle never ending
>   did I do it all in vain
>
> keep holding on my dear
>   you don't have to feel the fear
> take a breath, just slow down
>   I promise you'll be found

For us, truer words have never been spoken.

PART I HAS BEEN about self-reflection. In sharing my story and by describing some of the ways we all get sucked into traps that society sets for us, I hope I've helped you to uncover and expose the obstacles currently impeding your ability to achieve a higher quality of living. Here are a few key points I'd like you to reflect on before you move on to Part II:

- You can't achieve optimum wellness, happiness, and vitality without doing the uncomfortable work of looking within and challenging the notions you have about the way you live and function.

- Self-discovery begins with deep introspection and evaluation of your habitual behaviors and tendencies.

- Most people "boil to death" because they're intoxicating their body slowly with unhealthy food, lack of movement, poor emotional health, social media comparisons, toxic chemicals, and negative people. Some people are aware of their poor choices, while others are oblivious to them.

- If you're currently unfamiliar with or confused about the habits that cause low levels of health, then education must be prioritized.

- If your habitual behaviors are connected to a mental health condition, you should contact a trained professional and begin healing as soon as possible.

- If you avoid dealing with difficult-to-manage areas of your life (by overindulging in other areas), the health of the dimensions that you're ignoring will become progressively worse, which will require a steeper climb back to optimal.

- Our culture values breadth over depth; it will continue to ask more of you if you let it.

- Anticipation (of things like FFTs, commitments, and energy outputs), as well as the planning of work-to-rest output, is crucial to energy (physical, mental, emotional, and spiritual) renewal, accrual, and abundance.

- Your body is designed to handle episodic stress, not continual stress.

- The body is an incredible entity that's capable of rebuilding itself *if you let it*.

- If your body and/or mind has reached its limit, you've made yourself susceptible to your familial gene pool, which could cause the onset of an irreversible disorder.

- To build your capacity in a healthy way, you must build in rest and recovery after periods of stress (exercise, uncommon emotional output, illness).

- To achieve what most people crave—consistent and sustained energy—you must design a life that ensures that the energy is derived from within, from your own physiology.

- You might be only three feet from gold! By changing a few habits and routines, you may see a domino effect in the other areas of your life.

- Desperation can be a powerful motivator—so be desperate; be desperate for a vibrant, energetic, and beautifully present life!

Self-awareness, self-restraint, and the desire to follow a healthy road map to success are paramount for the achievement of consistent growth.

PART II

Exposing the Root Cause

"When solving problems, dig at the roots instead of just hacking at the leaves."

—ANTHONY J. D'ANGELO

MY TOP PRIORITY for you is progress—in terms of your energy, happiness, and immunity. But for those who want optimal, you must create a higher ceiling. To reach new wellness heights you'll need to give your body and mind a spring cleaning before you begin.

Exposing the root is all about digging deeper than you have in the past. You must be comfortable with critical evaluation and be willing to answer difficult questions that are designed to reveal the true cause of your obstacles, behaviors, and previous setbacks. With honest personal assessment you can help to zero in on the target (energy, fulfillment, happiness, and so on) and save time spent on unnecessary trial and error. And remember, previous "failures" are only in vain if you don't learn from them; otherwise they show you the incorrect path to sustainable change, and that, in itself, is a victory. You can use the knowledge from previous experiences to alter your approach, which may bring you closer to the optimal life you seek.

You may find that it's daunting to discern the root of all your obstacles. Rather than trying to focus on all of them at once, try to determine the larger ones that may have a domino effect. For instance, I used to be a "yes man" when it came to opportunity—this was a major root for me. When opportunity came knocking, I'd always let it in.

But instead of cutting something out of my life to make room for the new workload, I eliminated nothing. Well, that's not entirely true—I successfully eliminated my social life, sense of calm, physical health, sleep, and sometimes my sanity. I craved energy to propel my days but then had to rely on outside sources of "energy" (e.g., caffeine) to make it from task to task. A successful day for me was marked by the checking of boxes on a long to-do list. I lived in that state between fully awake and asleep. This became my new normal. And since it was my new normal, I had forgotten what optimal health felt like.

By learning to say no to certain opportunities, I was rewarded with more time. That additional time had a positive domino effect in other areas of my life, rewarding me with more time for sleep, exercise, meal prep, and socializing. Learning this one habit of saying no created the space for many wonderful things.

Consider these questions:

- Can you identify any behaviors or tendencies that, when altered, will bring positive change in other areas of your life?

- If you had the level of energy you desire, how would this impact the people in your life? Would you be more present with your partner? Your children? Your friends?

- If your brain fog was gone, would you write that book you've been talking about for years? Would you invent something? Would you finish work projects sooner and thereby free up more time to do the things you love?

- If you challenged your comfort zone more often, would you travel to an exotic destination? Ask your crush on a date? Request a promotion?

If you engage in critical (but nonjudgmental) evaluation of yourself, implement the strategies in this book, and complete the activities I've included, those all become possibilities. With an upgraded subconscious, a clear mind, and a healthy body, you can achieve even your wildest aspirations!

You must first recognize and be willing to face your fears, adjust your relationship with anxiety, and determine which stressors in your life are advantageous and which ones are not.

CHAPTER 4

Fear, Worry, Anxiety, and Stress

"The greatest weapon against stress is our ability to choose one thought over another."—WILLIAM JAMES

CONSISTENT FEAR OR worry is the antithesis of optimal living. That's not to say you can, or should, eliminate fear and worry from your life—that would be a futile exercise. Your priority should be understanding when fear and worry are persistent emotions that dominate your thoughts and actions, and therefore adversely affect your psychology and physiology.

Fear and worry typically lead to unwanted levels of stress and anxiety, which, if not properly managed, may lead to chronic mental exhaustion and physiological overwhelm (such as an unhealthy amount of cortisol being released daily[1]). When the body and mind are subjected to continual overwhelm, the result can be burnout and disease that could have been avoided.[2]

The cycle of mental and physical burnout is a too frequent occurrence in modern society.[3] Developing a healthier approach to life requires the curation of sustainable habits that steadily bring you back to mental clarity and physical abundance (in terms of the resources that are available to help you perform optimally).

The obstacles preventing you from living optimally may be either apparent or unknown to you. Lack of depth and accuracy in identifying and eliminating obstacles is frequently driven by fear. You may not recognize it as such, but deep within your subconscious something is holding you back.

If your desires for your body, mind, relationships, and career aren't where you want them to be, it's time to make a change. You need to overcome your fear and become the person your younger self would be proud of. If people never faced their fears (of failure, rejection, change, confrontation), who knows what today's society would look like? What inventions would never have been made? What life-saving medications would we be without? What books would remain unwritten?

Face Your Fears

Dr. Viktor Frankl, a psychologist and the author of *Man's Search for Meaning*, coined the phrase "paradoxical intention."[4] Dr. Frankl was a survivor of World War II and the Holocaust. During his imprisonment in concentration camps, he observed people in drastic situations. Using observational psychology, he became acutely aware of how people respond when fear is present. Although the level of fear that most people experience regularly pales in comparison to what people felt during the Holocaust, he discovered a trend that occurs when fear is justified and imminent, as well as when it is not.

Frankl noticed that when people are afraid of something, they want to avoid it. This is not surprising. However, the problem he surmised was that when people try to avoid something (a fear), they often make the situation worse. You have undoubtedly experienced this in your own life. Whether the fear is big or small, the more you attempt to avoid it, the larger it gets.

This is especially problematic for people who are prone to worry—typically, their fear grows disproportionate to the reality. As an example, if a person prone to worry has a loved one taking a flight, he or she might believe that the plane will crash, when in all likelihood it will land safely. When one has an outsized fear like this, the neural connection for the fear firmly roots itself in the worrier's brain.[5] It is almost as if it cannot be turned off. In our example, the only relief for the person is likely a message from the loved one saying they have landed safely. When people worry like this, the stress on the body is enormous, and it tends to sap one of our most precious resources: our energy!

Here's another, lighter, example of our fears taking root in our brains in a disproportionate way.

Do you remember your high-school crush? Perhaps you thought about asking them out at one point but you had a slight fear of rejection and so you said to yourself, I'll do it tomorrow. That little seed of fear, and the worry about rejection, likely began to grow roots that day. Then day after day the roots grew thicker and stronger, to the point where you wouldn't even consider asking the person out on a date. Your fear of rejection likely expanded to your being certain that by asking them out you'd be humiliated, and that would be too much for you to handle. If this sounds like you, I'm willing to bet that it spread to other crushes later in life, causing you to avoid taking that leap of faith and asking anyone out on a date.

Every time you failed to take a chance or to take courage in the face of uncertainty, you poured more water onto that seedling of poor behavior. Eventually it grew bigger and stronger. Thank goodness for internet dating—it will ensure that humanity continues! Although there are still plenty of no's in the virtual world, they are just words on a screen. You don't have to build up the courage to walk up to someone, look them in the eye, ask them out, and awkwardly walk away if they say no.

If you imagine a lack of bravery in the face of possible rejection as the pouring of water on that seedling, you should also imagine that if you begin to take chances it's as if you're beginning to cut down the plant that the seed has grown, and with repeated action you may rip it from the ground, roots and all.

Rarely in life will our behaviors and tendencies be situationally segregated. If you're afraid to walk up to someone and ask them out on a date, the fear is likely transferable to other areas of your life. The fear of humiliation and rejection that you've built up likely causes you to avoid asking for a raise, debating with someone you disagree with, or confronting someone who has wronged you. Perhaps for you it's situational, but I doubt it. It's been proven that people will do as much to avoid pain as they will to gain pleasure.[6]

Consider this: twenty seconds of bravery may be all it takes to positively change things. It may be enough time to get that promotion, stand up for yourself, protect someone, or make an impact in some way. So it may be useful for you to think back on your life: What are some moments where you didn't seize the opportunity or take the risk? After all, what's 20 seconds? You can take a deep breath and summon the courage for just 20 seconds, right?

Twenty seconds of bravery may be all it takes to positively change things.

This is a life approach I'll instill in my children. Although they'll grow up in a digital world, I'll impart to them the importance of face-to-face bravery.

So, then, to overcome fear, according to paradoxical intention, you must embrace the person, place, or thing that you fear. For instance, let's say you have a phobia about big spiders but you're required to travel to a place that has some of the biggest in the world. If you don't face the fear and rewire your brain, then your entire trip will likely be consumed by worry, fear, and lack of sleep. When dealing with a phobia, therapists use systematic desensitization to progressively help their patient to overcome it.

If spiders are your issue, the therapist might begin slowly by trying to make you comfortable looking at a picture of a spider. They might progress to having you watch a video of a spider. Then they might try to make you comfortable being in a room with a large spider. While the time frame is different for everyone, they may even work with you until you're able to touch or hold a spider. Through this process, you're "rewiring" your brain so that it no longer associates spiders with danger.[7]

Through each phase of desensitization, you'll feel the flight response in your mind and body. You'll feel the surge in adrenaline, the rise in heart rate and blood pressure, and the increase in perspiration and breathing rate. But eventually these sensations will level off and there'll be a return to resting or near-resting levels. You see, when people are faced with their fear or phobia they tend to retreat quickly, which denies them the experience of feeling their body return to its baseline homeostatic levels.

Overcoming fear requires repeated exposure and preparation. That's what paradoxical intention is all about. Over time you'll learn to see your fear for what it really is—no bigger and no smaller. This is easier said than done, of course. In some cases you might be able to do it on your own and in other cases you'll need the help of someone who's professionally trained. Your recovery time will depend on a multitude of factors (how long you've had the fear, whether or not you know its origin, whether or not you have access to quality care by a trained therapist, your motivation level to rid it from your life, etc.), so be patient, nonjudgmental, and kind to yourself during the process. As Tony Robbins has said hundreds (perhaps even thousands) of times in his life, "Progress equals happiness."[8]

In the end, the important thing to remember is that if you want to tap into your optimal self, uncovering the root of your fear and worry will be a key step in moving forward. Without this step, you'll never experience complete self-actualization—the full realization of your potential.

Identifying Your Fears

Do you believe you're capable of doing more than you're currently doing? If your answer is yes, then start thinking about why you haven't progressed farther in that area. A coach or mentor can help with this—they can help you to see that you don't have to settle for a life of mediocrity. With preparation, repetition, and willpower, you can take your life to the next level.

To start, list any fears, phobias, or anxieties you have and how they impact your life. Getting to the root of these issues will help you strategize how to deal with them.

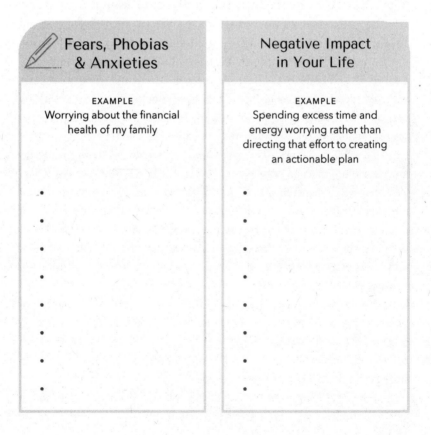

Fears, Phobias & Anxieties	Negative Impact in Your Life
EXAMPLE Worrying about the financial health of my family	EXAMPLE Spending excess time and energy worrying rather than directing that effort to creating an actionable plan
•	•
•	•
•	•
•	•
•	•
•	•
•	•
•	•

FEAR OF DEATH

Many people live with denial around death. Intellectually they know that death is a concrete truth, but for them it's not going to happen for a very long time. Because people often project death far into the future, they don't fully grip the reality of their mortality—the fact that they could die at any moment.

Because of people's failure to accept death, in terms of themselves or their loved ones, they're improperly prepared for reality when death is imminent. Additionally, without a healthy understanding of mortality you may spend an inordinate amount of time on things such as work and worry—and end up regretting it. My suggestion isn't that you spend your days ruminating about death, but that you fully accept its inevitability—for doing so will reduce the fear (conscious or subconscious) that has a hold over you.

Unfortunately, the flip side is also true: many people spend an inordinate amount of time thinking about death, to the point where it develops into an obsession. "Thanatophobia" is a term used to describe people who have an intense fear of dying or of the dying process.

It's natural for people to fear death, but when this fear consumes them and negatively impacts their daily life, it's a phobia, and, as with any phobia, you should endeavor to have it rectified in order to live a full life.

Thanatophobia can affect both adults and children, and the fear doesn't have to be about the fear of you yourself dying; it can be excessive worry about a loved one passing away. As a child, I had this fear. Before my dad gave up smoking, I was excessively worried that he was going to die. Each morning I'd wake up, go into his room, and check to make sure he was breathing. As soon as I realized he was, I'd carry on with my day. It became an ingrained part of my routine, one that was not serving me.

Do you have a fear of death that innervates your thoughts more than you'd like? If so, there's hope—but it's likely going to take paradoxical intention and the facing of your fears.

There's now something called the "death positive movement," a term coined by The Order of the Good Death, an organization committed to helping people to make death a part of their life by facing its inevitability without fear—to accept that "death is natural, but the death anxiety and terror of modern culture are not." [9]

The objective of the death positive movement isn't to make death obsolete but to help people understand that "cultural censorship" regarding death isn't serving us. Understanding and accepting death can be beautiful and can help people to live more fully—more in the present.

If you're excessively worried about death, there are many ways you can reduce your fear. Cognitive behavioral therapy (CBT), psychotherapy, exposure therapy, relaxation techniques, and perhaps medication if it's deemed necessary are all possible ways you can begin reducing the fear that death holds over you.

Additionally, if mortality is feared by you or a loved one, or if it's potentially imminent, you could hire an End-of-Life Doula (also called a Death Doula) for support and navigation through the difficult and complex emotions you may be experiencing. End-of-Life Doulas can be a tremendous support to individuals and their families.

Even for physically healthy individuals, if they experience excessive worry and fear regarding death or the dying process, an End-of-Life Doula may help them to face reality in a way that reduces the worry and fear by providing support, resources, and education.

Worry: The Destructive Cousin to Fear

Worry and fear are often passengers on the destructive highway to exhaustion. Worry plants scenarios in your subconscious of what you don't want to happen. Additionally, worry is often emotional and very repetitive. And since your subconscious doesn't know the difference between real and imagined,[10] your body will react as if the worry is real.

Worry (or "concern") can be useful at times, but, as discussed above, most people's worry tends to be overblown and they expend energy on a negative event that never materializes. When a worrisome event or circumstance is inevitable, then it's appropriate to use your emotion to effectively problem-solve—but once you've resolved the issue, stop worrying. Failure to do so will drain your overall energy tank, since worry is an exhausting emotion.

When I was a kid and had to give a presentation, I'd worry so much about it that I'd begin to shake long before I got up in front of the class, which would then plant another worry in my mind: that the class would see my nervousness. It was a vicious cycle. And all my worry did was fuel my fear and feed my exhaustion.

As is typical, most of my worries were overblown: the object of my worry never materialized. The incessant worry caused me to waste precious time and lose precious moments (by not being present). If I envisioned the end of my life, and I reflected, I was sure I'd prefer a life of contentment, relaxation, and being fully present. But since I had worry rooted deep in my subconscious, it wasn't easy to change. I now use daily affirmations, incantations, healthy routines, and mindfulness to ensure that my days are slow, present, and largely worry-free.

One of my favorite pastors, Dr. Tony Evans, once said, "Worry is concern on steroids. Worry is concern that's gone haywire. There is a difference between concern and worry. Concern is, I have an issue in my life that is troubling me, and I am setting forth a plan as best I can to address it. That is legitimate concern. But worry is where the concern controls you. It is where, because of the concern, I can't sleep; because of the concern, I can't control my temper; because of the concern, I am losing my ability to cope."[11] Dr. Evans goes on to clarify that he isn't talking about a chemical imbalance that requires intervention and possible medication. He's addressing what's an issue for a lot of people: that there are situations in your life that control you because of excessive worry.

Whether you follow the teachings of Christ, or your spirituality comes from somewhere else, the following message from Matthew 6:25-27 is valuable: "Therefore I tell you, do not worry about your life, what you will eat or drink; or about your body, what you will wear. Is not life more than food, and the body more than clothes? . . . Can any one of you by worrying add a single hour to your life?"[12]

Ask yourself: What has worry cost me?

I'm guessing that at times it has cost you time with the ones you love, the joy of new experiences, being fully present, and a sense of peace. Eliminating excessive worry and transitioning to contentment is possible—and once this is achieved not only will you be happier, but you'll have a lot more energy, because you'll be plugging up the energy leaks that worry and fear cause.

You may be wondering, How does worry drain us of energy? If you've ever heard the saying "you'll catch more flies with honey than with vinegar," then you've essentially heard of the spiritual hypothesis of the perpetual transmutation of energy. Spiritually it's hypothesized that our emotions are energy,[13] and as such will manifest themselves through our physical actions, which, when carried out repeatedly, will require an excessive number of bodily resources.

Think about a recent time when you were worried and stressed. What began in the mind eventually manifested physically (sweating, trembling, increased heart rate, and so on). The greater the worry or nervousness, the more prominent the symptoms.

So, if worry isn't serving us, where does it stem from? It likely has to do with our ancestral heritage. Early peoples weren't concerned about happiness and joy like we are today—they were interested in food, shelter, and safety. Today our brains are still wired to be on the lookout for danger—and, without conscious control and the reprogramming of our subconscious mind, our reticular activating system (RAS; located within our brain) will continue to notice what's wrong and alert us to where perceived dangers are. This in turn will lead to consistent worry and fear.

For many, our modern dangers aren't the same as those of previous generations. Danger today might be represented by a lack of social media Likes, not having the right clothes, being judged by others, or being unhappy with our job. While we can't rewire the circuitry running our brains (because fear will always induce certain chemical reactions), we can condition our brains to change what's identified as fearful.

EMOTIONAL STRENGTH

My brother Brian might be the most positive person I know. Just like everyone, he has been presented with many challenges throughout his life, but his ability to live with levity and humor has never ceased. Most recently, he was diagnosed with stage 4 terminal cancer and subsequently given the grim mortality statistics that accompany such a diagnosis. His positive demeanor continued through all his treatments. This wasn't a "fake it until you make it" scenario; he embodied it. He knew in the depths of his being that he would beat the odds. He even went so far as to tell the doctors on multiple occasions that the statistics didn't matter or apply to him, so he didn't want to hear them.

I would be remiss if I didn't provide you with a few more details about Brian that will further emphasize the power of our emotions. While he may be someone who does an incredible job of living with humor, levity, and confidence, he lacks other traits and habits that doctors and health experts would agree are necessary to overcome a poor cancer diagnosis. During treatment, he still ate sugar, had the odd beer (and the cancer had already spread to his liver), and enjoyed a periodic cigar. He didn't engage in regular exercise, and he continued his late-night card games with his buddies. Essentially, he wasn't vigilant about his dietary or lifestyle choices. He took his cancer seriously but didn't let it dominate his decision-making or his life. Brian has something most don't: a subconscious mind that doesn't flounder.

Cancer is knocking on the door for a lot of people. How people respond when cancer stops knocking, opens the door, and walks in is very different. Some people let cancer occupy their entire home; they think about it relentlessly and focus on the fear of the destruction the disease is wreaking within themselves. This is completely normal, and anyone who hasn't been through a similar diagnosis can't tell those people that they are acting or thinking incorrectly. But even though such thoughts of fear, doubt, and worry are completely justifiable, they aren't serving to improve the reality.

Although Brian had cancer living in his home (specifically, his colon, liver, lungs, abdomen, and chest), he didn't give it a prime seat at the table. He told cancer to hang out in the basement and to not get too comfortable, because it wasn't going to be staying long. One of the things that doctors marveled at was how Brian showed up to his chemotherapy and radiation treatments. He would stroll in, whistling and joking with doctors because that's just who he is. Every time they would ask him, "How? How do you have so much energy? How are you so happy? How are you still playing golf every day?" To Brian, the diagnosis wasn't a life sentence; it was an inconvenience.

Too many people take what doctors say as sacrosanct, never questioning or challenging the diagnosis or prognosis. You should seek a second (or even a third) opinion, do your own research, and decide which person you're going to be—the optimistic one or the pessimistic one. Remember, when life presents a challenging situation, it's best to stack as many chips in your favor as possible: a positive mindset, healthy food, regular movement, unwavering faith, and medications (when necessary). This approach, taken over a long period of time, can have an impact on the expression of your genes and therefore your potential medical outcome. Today, I'm elated to report that he is currently tumor-free ☺

Stress, Evolution, and Ways to Reprogram Our Perceptions

"The primary cause of unhappiness is never the situation but your thoughts about it."—ECKHART TOLLE

The excessive demands of twenty-first-century society have done a great disservice to the way our bodies are programmed. We're designed to handle episodic stress, not continual stress.[14] When faced with a threat—real or imagined—your sympathetic nervous system releases adrenaline and cortisol from your adrenal glands, which increases your heart rate, blood pressure, respiration, perspiration, and blood sugar to provide you with the highest degree of clarity and resources possible to face the situation head-on (fight) or run away (flight).

The ability of our bodies to deliver this rapid response certainly helped to ensure our survival. But this programming hasn't had enough evolutionary time to meet the demands of today's stressful lifestyle. The result? There are millions of people sleepwalking through life because they're exhausted from the overwhelming demands placed on them each day.

Aside from ensuring that your resources aren't being continually drained, you should take a proactive approach to stress, energy, and fatigue. Although you may not be able to change all the people or daily events in your life, what you can change is how you let them affect you.

You see, something is stressful only if you perceive it to exceed your ability to cope with it. That's why the same life event can cause anxiety, stress, and eventual fatigue in one person and have no negative effect on another person.

Eustress, as opposed to distress, is a type of stress that is interpreted as beneficial. Two people can experience the same event but their thoughts, and therefore their experiences with it, can be very different. For instance, when you find yourself in a summer rain, one person might perceive it as stressful, uncomfortable, and a nuisance while another person might enjoy the feel of rain on their skin and be grateful that the plants and flowers are getting nourishment.

I see the varying degrees of eustress versus distress play out in the classroom when I administer an exam or when I ask my students to present in front of the class. The level of anxiety for some is palpable—they're almost vibrating from frenzy—which will quickly drain their resources. Conversely, there are students who remain calm and prepared during the entire semester—they know they have the ability and the knowledge to cope with all the demands I'm placing on them.

Do you identify with the individual who has an excessive amount of daily stress?

If you quietly (or emphatically) nodded your head as a yes to being overly stressed, there are many things you can do to begin reducing your mental and, by default, physical load. When you find yourself ruminating for too long, the ability to refocus can help to clear the inner chatter and allow you to return to the present moment or task. I discuss this further in the chapter on paradigms (see page 271). For now, however, here are some additional tips, as provided in *Biohacker's Handbook*,[15] on how to calm the mind:

• Music—especially classical music, calming ambient sounds, nature sounds, solfeggio frequencies, binaural beats,* isochronic tones

  Note: Binaural beats are a type of brain-wave entrainment that involves two different tones, one in each ear. Your brain will then combine the frequencies and recognize the difference between the two. For instance, to induce more relaxing and meditative alpha waves, you want the difference to equal the frequency associated with that brain wave. There are apps that can help you to choose which brain wave to induce.

- Scents and aromatherapy: lavender, rosemary, jasmine, cedarwood, lemon, chamomile, peppermint

- Acupressure mat (or spike mat) is designed with hundreds of plastic points to produce results similar to those of acupressure massage (which helps to boost oxytocin and endorphins)

- Yoga, massage, and stretching, which help by boosting our circulation

- Reducing sensory stimuli (sensory deprivation) through the use of deep breathing exercises, an isolation tank, and/or silence exercises

---

There are millions of people sleepwalking through life because they're exhausted from the overwhelming demands placed on them each day.

GOT A SPARE TIRE?

Change occurs in an instant. I believe it's part of my job to create light-bulb moments to expedite people's decision-making—this requires the ability to alter the delivery of a message to meet the individual's predominant decision-making state. Some people base their decisions on emotion, while others might rely on facts, analytics, and percentages. That said, if you're still not convinced of the need to change your daily stress response to the inevitable stressors that invade your day-to-day life, then I want you to reach down to your stomach and grab as much fat as you can around your belly button . . . I'm willing to bet that you'd like that handful to be much smaller.

That excessive fat is partially due to the stress you experience daily. Have a look at the graphs shown here. Imagine that two people are presented with the exact same number of "stressful" events throughout their day. Compared with person 1, person 2 perceives twice as many of those events as exceeding their ability to cope with them. Person 2 therefore has more adrenaline (sympathetic) spikes and a rising level of cortisol.

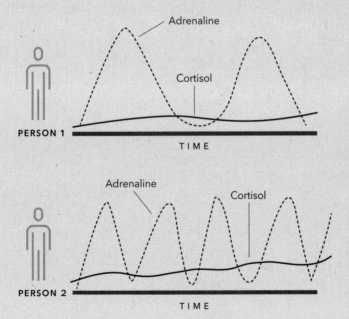

When we encounter a traditional stress (e.g., being physically attacked) or a modern-day stress (e.g., being stuck in a traffic jam), there's an initial release of adrenaline that arms your body and brain with the resources to fight or escape. After the initial adrenaline release, there's a release of cortisol, which helps to ensure that you're prepared if the "threat" takes longer to remedy. What you'll notice in the graphs is that adrenaline spikes quickly and declines quickly whereas cortisol rises slowly and returns to baseline slowly.

One of the primary responsibilities of cortisol is to release stored glucose (sugar) from your liver.[16] The glucose that's released is sent to your bloodstream. Having access to this additional blood sugar is advantageous *if* you are faced with a traditionally stressful situation that requires the physical movement of your body (since your body uses glucose to power your ability to endure high-intensity movement for short periods—about 1-2 minutes).

Due to the repeated "stressful" events, the cortisol level for person 2 is unable to return to baseline. The unused blood sugar must be sent to another region of the body (since it wasn't used for physical activity). According to an article by Epel and colleagues, "stress-induced cortisol secretion may contribute to central fat."[17] This occurs because the additional blood sugar causes the release of insulin, which is secreted to reduce blood sugar levels by depositing them in regions such as the abdominal area as adipose tissue[18] (fat, or "spare tire").

So, the next time you encounter a modern-day stress, remember that you're operating new software (modern stress) on an old operating system. By letting too many modern stressors impact your sympathetic nervous system, you're not just exhausting your overall energy resources but also contributing to the spare tire that you so desperately want to eliminate!

In time, perhaps, our evolution will progress to the point where we know the difference between a physical threat and an emotional one, but that could take millennia. In the meantime, sit back, take a few deep breaths, and shift your focus from a negative emotional state to a positive (or at least a neutral) one.

Reforming Your Relationship with Anxiety

Anxiety is normal; we all experience it nearly every day. The goal in life shouldn't be to eliminate anxiety—that would be futile. The goal should be to re-establish a relationship with anxiety that's healthy, has boundaries, and can help you to grow. Oftentimes people associate the word "relationship" with the healthy, or unhealthy, interaction between individuals. It's important to keep in mind that you have a relationship with so many other things in your life. And just as a relationship between two people requires attention so that unhealthy habits aren't formed, so too does your relationship with anxiety.

Far too often, the activities we engage in to reduce our stress or anxiety are unhealthy. While they may provide temporary comfort, the negative effects can add up and cause problems if they're overused. For instance, if you have a stressful and anxiety-inducing day, perhaps a glass of wine or some of your favorite guilty-pleasure food will help you settle into a better mindset. Conversely, if this strategy is overused, the negative effects will compound your issue (and may give rise to other issues, likely increasing your anxiety).

Similarly, many people resort to retail therapy when stress and anxiety levels rise. Spending money periodically to help ease anxiety may be okay, but if you begin to lean heavily on it you may find yourself in financial trouble.

On the next page is a chart of some anxiety-reducing strategies I use either daily or periodically. I'm fortunate to have access to things like a sauna and hot tub, and I'm eternally grateful for that. However, there are many other strategies I include that are easily accessible and just as calming.

As we've discussed, anxiety is a normal part of life. You'll never completely eliminate it, nor should this be a goal. In many circumstances a certain level of anxiety may be beneficial. That said, anxiety, and anxiety-related disorders, have risen dramatically and resulted in negative physical and mental conditions for those who are afflicted by anxiety.

Joseph's Strategy	Daily (D) or Periodically (P)
Mindfulness	D
Infrared sauna	D
Going in a hot tub	P
Sitting by a fire	P
Exercise and physical activity	D
Watching a relaxing movie	P
Getting some alone time	P
Acupuncture	P

Complete the chart with as many strategies as you can think of that will reduce the intensity and/or frequency of anxiety-inducing circumstances.

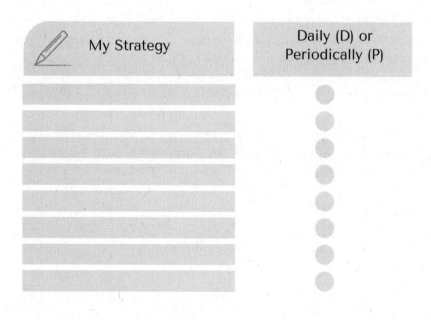

My Strategy	Daily (D) or Periodically (P)

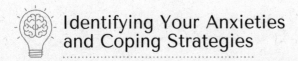

Identifying Your Anxieties and Coping Strategies

In order to reform your relationship with anxiety so that its negative effects, especially when there's elevated exposure over a long period, are minimized or eliminated, you first need to identify the things that cause you anxiety. It's important to note that some people have anxiety-related issues that may require medical attention or therapy. If your anxiety is provoked by something that's a part of your everyday life, then it must be addressed by a qualified health professional. For instance, if you have a phobia about enclosed spaces (such as elevators), then avoiding elevators shouldn't be the solution. To enjoy a full life, you must address anxiety-provoking situations directly or your quality of life could suffer.

In the next chart, fill in the following columns:

1. Identify the people, places, things, and/or events that cause you anxiety.

2. Indicate whether you believe the source of your anxiety can be eliminated (E) or reformed (R). For instance, if you have a personal relationship that's causing anxiety, should you extricate yourself from it completely? Or should you attempt to reform the relationship as it pertains to your anxiety?

3. List the ways you currently address this source of anxiety and identify alternatives if your strategies might be causing more harm than good. Be nonjudgmental of yourself—remember, it's not necessarily bad to use strategies such as alcohol or food for stress reduction; these strategies become harmful only when overused. Be realistic about the strategies you might use—the goal is not perfection but improvement.

I want to give you examples of my anxiety-provoking situations as well as the coping strategies I use. I hope this provides insight or encouragement regarding your approach. I also include a justification for each strategy or scenario, something you may or may not choose to do. My entries here are broad for the purpose of providing insight; yours should be more specific.

Person/Place/ Thing/Event	E or R	Current and Future Coping Strategy
When my kids are sick	R	As a result of the very stressful journey to bring our kids into the world safely, my wife and I would conjure up stressful scenarios for what most people would consider a normal cough or fever. Reforming our relationship with their symptoms required the help of a trained psychologist; she helped us to cope and rewire our response to the kids' symptoms.
Rushing	E	My wife and I were prone to this for years, typically because we'd packed our days with too many commitments. Reducing commitments and undertaking proper preparation (meal prep, laying clothes out the night before, getting up earlier, etc.) helps to ensure that our days flow at a relaxed pace.
Onset of depersonalization symptoms	R	Depersonalization is something that I live with. Although it can't be completely eliminated, I've learned to view the onset of symptoms as a blessing. It's my warning sign that if I stop I'll recover quickly and therefore won't risk exhaustion or burnout. When I feel the symptoms emerge (usually from anxiety or overworking my brain), I step back from whatever I'm doing and slow everything down. I incorporate mindfulness and pull myself back to the present moment; eventually the symptoms subside.
Toxic people or relationships	E or R	There've been people over the years from whom I've had to distance myself to preserve my mental health. Many people choose to leave toxic romantic relationships without considering the other people (family and "friends") who contribute to their anxiety. *Note: Separation wouldn't be my first choice; trying to reform the relationship with open discussion of feelings is typically my initial instinct.*

FEAR, WORRY, ANXIETY, AND STRESS   69

Now it's your turn to ruthlessly consider everything that brings you unwarranted anxiety—and discover ways you can remedy the issue.

Person/Place/ Thing/Event	E or R	Current and Future Coping Strategy

It's possible that your anxieties are deeply rooted within your subconscious; this will make their resolution more challenging. Educating yourself on how subconscious programming influences behavior and our emotional responses may be necessary to spark a shift in your programmed response to situations or people.

CHAPTER 5

The Subconscious Mind

"Whatever we plant in our subconscious mind and
nourish with repetition and emotion will one day become reality."
—EARL NIGHTINGALE

FOR MOST PEOPLE, the physical brain is an easy concept to grasp; what's tougher is the understanding of our mind, which is composed of our conscious mind and subconscious mind. Neuroscientists estimate that our conscious mind is responsible for only 5 percent of our cognitive activity, which leaves the other 95 percent of our decisions, actions, emotions, and behavior to our subconscious mind.[1]

Have you ever been driving to a destination that you've been to many times before and suddenly said to yourself or to your passenger, "Whoa, where did the last 20 minutes go?" You "zoned out" and don't recall putting any conscious effort into driving. This might seem extremely dangerous considering that you're operating a very heavy, potentially lethal vehicle. The only reason why you're able to zone out and not crash is that you've driven that same stretch of road dozens if not hundreds of times—your subconscious knows all the landmarks and it knows the speed at which you need to travel.

Conversely, if it's your first time driving the route, everything is new to you and you can't go into "autopilot," since your subconscious doesn't recognize any of the surroundings. Zoning out in this case would exponentially increase your odds of crashing.

Your subconscious mind can perform an incredible number of tasks at the same time. It contains all the software needed for your involuntary functions, emotions, and habits.[2] Fortunately, or unfortunately, most of these functions, emotions, and habits were formed in early childhood[3]— which helps to explain the repeated behavioral patterns that some people exhibit despite their desire to rid themselves of a negative habit, routine, or behavior.

Our subconscious mind has no ability to reject—it will accept whatever is impressed upon it.[4] The reason why it doesn't accept everything that every person says to you is because during your waking hours you're able to use your conscious mind to filter the information. The conscious mind can accept or reject the message before it's rooted in your subconscious. If someone says something negative about you, you can choose not to internalize it.

Our subconscious mind has no ability to reject—it will accept whatever is impressed upon it.

Our conscious mind is logical.[5] It filters the input (decides what the information means) into the subconscious, which is good because everything gets into the subconscious[6] and we must filter the informational garbage (negativity, unjust criticism, etc.) that comes our way every day.

The subconscious mind isn't logical.[7] It's the feeling mind—the source of love, hatred, fear, sadness, jealousy, et cetera. For instance, if you say the word "father" your conscious mind hears the word objectively. Conversely, when the subconscious hears the word "father" there are various feelings that arise. The subconscious might associate the word with love, abandonment, sadness, happiness, and so on. It all depends on the experiences you've accrued up to this point.

Put another way, our conscious mind thinks, and our subconscious mind executes—the subconscious takes the information that it's given, then formulates a response and behavior that align with the operational paradigm it's accustomed to.

Unfortunately, logic and critical thinking of the conscious mind don't begin to develop until you're about seven years old,[8] and it isn't fully developed until you're an adult.[9] This means that the people who populate your life have an enormous impact on your habits, self-esteem, attitudes, behaviors, and so on. Since the subconscious brain doesn't have the ability to reject, if you tell a child they're worthless, stupid, or clumsy, that message will begin to grow roots.

Additionally, your subconscious doesn't understand sarcasm,[10] so without a fully developed conscious mind to filter the information, any sarcastic statements may be held as truths to the person to whom they are being directed.

The bottom line is to be careful regarding the people and information you let into your life. This is relatively easy to do as an adult, but during a child's formative years the critical mind is formed by the environment, social settings, and the primary caregivers to whom the parents expose their child. So, when raising children, we need to surround them with safe environments and positive role models.

Going forward, our focus will primarily be on the subconscious mind, since this is the source of lasting change. To further illustrate the power of the subconscious, I'd like to talk to you about expectation.

Expectation

What do you expect of yourself? Although most people won't admit it, they're settling for a life of mediocrity. They continue to delay their dreams, content to talk or ruminate about them but never act. Their dreams perpetually live as fantasy, never coming close to reality.

If you're honest about yourself, do you *expect* to see success, growth, and achievement in your future? Or do you believe that talking about your dreams is enough of a self-preserving Band-Aid to carry you through to the next day, only to talk about them more, without taking any action?

In my line of work, expectation bias (or confirmation bias) refers to the bias of researchers that makes them believe and publish data that are congruent with their expected outcome, and disbelieve or downgrade corresponding evidence that conflicts with their expectations. This doesn't happen in academic settings only; it happens to humans every day.

My wife may cringe when she reads this, but she told me that when she was in high school her teachers had great expectations for her as a student because she was polite, helpful, and involved and she began each semester diligently. She noticed that as the semester would go on, she was able to get away with more time away from class and was shown more leniency with regard to work that was due because the teachers viewed her as a great student.

We all form expected outcomes in our head, which is why first impressions are really important. This doesn't mean that you can't change the view that others have of you or their opinion about you, but it's much easier to begin with the character traits you want people to remember you as having. Fortunately, and unfortunately, expectation can be self-fulfilling.

History books are filled with proof that our subconscious drives the way we think and behave. Back when I was doing my undergraduate degree, my friend Andrew enrolled in a psychological experiment at the university (to earn a little extra money, we both enrolled in as many studies as we could). This study seemed to be perfect—almost too good to be true. He met a couple of graduate students at the on-campus pub. They were studying the effects of alcohol on decision-making (or something along those lines). He was asked to complete a questionnaire and then have a pint of beer. Then he'd complete another questionnaire and consume another pint. He did this a few more times until he was, in his words, "hammered." He said that by the fourth pint he was really drunk when he filled out the last questionnaire. That's when the real study was revealed to him. The researchers told him he had been drinking non-alcoholic beer the entire time. *Boom!* He instantly went from intoxicated to sober. When he came home to our house to tell me, I was blown away! His conscious mind had no reason to think that he was drinking non-alcoholic beer, so his subconscious mind acted as if alcohol were being consumed. Remember, your subconscious mind has no ability to reject what is impressed upon it—if it believes you're drinking alcohol, then it will behave accordingly.

Similarly, if your subconscious doesn't believe you'll be successful in reaching your goals, it will behave accordingly (and do nothing). However, if success has been a staple of your life blueprint (if you've continually set and achieved goals), your subconscious will take the steps needed to drive you toward the achievement of your goals. Even if it doesn't fully understand the entire path, it will have the confidence necessary to obtain the answers by asking the right questions, taking the right steps, and finding the appropriate resources.

The Placebo Effect and Your Expectation

Placebos don't mechanistically act to accomplish tasks such as reducing cholesterol or shrinking tumors; they're effective because of an individual's expectations. If you believe the pill or injection is real, your brain may induce a response from your own body chemistry to cause a reaction similar to what a medication might.

To bolster the effectiveness of a placebo, administrators should be cognizant of *how* placebos are administered. For instance:

- A big pill is better than a small one.[11]
- A bitter pill is more effective than a bland one.[12]
- Two tablets work better than one.[13]
- Capsules are stronger than tablets.[14]
- An injection is more effective than a tablet.[15]

Even color plays a role. For example, red, yellow, and orange pills are associated with a stimulant effect, while blue and green ones have a stronger tranquilizing effect.[16] Additionally, it's surmised that medication administered by a doctor is more effective than medication administered by a nurse, and that a doctor in a white coat is more effective than a doctor in street clothes. Incredible, isn't it?

The ability to tap into and influence someone's subconscious is a powerful skill—a skill that's used by people every day to have others "buy" what they're selling, be it a product, a belief, or a worldview. This power can be very dangerous and manipulative if used deceptively for personal gain.

On a lighter note, think of a hypnotist's ability to make people act, think, and behave in atypical ways. Hypnotists are able to make people act like animals.[17] They've made people eat a raw onion because they had them believe it was an apple.[18] They've made people act in ways they never would have if they consciously knew what they were doing.

The ability to hypnotize people can be fun when used for entertainment. Although you might think of hypnosis as a comical way to entertain a crowd, practically speaking, before the invention of anesthesia some surgeons used hypnosis (also called clinical hypnosis or hypnosurgery) and had better outcomes (such as reduced pain perception) with their surgeries.[19]

According to the American Psychological Association, hypnosis involves "focused attention and reduced peripheral awareness characterized by an enhanced capacity for response to suggestion."[20] If you've ever seen a hypnotist, you know the power of subconscious manipulation. Hypnotists are very skilled at getting you into a mental state where your conscious mind is resting and therefore not filtering (similar to when you're very tired or in a deep meditative state). Hypnotists are keenly aware that if they can get you to let your guard down in terms of your conscious mind, they can implant suggestions in your subconscious.

Understanding your subconscious mind can help you to learn about your behaviors, your self-imposed limits, and the possibilities for the future (both positive and negative). If harnessed correctly, it can be a force that propels you toward a better, more fulfilling life.

There's another level available to you, another gear you can shift into whenever you want. However, to improve your life you must be willing to say goodbye to your old life. **Is that a trade-off you're willing to make?** I like to believe that by choosing to read this book you're motivated to make the necessary changes. Don't become overwhelmed by thinking you have to overhaul your entire life at once. If you move the needle little by little each day, you'll realize that the mind, body, and life you desire are closer than you think. Remember the story of the resourceful junkman?

Your Internal Barometer

The limits of your subconscious may have been set at a very early age. If your subconscious believes that something is impossible to achieve, then you'll never achieve it. For instance, it was a long-held belief that running a mile in under four minutes was physiologically impossible. However, on May 6th, 1954, at the Iffley Road track in Oxford, Roger Bannister did the "impossible"—he ran a mile in 3 minutes and 59.4 seconds. He did it!

He broke the world record and accomplished what most people believed to be an impossible feat. Was he superhuman? No. He just believed that it could be done and then did everything possible to make what he believed come true.

Most of the information you're subjected to on a regular basis, both good and bad, is repetitive. Your conscious brain builds rules and beliefs to create a filter that your critical mind can use to process the information coming in. Information that mirrors your formed beliefs will be quickly accepted and received by your subconscious mind. Thoughts that don't match your blueprint, or what you believe to be true, will be challenged.

Some people stand by their beliefs, their political party, or their position on religion, for example, without ever questioning whether there could be an alternative truth. And since, for many people, their beliefs are the foundation of their being, they often close the door to any other possibility. This way of thinking is dangerous and can lead to blindly walking in a direction that is incorrect, irresponsible, or even perilous.

Roger Bannister's amazing accomplishment shattered the belief of so many runners that breaking the four-minute record was impossible. Now that their conscious and subconscious knew it could be done, the glass ceiling was removed and other runners began to break the four-minute barrier as well. Just 46 days later, John Landy broke Bannister's record. Soon after that, more and more runners accomplished the sub-four-minute mile.

Ultimately, you determine what's possible for your life. If you have negative behaviors or negative beliefs about what's possible, they may have come from how you were raised and the people who were around you as a child—but change *can* happen. It requires a lot of self-discipline and a willingness to discover the root of your limitations. Competently trained therapists can help you reach this objective while providing a safe environment for you to do so.

You determine what's possible for your life.

Thoughts, Behaviors, and Ripping up Long-Held Beliefs

Imagine your brain as a garden. If you want it to be filled with beautiful flowers, you must first eliminate the weeds that have taken over its soil. Failure to do so will leave you with a landscape that has flowers and weeds competing for space and resources.

Since you're now better informed on the power of the mind, you must become privy to all the limitations, personal and professional, that reside within your subconscious—these represent the weeds in your garden. Knowing your subconscious constraints will allow you to prepare for their elimination. Once they're removed, you'll be able to populate the new belief structure, which will dictate future thoughts, behaviors, and outcomes. And once you've planted your new belief within the soil, you must nurture it daily to ensure that it will prosper.

Over time, with adequate nutrients (incantations and visualizations performed with absolute clarity; regularly taking actionable steps) and your persistence (in developing a routine), that seedling will develop a deep and robust root structure—it will bloom and become bigger, stronger, and more resistant to a harsh environment (negative people and occasional self-doubt). Think about it. A weak and negative person can easily crush an acorn, but even the strongest person can't get a strong, stable, mature oak tree to budge.

If your weeds stem from your environment, you'll be happy to know that with repeated action you can alter the way your body reads its DNA sequence[21]—which can help you to engage in sustainable change toward the person you want to be. The field of study dedicated to exploring the correlation between our behaviors and our environment, and how our genes work, is called epigenetics.

Epigenetic changes don't affect our DNA sequence, but they do impact how our body reads our DNA sequence.[22] This is a field of research that I'm particularly interested in because I have identical twin boys who act anything but identically despite having the same DNA. Since birth, they've had the same upbringing, the same food, and the same opportunities, but when they were in utero their experiences were anything but similar.

Since identical twins share a placenta and have interconnecting blood vessels, there's a risk they'll develop what's called twin-to-twin transfusion syndrome (TTTS). When this happens, one of the twins (the "donor") sends his or her nutrients to the other (the "recipient")—which essentially means that one of them can starve to death and the other can receive too many nutrients and end up with heart damage.

As you have probably guessed, our boys developed TTTS—but thanks to our surgical heroes, Dr. Ryan and Dr. Norgaard, they are here, and they are healthy. We also did a heavy dose of praying and we thank God for their safe arrival each and every day!

Even after surgery (which was carried out at 17 weeks' gestation), the body and brain of our "donor" son, Elijah, was under extreme stress, and remained so for the rest of the pregnancy. This epigenetic difference between the twins is one of the reasons why their personality traits are so different.

Curious about how epigenetic changes work and how you can take advantage of this extraordinary phenomenon?

According to a study conducted by researchers at Harvard University, "During development, the DNA that makes up our genes accumulates chemical marks that determine how much or little of the gene is expressed. This collection of chemical marks is known as the epigenome. The different experiences children have rearrange those chemical marks. This explains why genetically identical twins can exhibit different behaviors, skills, health, and achievement." [23]

The authors of the study explain that "Recent research demonstrates that there may be ways to reverse certain negative changes and restore healthy functioning." [24] This is positive news for anyone wanting to make a change. And, according to what I've read, the change must begin in your psychology, for that is what determines your behaviors and your actions.

Ben Greenfield, a *New York Times* best-selling author of 13 books, including the very popular *Boundless*,[25] addresses the power of the mind and how our emotions affect our physiology. He explains that the shape of our bodily proteins (of which there are tens of thousands of varieties) can change as a result of electromagnetic fields (which are generated by thoughts and emotions), and when this occurs it can alter the expression of our genes. In his book he explains that "Beliefs, true or false, positive or negative, creative or destructive, influence the very cells of your body . . . harnessing the power of your mind can be just as effective or even more effective than pharmaceuticals, supplements, and biohacks." [26]

In *Boundless*, Greenfield references a 2007 Harvard study by Kubzansky and Thurston[27] that followed more than 6,000 men and women aged 25 to 74 over a period of 15 years. It was determined that "emotional vitality—a sense of enthusiasm, hopefulness, engagement in life, and ability to face life's stresses with emotional balance—significantly reduces the risk of coronary artery disease, even when accounting for healthy behaviors such as not smoking and physical exercise." This adds a great deal of credence to the words of Buddha (who lived way back in the fifth century B.C.): "What we think, we become."

There are many other scientific publications linking mindset and emotions to positive or negative physiological outcomes.[28, 29, 30] According to a 2014 study, "A growing body of research shows that mindfulness meditation can alter neural, behavioral and biochemical processes." [31] The authors comment: "Most interestingly, the changes were observed in genes that are the current targets of anti-inflammatory and analgesic drugs." [32]

Dr. Bruce Lipton, a stem cell biologist and the best-selling author of *The Biology of Belief*,[33] works diligently to spread the idea that our thoughts have a tremendous impact on our physiology. Elsewhere he states that "your mind will adjust the body's biology and behavior to fit your beliefs. If you've been told you'll die in six months and your mind believes it, you most likely will die in six months. That's called the nocebo effect, the result of a negative thought, which is the opposite of the placebo effect, where healing is mediated by a positive thought."[34]

Dr. Lipton says that he was "exhilarated by the new realization that I could change the character of my life by changing my beliefs. I was instantly energized because I realized that there was a science-based path that would take me from my job as a perennial 'victim' to my new position as 'co-creator' of my destiny."[35] The question is, How do you achieve this? Can you "will" it to happen through positive affirmations, or are the effects realized only if you dig deeper into your personal paradigm and long-standing belief system?

Although your conscious mind may want something (such as a promotion) or not want something (such as a mortality diagnosis), it is your subconscious mind that typically controls the outcome. Learning how to influence the subconscious mind is a staple of this book, because without this ability you'll continue to get the same results over and over.

Additionally, although it's been proven in science that we impact our genes and how they're expressed based on our beliefs and emotions, I do believe that some people will fall victim to their genetics even though they've done everything right. But we must recognize that it's a very small percentage of people who are at the mercy of their genetics. Most people, especially adults, can have a significant impact on their health and longevity. This book is designed to stack the odds in your favor—it will help you achieve an optimal life that is rich in fulfillment, passion, and growth.

I know you want more for yourself—and I know it's not a lack of desire that's brought you to your current physical and mental condition. There are vices and distractions everywhere, but that's not the primary issue keeping you from the outcome (personally and professionally) you desire.

Success begins
in the mind—
deep within your
subconscious.
If you can learn
to alter this, you'll
have limitless
potential.

Changing Your Paradigm and Engaging Your Reticular Activating System (RAS)

To challenge and change your paradigm you must have very strong conscious control over your thinking; this is the biggest barrier when it comes to achieving the life you want. First, you must spend time objectively looking at yourself—looking at your strengths, weaknesses, dreams, and current circumstances. You must find out what your emotional home is (anger, fear, jealousy, or regret), what the story is that you've been telling yourself (I'm not good enough, others are lucky, I'm never going to leave this town, etc.), and then begin the journey of changing the narrative to one that makes you smile, makes you fulfilled, and makes you take control of your life. The path to sustained change isn't necessarily easy; to be successful you must resist the urge to retreat into "comfort" and "safety"—that will keep you tethered to your old life.

Money, health, and happiness are not reserved for a "lucky" few. What you desire is possible, but it's going to take a full and unwavering commitment by you. Period.

Thankfully, we have an internal tool we can use to help us rewrite our subconscious narrative—it's our Reticular Activating System (RAS). This network of neurons located in our brain stem helps to decide which information we notice and which information can be ignored. If it weren't for the RAS, we'd be mentally exhausted by the sheer amount of information that's projected onto us every day. Fortunately, the RAS narrows our focus.

Think about a time when you were preoccupied with something, and chances are you noticed just about everything that relates to it. For instance, when you buy a new car, you suddenly notice the same car on the road every day; before buying it you never noticed these cars. When you're moving, suddenly you notice boxes everywhere; because you know you need a lot of them, your RAS is primed to be on the lookout for them.

Similarly, we can prime our subconscious by repeating positive, powerful phrases. "I am" is one such powerful phrase that must be used with caution. Each time you utter the words "I am" followed by how you're doing, you're communicating this with your subconscious. That doesn't mean you need to quash the negative emotions or problems you're currently facing. When situations arise that require attention you need to be honest about how you feel so you can effectively manage those emotions and/or problem-solve to remedy the situation.

That said, your average day isn't filled with dramatic highs or lows; most of the time your life is very repetitive. In knowing this, you must effectively communicate with the words and emotions that you want to embody. So, when someone asks, "How are you?," instead of your typical "I'm good," try substituting "good" with a word that better describes how you want to regularly feel. You could say, "I'm great!," "I'm fantastic!," or "I'm grateful."

Additionally, use positive vocabulary when describing yourself or who you want to be. For instance, instead of saying, "I'm not afraid" say "I'm assertive and confident" or some other combination of positively charged words. And be wary of the word "try." In a lot of circumstances, to try means to fail. You want to always think of yourself as you want to be. I won't try to become a more patient person; I *will* become a more patient person. I won't try to overcome my fears; I *will* overcome my fears. With a little thought you'll begin to see how often you can use "I am" and "I will" to your advantage. It's time to be more confident, direct, and assertive—don't let your mind entertain anything that isn't serving you.

So, if your mind is focused on "why me?" or you have a glass-half-empty attitude, then your RAS is primed to prove you right. Conversely, if you have a positive attitude, you'll notice all the positive things in your life. We all have good and bad in our lives; which of these do you want your mind to focus on?

For optimal it is imperative to have your RAS working for you. Try the tactics above for a few weeks and see if the repetitiveness of telling your subconscious that you're in an elevated state (from your typical "good" state) and using positively charged words (instead of neutral or negative ones) makes a significant improvement in your overall mood and sense of wellness. I'll bet it does.

Have your RAS confirm why your life is great, why you're so blessed, why today is going to be a great day! If you believe something is important, your RAS will be primed and ready to notice any time it's present.

Here's a novel approach: Why not begin viewing the world like a comedian? New, fresh, and funny material is like gold to a comedian. Comedians understand that there's humor happening all around us, every day. Their RAS is much more primed than ours to notice what's funny, ironic, silly, or smile-inducing. For many of them this becomes their dominant view of the world. They're human, so of course they get sad, angry, and frustrated, but I'm willing to bet that they seek out the humor in life more than you or I do.

What's the dominant lens through which you view life?

Choose from the options in the table. If your RAS is being governed by the negative words, rather than the positive words, it's time to make a conscious change in order to engage your subconscious messaging.

Humor	Gratitude	Misery	Excitement
Opportunities	Blessings	Fear	Contentment
Problems	Hopelessness	Nervousness	Guilt
Annoyance	Anger	Regret	Shame
Melancholy	Cynicism	Enthusiasm	Serenity

When you become successful at shifting the dominant lens through which you view life, you'll be better equipped to continually set and achieve goals. Consistent self-improvement isn't easy when you spend most of your time in a negative state. If you value growth in your life, begin by shifting your outlook and dominant emotions, then get smart about your goal-setting.

Goal-Setting and Visualization

You've likely heard about the importance of setting S.M.A.R.T. goals. If you have, you'll know that for goals to have a chance of succeeding they must be Specific, Measurable, Attainable, Relevant, and have a Timeframe associated with them. When your goals lack clarity and focus, their chances of coming to fruition are extremely low. Your RAS is a powerful tool; you want it to be on the lookout for anything that might move you closer to your goals. Without specificity in what you want, the opportunities, people, or moments that could move you toward your goal could easily go unnoticed.

To help make your goals stick, you should set up a system whereby you consistently take small but actionable steps toward their realization. Also, make sure you think about and talk about your goals regularly—this will help to impress them onto your RAS. But be sure to engage with people who'll be supportive; otherwise you'll be inviting doubt to creep in. As Mahatma Gandhi said, "I will not let anyone walk through my mind with their dirty feet."

When it comes to discussing your ambitions, you should learn to distinguish the difference between constructive feedback and unjust criticism. You must be open-minded and willing to learn from the education and experience of others. However, if you're doubtful that your inner circle of people will support your goals, then you should focus more on visualization. And if you can afford to do so, hire a performance coach who'll listen to you and guide you.

"The mind is everything. What you think you become." –BUDDHA

It's not cheesy to visualize what you want out of life—what you focus on tends to expand. You can use this awareness to your detriment or to your advantage. An analogy that demonstrates this power is my experience on the golf course. I know I shouldn't, but as I stand over my ball while looking forward, if there's a sand trap or water I sometimes can't help but focus on where I don't want the ball to go. And guess where it inevitably goes?

Visualizing what you want out of life, and how you want situations to unfold, is an art form. If you can combine visualization with the willpower and motivation to make steps toward your goals, this will produce powerful results.

Here's an example of how it works. Australian psychologist Alan Richardson took a group of basketball players who'd never practiced visualization and separated them into three groups:

- Group 1 practiced free throws for 20 minutes per day for 20 days.

- Group 2 practiced free throws on Day 1 and Day 20 and did not do any visualization.

- Group 3 practiced free throws on Day 1 and Day 20 and spent 20 minutes per day visualizing free throws.

The results showed that Group 1 had the most improvement and Group 2 had no improvement; Group 3, however, had significant improvement, with results that were almost as good as those for the group who practiced shooting free throws for 20 minutes per day.[36]

Visualization in sports works because the process activates the same neural network in the brain as physical training.[37] It's been proven that when an athlete participates in both physical training and ideomotor (ideo = thought; motor = muscle activation) training, the results are better than those for physical or visualization training alone.[38]

In Part IV of this book, I'll provide you with activities and pathways to help incorporate goal-setting and visualization into your daily routines. Implementing these two powerful tools will enable you to rip up the roots of any belief structure that isn't serving you—while planting the seeds for the beliefs that will enable you to realize the life you desire.

Before you move on to the next chapter, ask yourself the following questions to help determine your current level of self-confidence. If it's high, you're more likely to take the risk of making a change. If it's low, you can follow the steps in Part III to improve your subconscious confidence and reduce fear. Remember, we're still uncovering your patterns—knowing where you are is a vital part of ensuring positive and sustainable growth.

 ## Determining Your Self-Confidence

1. When you see someone else achieve a goal you want to reach, what is your thought?

   If they can do it, so can I / I couldn't do that

2. Are you a leader or a follower?

   leader / follower

3. Do you speak up or keep quiet when you have an opinion?

   speak up / keep quiet

4. Are you more likely to retreat into safety or, when appropriate, take a risk?

retreat / take a risk

5. Do you have an excessive fear of being judged?

yes / no

Self-confidence and the ability to accept judgment are key components of successful behavior modification. True confidence starts from within—it's developed by challenging yourself—and is reinforced each time you endure whatever is necessary to succeed.

With enough repetition, your subconscious will begin to expect success because you've conditioned it to know that you'll always find a way to prevail.

VISIONARIES

"The opposite of courage in our society is not cowardice, it is conformity." —ROLLO MAY

Visionaries go beyond traditional thinking and elect to operate and think of ideas that challenge what most people believe to be real or true. For instance, when U.S. president John F. Kennedy asked aerospace engineer and space architect Dr. Wernher von Braun what it would take to build a rocket that would carry a man to the moon and return him safely to Earth, von Braun's answer was simple and direct. He said all it would take was "The will to do it."[39]

While you may have set unnecessary boundaries for what's possible in your life, some people have two very important beliefs:

1. It is *possible* for them.

2. They have the *will* to ensure that it happens.

Self-help author Bob Proctor often talked about the importance of seeing yourself as the star of your own movie.[40] He would say that most people have relegated themselves to extras or supporting cast members.

Are you the star of your movie? If not, you may be living a life of quiet desperation, trudging through your days and counting the minutes until you can sit on the couch and watch television, only to get up and do it all over again.

The world as we know it has come to be because of people who decided to challenge the status quo. Whether it be in business, politics, religion, human rights, healthcare, climate, or sports—you name it—our world didn't just wind up this way. It was made this way by visionary people!

If you're looking for inspiration, you need only to consider what you're holding. If not for Johannes Gutenberg inventing the printing press, would we have the books we do today?

To live a fulfilled life, you don't have to set out on a mission to change the world (though kudos to you if that's your dream!), but you do have to challenge and transform yourself into a person who's less averse to risk. By doing so you will gift yourself the capability of continued growth and the ability to live a self-actualized life.

Best-selling author and motivational speaker Les Brown succinctly describes what's at stake if we fail to challenge ourselves:

> The graveyard is the richest place on earth, because it is here that you will find all the hopes and dreams that were never fulfilled, the books that were never written, the songs that were never sung, the inventions that were never shared, the cures that were never discovered, all because someone was too afraid to take that first step, keep with the problem, or determined to carry out their dream.[41]

CHAPTER 6

A Spiritual Journey

"It is in your moments of decision that your destiny is shaped."
—TONY ROBBINS

A FRIEND ONCE told me that she really struggled with decision-making, that she worried and second-guessed herself, and that she was unsure of her purpose in life. This lack of a framework from which her decisions were drawn caused her to flounder from one day to the next. For her, the lack of a spiritual center was a root cause of her energy leaks and unhappiness.

Have you ever considered one of your "roots" as being spiritual?

Everyone is on a spiritual journey—and your journey is unique to you. For some people it may be a relationship to a god or some other higher power but for others it could be just a set of principles they choose to abide by. For instance, a friend of mine is a self-described atheist but his spiritual guide is karma: he believes that the good (or bad) you put into the world will come back to you. For him, decision-making is drawn from the belief that if you do good you'll attract good things or outcomes and if you're bad you'll attract bad things or outcomes.

Whatever your journey, and whatever the moral barometer you choose to guide you, consistency and clarity will help to shape your life. I use the teachings of Jesus as my guiding force: I aspire to follow his message of love, acceptance, and treating others as I'd want to be treated.

Whether you ascribe to the teachings of a world religion, follow the collected wisdom of your people as passed down from community elders, or follow your own moral compass, what's clear is that it's important to live your life for a greater purpose than just your own. It could be, among many other things, feeding the needy, advancing God's kingdom, or working to save the environment. There's no right or wrong answer, and not knowing the reasons or the forces that motivate and inspire you is okay—many people don't know—but a more connected, more fulfilled life awaits if you can tie yourself to something beyond just you.

Stop Dabbling and Go All In

Do you have a clear vision for each day? I'm not talking about the things you're going to do during each day (eat breakfast, go to work, eat dinner), but, rather, a guiding structure in which to ensure that you're aligned, focused, and purposeful in the decisions, conversations, and outcomes you aim to achieve. In other words, what guides you? Is it a desire to make money, pay bills, and go on one trip per year—or is your life map designed to increase connection, develop deeper bonds, and improve the lives of those around you?

Fulfillment doesn't come from a monotonous life that is focused on the end of the workweek so you can watch TV and scroll your social media apps. There's more to life, especially if you value connection and contribution.

My spiritual journey hasn't always been clear—for years I lacked a distinct path. However, when I stopped dabbling in my faith and went all in, it changed my life in profound ways. But getting to this alignment took much longer than I care to admit.

I've personally come to believe that all the ups and downs I've experienced were God's way of nudging me to discover my guiding principles and force. You may not believe in God the way I do—you may believe in Allah, Buddha, or Shiva—or you might simply believe in the greater concept of the Universe. Whatever it is, there's a certain amount of faith you must give to the idea that you can't control every outcome. Life is a journey that's meant to have meaning. Some call it fate, others kismet, karma, or destiny. The idea is that there's something in our lives that's beyond us and within us, all at once.

For me, I had to come to the realization that there are certain circumstances that are beyond my control, that can't be solved with research and determination. My final reckoning with that idea came on September 11th, 2017. That was the day we received the news from our doctor that our in utero boys had developed TTTS. We were watched closely for the next three weeks, until September 28th. On that day, Drs. Ryan and Nor-gaard came to tell us that surgery was needed—the next day. They were direct but caring when they told us that we had two options. Option one was to "selectively terminate" one baby to almost guarantee the survival of the other (typing that makes me want to vomit). Option two was to have them perform a procedure called laser ablation surgery whereby they would essentially remove communication (blood transfer) between the boys. This meant that the babies would each receive blood independently from the placenta. There were, however, a few complicating factors that made the success of the operation less than likely:

- Lauren could go into spontaneous labor (which at 17 weeks' gestation would be devastating).

- Our "donor" (Elijah) had an extremely small part of the placenta, and an equally tiny umbilical cord, meaning that even if the surgery was successful he would be in for a tough time.

- Lauren had an anterior placenta (which, as Dr. Ryan explained to us, would make him feel as if he were performing the surgery "on the ceiling").

All these additional issues meant that after the surgery the boys would have about a 32 percent chance of survival. When it came time for us to give our answer, there was no hesitation: we were going to have two babies.

To provide even more context to what was happening in our lives at the time (beyond the obvious mental and emotional strain of wonder-ing whether our babies would survive), in the span of 13 months, from December 2016 to January 2018, we were tested physically, emotionally, and spiritually. That time frame included an engagement (an exhausting and elaborate one), the first Christmas without my mom, a mysterious head condition (discussed previously), two ruptured ligaments, two torn ligaments, an impact fracture, MRIS, physiotherapy, laser therapy, a bear "attack" (yes, you read that correctly . . . a story for another time), a wedding, a pregnancy, the news of twins, weekly ultrasounds, hypo-thyroidism, surgery for the boys, and a five-week labor strike at my work.

I don't say any of this to elicit empathy from you; I tell you to provide context: the deep level of exhaustion and burnout we were feeling. What carried us through was spiritual alignment and faith. We stopped dipping our toe into the faith pool; we made the decision to go all in.

Regardless of our spiritual calm, we felt like zombies, slogging through our day, going from task to task. But at the end of those crazy 13 months, on January 30th at 10:17 p.m. and 10:19 p.m., we were blessed with two beautiful baby boys, Jakoby and Elijah.

My eyes were open wider then than at any other point in my life to the power of giving yourself over to something greater than yourself. From that point onward I was no longer dipping my toe into the faith pool; I had jumped in and was enjoying the comfort and guidance that it provided.

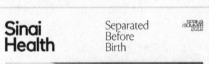

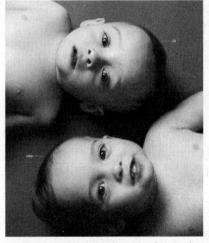

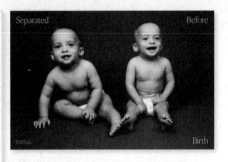

It seemed he was destined to die: At 17 weeks in his mother's womb, Elijah Gibbons was far too small. His umbilical cord was extremely thin; he had fetal growth restriction and, worst of all, he was donating most of his blood and nutrients to his identical twin, Jakoby.

Believing, having faith, and aligning yourself with a life principle that resonates with you doesn't mean your path will be easy. After a month in the Neonatal Intensive Care Unit, we were able to bring the babies home, but for many months we experienced the exhaustion and challenge of colicky boys and sleepless nights. We had multiple appointments per week with specialists to make sure they were staying healthy and on track. And we did it all happily because our kids had arrived safely. But the human body and mind can handle only so much.

My amazing wife and I had been passengers on a ride that seemed more like fiction than reality. It was as if we were edging toward a cliff. The inevitable last step could have us falling into an abyss. The struggle was daily. But I believe that in 99 percent of scenarios there's a lesson to be learned, sometimes multiple lessons.

When it comes to faith, in whatever form, it's useful to reflect on what that means to you. I grew up Catholic, and as a child I heard a lot of the people around me identify as such, but how many of them questioned their belief or the reasoning behind this self-identification?

When you tie yourself to a religion, spiritual teaching, or political party, for instance, you'd benefit from investigating *why* you have aligned yourself in this way. Was this path chosen by you, or was it instilled into you as a child?

Being a follower isn't innately bad, but being a blind and uneducated follower is. I was this way as a child—never questioning the values and institutions I was led to by my parents. If I was asked why I had beliefs in certain areas, I never had a well-formulated response that aligned with my true beliefs. Thankfully that has changed. However, becoming an adult with a fully formed conscious brain doesn't mean you'll automatically reflect on your belief structure and come to your own conclusions.

The questions in the following exercise are ones that helped me determine how I wanted to align my faith-related dimension of health. In doing so I became much more connected to my spiritual self, which in turn made me feel more aligned than ever before. I hadn't realized how much I needed this clarity to feel grounded and self-assured.

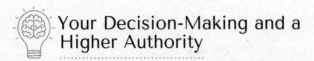 Your Decision-Making and a
Higher Authority

QUESTION 1: Are the decisions you make influenced (even in part) by your belief in a higher power or universal principle (Allah, Karma, Tao, Buddha, Christ, Holy Spirit, Infinite Spirit, Krishna, Shiva, etc.)?

QUESTION 2: What are the basic teachings or beliefs that define that power or principle?

Note: If you don't know the answer to this question, you will need to educate yourself in order to determine your level of alignment with the teachings and principles.

QUESTION 3: Does your day-to-day decision-making align with your beliefs? If your answer is no, what are some of the ways you can better align yourself with your belief structure?

AS YOU'VE LIKELY noticed, the first half of Part II was devoted to your psychology. As we move to Chapter 7, the focus shifts to your physiology, as this may be where your main obstacle in the pursuit for optimal resides. If your daily energy levels are hijacked because your body has been inundated with toxins derived from your food, water, and environment, it's going to be much harder to push through on the days when your motivation is lower than usual. If you can reduce your toxic exposure, the other behavioral dominos might easily fall into place. Let's find out!

CHAPTER 7

Toxic Overload, Immunity, and Your Detoxification System

"To keep the body in good health is a duty . . . otherwise we shall not be able to keep our mind strong and clear."

—BUDDHA

TO ME THERE'S little worse than having negative, unexplained health symptoms. If you don't know the etiology, resolving the issue is akin to closing your eyes, spinning in a circle 10 times, then throwing a dart and hoping to hit the bull's-eye. Although finding the exact answer may require expensive medical or naturopathic tests, repeated visits to specialists, and/or tedious and time-consuming food-elimination dieting, there's an option that, if implemented in tandem with these measures, could expedite your search.

First, cleanse your body of unwanted and foreign physiological disruptors such as toxins. A toxin is anything that interferes with your normal physiology and therefore negatively affects your bodily functions. One of my priorities in writing this book is to get your physiology working as it once did, with better communication between organs, less toxicity impeding the healthy growth and recycling of bodily tissues, and an elevated sense of calm, clarity, and mental focus. You're likely aware of the more obvious dangers (poor diet and lifestyle decisions) that disrupt a healthy internal system, but it may be the hidden dangers that are holding you back.

Toxins

An exotoxin is something made by humans (chemical cleaners, vinyl, etc.) that causes a disruption in our internal physiology. There are thousands of chemicals in our world, most of them used by companies looking for ways to make their product more effective while ignoring the fact that these chemicals make their way through our skin, into our water supply, and into our food. And when toxins accumulate in the body, they can cause inefficiencies in our internal chemistry.

Are you aware of the physiological disruptors that enter your body daily?

Most people are likely not aware of their exposure to toxins, because they can't see them—and they aren't educated to know which substances are harmful to our body and which are harmless.

Before I provide you with some strategies you can use to safeguard yourself and your family, let's have a look at the ways these substances find their way into your body.

1. **Through your mouth.** Most people ingest toxins daily. Whether it's from harmful dietary ingredients, the leaching of chemicals into your food or drink (such as BPA from plastic water bottles), or the residue left on food (such as pesticides), you likely consume dozens of toxins per day through your mouth.

2. **Through your skin (the epithelial cells).** The toxins that usually get into your body via the skin are those found in cosmetics, toiletries, and in your clothes. Once in the body, they end up circulating in your blood. There are many ways these substances can negatively impact your internal physiology. For instance, parabens (a preservative commonly used in beauty products) can cause endocrine dysfunction,[1] and most deodorants contain aluminum, which is known to cause DNA alterations and epigenetic effects.[2] Additionally, aluminum blocks your sweat pores and therefore inhibits proper toxin elimination from the sweat glands in the underarm region.[3]

3. **Through your respiratory system.** We breathe in a lot of toxins. Vehicle and factory emissions are a huge contributor, but according to the Environmental Protection Agency (EPA) indoor air is more polluted than outdoor air.[4] This pollution is typically caused by emissions from furnishings, paintings, foam, insulators, fire retardants, floorings, and carpets.

DID YOU KNOW . . .

Most new shower curtains have a distinct smell, which is caused by chemical off-gassing from polyvinyl chloride plastic.[5] This is one of the most hazardous consumer products ever made, and the off-gassing, which can persist for up to a month, releases as many as 108 volatile organic compounds (which negatively affect the liver, central nervous system, and the respiratory and reproductive systems).[6] Don't go the cheap route when purchasing this item: buy an organic cotton curtain and help to reduce your toxic load.

How Toxic Are You?

The EPA is an independent executive agency of the U.S. government whose purpose is to protect people and the environment from health risks. The EPA estimates that there are over 80,000 chemicals used in everyday products,[7] so it's impossible to escape them. And with growing evidence that many of these chemicals are unsafe, the "safe until proven otherwise" stance that many governments take is causing a tremendous amount of harm to the citizens they are supposed to be protecting.

Worse still, the chemical pollution that we're exposed to begins in the womb (through the placenta and into the fetus). A recent study by the Environmental Defense Fund found that 232 different toxic chemicals had found their way into the umbilical cord blood of babies born in the United States.[8]

The dangers of certain chemicals (such as mercury and lead) are well established,[9, 10] but there are thousands of other chemicals that can cause disruption in our endocrine system. According to Cancer Council Australia, in the past 30 years the incidence of testicular cancer has risen by over 50 percent in that country.[11] This spike in cancer cases has been too rapid to be genetic, so the cause must be environmental. And although most men are diagnosed at around 30 years of age, the initial cause can be traced back to the womb.[12] Since bisphenol-A (commonly known as BPA) mimics the hormone estrogen,[13] if a fetus is exposed to BPA during the development of the testes, it could cause health challenges (testicular cancer) that don't manifest for decades.

The Endocrine Society, whose mission is to advance hormone research and improve health and well-being worldwide, set out to update all the scientific evidence that links chemicals and endocrine-related disorders. In the report of its study (titled "Endocrine-Disrupting Chemicals: An Endocrine Society Scientific Statement"), Dr. Andrea Gore from the University of Texas, a toxicologist, notes that "there were increases in infertility, there were disorders of puberty, people were noticing their girls were going through puberty at nine and ten years old, instead of eleven, twelve, thirteen years old – which is when they used to go through puberty. And the society began to wonder, and the endocrinologists began to wonder, whether there were chemicals in the environment that may be responsible for that change."[14] And since puberty in girls is stimulated by a large amount of estrogen,[15] which is typically produced right before puberty, if there's an agent that mimics that hormone (such as BPA)[16] it may stimulate early puberty (also called precocious puberty).

It's very evident that we can't avoid toxins. However, with a little insight you can make decisions that will reduce exposure—which may provide the immune system with the break it needs to tend to other bodily issues.

Here are just a few examples of toxins that many people encounter every day:

- Many baby books are full of chemical plasticizers.[17] These are intended to protect the books from slobbering babies, but if those babies handle the books or, worse yet, chew on them when teething, they're exposed to the plastic products that make the books durable.

- Shopping receipts use heat-sensitive paper that contains a lot of plastic products (BPA and phthalates).[18] One study measured the levels of BPA in cashiers before and after their shift and found a notable increase in urinary BPA concentration.[19]

- Gasoline vapors contain benzene and toluene (among other hazardous chemicals), which are very toxic.[20] Benzene is known to cause cancer (particularly leukemia)[21] and toluene is a central nervous system depressant.[22] Inhaling these toxins through gas fumes can increase your likelihood of experiencing health problems.

- Bug sprays typically work because they contain the pesticide diethyltoluamide (DEET)—which also contains toluene.[23] Spraying this chemical on your skin will allow it to get into your body. Although some countries have banned DEET concentrations that are greater than 30 percent,[24] you should choose less-toxic bug repellants.

- Plastic water bottles are not only terrible for the environment but may also cause disruptive physiological issues due to the BPA used to make them. We'll be discussing the dangers of soft plastics shortly.

- Your bed, pillows, and sheets may contain harmful toxins. Chemicals such as formaldehyde (used to make bedding wrinkle-free), aldicarb (an insecticide used in the growing of cotton), parathion (also an insecticide), and azo dyes (for coloring) are used by bedding manufacturers.[25]

- Dry cleaners use toxic chemicals (such as trichloroethylene, which can cause liver, kidney, and central nervous system issues)[26] to clean your clothes. If you must dry clean, let the items air out before you bring them into your home or wear them.

- Household cleaning products can be very dangerous to your health. A lot of cleaning products contain highly concentrated chlorine (which can cause respiratory issues),[27] petroleum distillates (linked to skin and lung cancer),[28] and trichloroethane (a nervous system depressant),[29] and some even contain hydrochloric acid (which can cause liver and kidney damage).[30] These are just a few examples of the toxic chemicals found in many household cleaning products.

- Cosmetics and skin-care products often contain ingredients (parabens, sodium lauryl sulphate, phthalates, among many others) that disrupt your physiology.[31] Some of the harmful chemicals are carcinogens and reproductive toxins.[32] Always read the label before buying shampoo, soap, sunscreen, nail polish, et cetera, because even though a product might be listed as having organic ingredients, it typically needs to be only 70 percent organic for the manufacturer to make that claim.[33]

When it comes to the toxins and chemicals in your life, remember: don't let perfect be the enemy of good. Even if you can't afford all the recommended foods, bedding, water filters, or cosmetics, you can still eliminate some of the burden. By cutting down on the chemicals that enter your body every day, you may reduce the burden on your detoxification system sufficiently for it to keep up with the demands placed on it.

Think of your kitchen tap. If the water coming from the tap represents the chemicals and toxins that enter your body, and the drain represents your detoxification system, then your goal should be to reduce the flow of water (the toxins) from the tap. Slowing it down allows the drain to easily expel the toxins so they can't accumulate and cause disruption in your physiology. If the flow of toxins into your body is too much for the drain to filter, the sink will begin to accumulate the excess. When this happens in our body, the "excess" that is allowed to linger negatively impacts our internal harmony. The result? You feel sick, tired, and lethargic.

Determining whether a product is healthy can be challenging because companies use terminology such as "naturally derived" or "plant derived" to deceive the customer—all this means is that the ingredient started out as a whole plant; it doesn't account for the processing of the ingredient that takes place. What began as natural may have been modified (through harmful ingredients) into a product that is no longer healthy for our body.

To expedite your decision-making and avoid toxic chemicals, look for labels such as MADE SAFE and EWG VERIFIED. These labels guarantee that the product meets very strict health standards and therefore contains no chemicals of concern.

Take a moment to walk around your home and look at the everyday items on the next page. Again, you can't completely rid yourself of chemicals, but there are some inexpensive shifts you can make (like using vinegar instead of countertop cleaner) that will begin to relieve the toxic burden on your system.

The toxic overload in your body may be extensive, so it's important to understand the warning signs indicating that your body is struggling with the demands placed on it.

Toxic Overload Warning Signs

Have you ever wondered why two people can get the same flu but one recovers within days while it takes the other person weeks?

The answer is simple: one of those people has a much more efficient and a much healthier immune system. When our immune system is operating as it's meant to, it uses the power of a sophisticated set of organs and bodily functions that work together to maximize detoxification capabilities and rid itself of foreign invaders such as toxins.

Item	MADE SAFE?	EWG VERIFIED?
Floor cleaner	◯	◯
Countertop cleaner	◯	◯
Window cleaner	◯	◯
Toilet bowl cleaner	◯	◯
Air freshener	◯	◯
Cosmetics	◯	◯
Antiperspirant (deodorant)	◯	◯
Shampoo	◯	◯
Conditioner	◯	◯
Mattress	◯	◯
Laundry detergent	◯	◯
Fabric softener	◯	◯
Dryer sheets	◯	◯
Dishwashing detergent	◯	◯
Non-stick cookware	◯	◯
Baby-care products	◯	◯
Shower curtains	◯	◯
Candles	◯	◯
Food-storage containers	◯	◯

Contrary to what you may think, not all toxins are derived from the outside world. Our body produces toxins as well—these are termed "endotoxins." Endotoxins are waste products (uric acid, ammonia, lactic acid, and homocysteine, among others) from the normal activity of cells. If these substances aren't eliminated by the body, and are therefore allowed to accumulate, disease can occur. For instance, when uric acid builds up it can cause gout.

"Immunotoxicity" is a term used to describe the adverse effects of agents, such as toxic chemicals, on the functioning of the immune system. Here are a few signs and symptoms that your body may be experiencing an overload of toxins that are negatively affecting your immune and detoxification system (of course, this is only one explanation, and you should consider all factors in your lifestyle when seeking remedies for the issues outlined below):

- **Trouble losing weight.** Some toxins, such as dichlorodiphenyltrichloroethane (DDT), dioxin, and certain pesticides, are attracted to fatty areas in your body.[34] These toxins are lipophilic (fat soluble) and are more difficult to eliminate from the body, which is why it's essential that you reduce your contact with toxins and keep your liver functioning properly.

- **Chronic exhaustion.** This is a primary concern for most people I've worked with, even when they reported having an adequate amount of sleep. If certain organs in your body are struggling, the amount of sleep, and even the quality of sleep, might not completely resolve the problem. For instance, your adrenal glands are crucial to your energy and vitality; if toxic accumulation is affecting these glands, the result will likely be consistent fatigue.

  There are many other reasons why you may be suffering from exhaustion (poor diet, consistent stress, etc.), but if you're living a relatively healthy lifestyle, then persistent low energy could mean your immune system isn't working very well.

  Imagine your immune system as an army inside your body. If your army is low in soldiers, or they're not very good at what they do, they'll take a lot longer to fight the foreign invaders that we continuously encounter. And since the immune response is considered a priority within the body, if your internal "army" is healthier and more capable, you'll spare energy each time it must eradicate an invader because it neutralizes and eliminates the threat more quickly, not allowing it to linger.

  According to the article "Stress, Energy, and Immunity: An Ecological View," "the immune system may have energy made available for it via reduction of other activities."[35] The author continues by stating that this situation "may change in energetically conservative ways when the protection it confers needs to be balanced with the energetic demands of other activities such as fight or flight, or may be suppressed when other activities are more important than immunity for total well-being."[36] Essentially, what this means is that the body sends resources to where they're needed. Your job is to ensure that it has those resources so it doesn't have to choose.

- **Frequent headaches**. An unwell physiological state can manifest in chronic headaches. Reducing headache triggers such as stress, alcohol, artificial sweeteners, and certain food preservatives can reduce the toxin accumulation so much so that your detoxification system is able to keep up with toxin removal.[37, 38, 39]

- **Mood swings**. Bodily hormones that are unbalanced could be contributing to your frequent mood swings. Toxins such as BPA, PCBs, and phthalates have been known to disrupt hormone balance.[40] One easy way to limit exposure would be to reduce or eliminate your use of plastics (such as disposable water bottles).

- **Chronic inflammation**. Some toxins (such as benzene and nitrosamines) have the capability to cause inflammatory states that may result in aches, pains, and overall discomfort.[41]

- **Slow illness recovery**. If you get the occasional cold (two or three a year), that's completely normal. It becomes a problem when it takes you a long time to recover (more than seven days). Dr. Nadia Hasan of Penn Medicine states that "it takes the immune system three to four days to develop antibodies and fight off pesky germs."[42] But if your immune system is weak, possibly resulting in accumulated bodily toxins, it may not have the resources to fight the infection as quickly. In addition to long-lasting colds, if you're catching them more frequently it could indicate the need for a boost to your immune system.

- **Slow wound healing**. The length of time it takes to heal from a burn, cut, or scrape may provide a clue as to toxic overload and the health of your immune system. Dr. Hasan explains that "your body works hard to protect the wound by sending nutrient-rich blood to the injury to help regenerate new skin. The healing process depends on healthy immune cells. But if your immune system is sluggish, your skin can't regenerate. Instead, your wounds linger and have a hard time healing."[43]

- **Excessive gas, constipation, or diarrhea**. A large multinational study determined that more than 40 percent of people worldwide live with gastrointestinal disorders.[44] Many people are unaware that their issues around fatigue, brain fog, unhappiness, and so on may be attributable to issues in the gastrointestinal system.[45, 46] Learning to speak the language of the gut, then appropriately responding through the elimination of its irritants, as well as the addition of what may promote healing and good health, will quickly result in positive changes.

In the article "Allergy and the Gastrointestinal System," the authors state that "The gastrointestinal system plays a central role in immune system homeostasis. It is the main route of contact with the external environment and is overloaded every day with external stimuli, sometimes as dangerous as pathogens (bacteria, protozoa, fungi, viruses) or toxic substances, in other cases very useful as food or commensal flora. The crucial position of the gastrointestinal system is testified by the huge amount of immune cells that reside within it."[47]

The researchers add that 70 percent of the immune system resides within the gastrointestinal system.[48] Given that the GI system plays such an important role in our immunity, if there are symptoms of a disturbance (gas, diarrhea, constipation, etc.) it likely indicates that there's some internal disharmony within your GI tract.

MY GI DISCOVERY

In 2014 I was visiting my naturopath weekly to determine why my energy was so low despite having many healthy habits (except working at a moderate pace . . . which you already know). After we had spent an extensive time working together, she was certain that I had an overgrowth of yeast in my body (candida albicans).

It's normal to have candida in the human body. It's a type of yeast that typically resides in the mouth, throat, gut, and vagina. However, if the levels of candida in the body are allowed to propagate, you'll begin to feel its adverse effects.[49]

Likely because of excessive stress and years of chronic antibiotic use, my GI system and the bacteria that reside within it were very unbalanced. In this environment, where the bad bacteria outnumbered the good bacteria, fungus (in the form of yeast) was able to proliferate. And just like you get hungry, yeast toxins also get hungry.

Yeast thrives on sugar, which is one of the reasons why some people crave it.[50] Here's how bad it got for me. I'd wake up in the middle of the night, walk downstairs to the kitchen, pop two Oreo cookies in my mouth, then saunter back up to my bed.

Disgusted? Lauren was too. I knew I was doing it, but I never felt fully conscious while I did it, if that makes sense to you. In the morning she'd remind me, and my cookie shame would then kick in.

When I wasn't in some sleepy, hypnotic sugar trance, I'd still feel the craving for sugar but could use my willpower to stop myself from eating it. I know what you're thinking. Why did you have Oreos in the house if you'd chronically sleep-eat them? Great question! But I don't have an answer for you.

So why is yeast, alternatively called small intestinal fungal overgrowth (SIFO), an issue? Because your unexplained health issues may stem from it.

Recently it's been found that approximately 25 percent of people with unexplained GI issues have SIFO.[51] Among the problems that yeast overgrowth can cause is a burden on the immune system,[52] stemming from the fact that yeast produces 178 different toxins, which your body must work to eliminate or you may experience symptoms such as brain fog and frequent infections.[53]

For myself, the dysbiosis within my gut was likely a key contributor to my issues around poor immunity and decreased sense of well-being. This was one of my core issues—discovering its root allowed me to design a strategy to eradicate it.

If you have classic GI issues like diarrhea or constipation—or additional symptoms like fatigue, brain fog, joint pain, or insomnia (to name a few)—consider speaking with a healthcare practitioner about your concerns.

LET'S HAVE A look at how your detoxification system works. By having a basic understanding of the organs involved, how they work to detox, and what you can do to support this vital physiological system, you'll be better equipped to expedite its optimization.

How Your Detoxification System Works

The word "detox" has attracted *a lot* of attention in recent years. The use of this word has been so watered down that people don't fully understand its true meaning. Don't get me wrong—there are terrific detox programs out there that can provide your physiology with the kickstart it needs to remove unwanted toxins; however, the change needs to be sustained or you're destined to repeat the same lifestyle missteps.

Ask yourself the following question: What can I do to get out of my body's way and let it do what it's been so beautifully designed to do: remove the unwanted intruders (foreign invaders and toxins) and rebuild (in a timely manner) what's useful to it (hormones, enzymes, tissues, and cells)?

The body uses the capabilities of your liver, kidneys, skin, intestines, respiratory system, lymphatic system, and immune system to keep itself as healthy as possible. Proper functioning of these organs ensures that your protection is at its peak. A weak link in any of them may result in the gradual accumulation of toxins, which will affect your physical and/or mental state.

Here's a list of detoxification organs, along with their role in detoxification and a few tips on how to support them through diet and/or lifestyle:

Organ	Detox-Related Role	How to Support
Liver	Alters the chemistry of toxins, making them easier to remove from the body	Foods: beets, garlic, leafy greens, green tea Supplements: milk thistle, turmeric, cysteine, vitamin C, vitamin D, vitamin E, alpha lipoic acid, dandelion root
Small Intestine	Distinguishes between foreign invaders (such as parasites) and the nutrients that you want absorbed	Drink a healthy volume of water and eat an adequate amount of fiber. Fiber (consumed through foods such as fruits and vegetables) aids in bowel movement and in ensuring good gut bacteria. Boosting your good bacteria via exogenous probiotics is also beneficial.

Organ	Detox-Related Role	How to Support
Large Intestine (colon)	Removes toxins and waste products through bowel movements; constipation causes toxins to remain in your colon, which if left long enough can be reabsorbed into the body	As with the small intestine, following a healthy, fiber-rich diet and drinking an adequate amount of water will support the functioning of the large intestine. Other ways of supporting this organ include stress management and exercise.
Skin	Through sweat and oil glands, provides a route for toxins to be removed from the body	Use healthy skin-care products and aluminum-free deodorant and slough off dead skin cells by regularly dry brushing and exfoliating. Exercise and saunas can also expedite toxin elimination, hence the term "sweat it out."
Respiratory System	Network of organs that eliminates waste and toxins through your breath and mucus expulsion	Ways to support your respiratory system include limiting indoor pollutants, reducing outdoor air pollution when possible, exercising regularly, and not smoking.
Kidneys	Filter the blood and remove its waste through urination	Proper hydration and a healthy blood pressure (managed through diet, exercise, and stress reduction) are essential for good kidney functioning.
Lymphatic System	Composed of lymphoid organs (bone marrow, thymus, lymph nodes, spleen, tonsils, and mucous membranes), it manages bodily fluid levels, reacts to foreign invaders, and removes cellular waste	Lymphatic fluid is stagnant when you are stagnant; moving your body regularly and rebounding are excellent ways to ensure that it circulates effectively. Also, dry skin brushing and massage therapy can enhance fluid movement.

Your detox system works best when you're in a relaxed, parasympathetic state as opposed to a sympathetic state. The parasympathetic nervous system is a network of nerves that aids your digestion and relaxes your body after stressful periods. Conversely, the sympathetic nervous system responds to stressful or dangerous situations by providing your physiology with the resources (elevated blood glucose, blood pressure, heart rate, respiration, and mental acuity) necessary to remedy (confront or flee) the situation. Using mindfulness breath work can support the transition from sympathetic to parasympathetic.

THE JARISCH-HERXHEIMER PHENOMENON (A.K.A. THE HERX REACTION)

After I'd spent thousands of dollars on naturopathy and the recommended supplements, my fatigue and signs of candidiasis were still prevalent. My naturopath then suggested something that would leave me bedridden for two days straight. She said it was time for me to take a more aggressive approach and cut out *all* sugar immediately. And not just your typical sugary snacks: if it contained sugar or could easily be broken down to sugar, it was now gone. I've always loved a good challenge, so I was all in . . . and then it all came out.

When I began starving the candida, I immediately felt its wrath. Remember when I said it could get worse before it gets better? Well, that statement sums up the Herx reaction perfectly. When your body is aggressively detoxifying, it's common to experience symptoms that mimic the flu. People often report having a headache, fever, sore throat, body aches, chills, nausea, and other flu-like symptoms.

When pathogens are killed in the body, they release toxins. If toxins are released slowly, and if your detox system is relatively healthy, you might not notice too many deleterious effects. However, when you take an aggressive approach to certain ailments there may be a sudden surge in toxins that causes the immune system to ramp up dramatically, which in turn causes the flu-like response.

When I stopped feeding the yeast, it began to die rapidly (this is called candida die-off). This resulted in a very high fever that lasted two days. Even though the shaking, sweating, and chills were very unpleasant, I welcomed the fever—it made me feel that change was happening. After two days of bed rest, the fever finally subsided. To me, the Herx reaction I experienced was confirmation of yeast overgrowth.

Although I don't recommend that everyone take an aggressive approach to toxic-waste elimination, it was my preferred method. It allowed me to expedite the rebuilding of my gut microbiome. And since 95 percent of your happiness hormone, serotonin, is derived from your gut,[54] it's crucial that you construct an environment that supports its production. For me, that meant rapidly killing off the unwanted yeast and dealing with the unpleasant side effects of massive toxin release and elimination.

Life Cycles in Your Body

Your internal chemistry has likely been subjected to years, perhaps decades, of improper treatment. The toll taken by this improper treatment is only partly your fault. It's impossible to live in the Western world and not come into contact with human-made chemicals and physiological system disruptors—they're everywhere. But as we'll soon discuss, there's a lot we *can* do to minimize our contact and to clean up our internal chemistry and have it run more efficiently.

Getting a cold sucks. Getting the flu sucks. Getting any kind of infection sucks! The goal is to do whatever we can to get out of the body's way and let it do what it's intended to do, which is to keep your system (all of your organs) working in flow. Proper organ flow means that your organs are symbiotically communicating with one another and constantly eliminating what isn't serving the body (while regenerating what the body needs). It's the most beautifully designed entity this world will ever see, so let's ensure that it can do its job.

According to a 2018 study,[55] you have approximately 37 trillion human cells (as opposed to bacteria cells, which are estimated to be 38 trillion[56]) in your body! Those 37 trillion cells are categorized into 200 (approximately) different types of cells (such as red blood cells, fat cells, and nerve cells).

Blood cells represent the highest percentage of human cells (more than 80 percent). Blood cells include red blood cells, white blood cells, and platelets. According to Jacquelyn Cafasso of Healthline (medically reviewed by Dr. Suzanne Falck M.D., FACP), "Cells are constantly dying, and new ones are being made simultaneously. . . . It's challenging to figure out exactly how many cells die in the human body each day. Cells aren't created equal when it comes to the length of their life cycles. For example, white blood cells only live for about 13 days, whereas red blood cells (RBCs) live for about 120 days. Liver cells, on the other hand, can live up to 18 months. Cells in the brain will stay alive throughout a person's life."[57]

The constant life cycle happening within your body should excite you! No matter where you currently are in your health journey, you always have the option of providing your ever-changing body with the tools it needs to grow healthy, thriving cells—ones that will provide you with the energy you've been craving for so long. Dr. Dean Bethesda of the National Center for Biotechnology Information estimates that "Every second, 2–3 million RBCs are produced in the bone marrow and released into the circulation."[58] This means that roughly 173 to 259 billion RBCs are produced per day!

So even if you're suffering from decades of neglect, it's never too late to flip the script. Minimizing your toxic burden, even a little at a time, will go a long way toward helping you to get on with optimal living. And given the constant life cycle happening within you, you should be excited about nourishing your body with fuel that will create the heathiest cells possible.

CHAPTER 8

Modern Food and Water

"Let food be thy medicine and medicine be thy food."
—HIPPOCRATES

DOESN'T IT SEEM backwards that companies that produce wholesome organic food must advertise it on their label to differentiate themselves? To me, if it doesn't say anything on the packaging, then it should be as close to natural as possible, and if there've been modifications, the law should require that this be on the front of the packaging to inform the consumer.

The reality, however, is that to get the good stuff, you need to put in an inordinate amount of time checking labels in grocery stores—and spend a lot of extra money for food that's considered premium. The alternative is to put yourself and your family at risk of consuming any number of harmful additives or chemicals. It's clear that our governments have failed society.

As for the root causes of the obstacles that stand in the way of optimal health, what you need to know is that much of our food is exposed to dangerous products at the growing and production stages.[1] And although there are branches of government—such as the EPA in the United States— that set limits for safe levels of chemicals such as pesticides, remember that just because your individual exposure (one meal, for example) might be low, if your detox system isn't working well, those dangerous chemicals may begin to accumulate and could become toxic in your body.

We could all be more vigilant about the screening process for the foods we eat. One of your primary goals should be to eliminate as much of the toxic burden placed on your body as possible. That said, you can only operate in the world in which you live. Try not to stress about the chemical load you might be battling, as additional stress will similarly deplete your system and have the opposite effect of what you want: resources that are available for the elimination of foreign invaders.

Do your best, and remember that eliminating a little is better than eliminating nothing. Take things one step at a time. If your budget constraints are such that you can't afford organic food, that's okay. Focus your attention on eating those foods, organic or otherwise, that we know to be healthy and concentrate on lowering your toxic burden in other ways, such as by eliminating chemical cleaners from your home. Where there's a will, there's a way.

The Dirty Dozen

In 2004 the Stockholm Convention ratified an international treaty to target chemicals that have a known impact on human health. The chemicals targeted by the treaty include pesticides (such as DDT) and industrial chemicals (such as polychlorinated biphenyls, or PCBs).

Each year, the Environmental Working Group (EWG) publishes a list of the 12 crops most contaminated by pesticides, along with the 15 crops that have the least amount of pesticide contamination.[2] It is reported that "More than 70 percent of the non-organic fresh produce sold in the U.S. contains residues of potentially harmful pesticides."[3]

Additionally, the EWG has begun testing citrus fruits for harmful fungicides. It is reported that "Imazalil, a fungicide that can change hormone levels and is classified by the EPA as a likely human carcinogen, was detected on nearly 90 percent of citrus samples tested by the EWG in 2020, and over 95 percent of tangerine samples tested by the USDA in 2019."[4]

The EWG has stated the following: "Whether organic or conventionally grown, fruits and vegetables are critical components of a healthy diet. However, many crops contain potentially harmful pesticides, even after washing, peeling, or scrubbing, which the USDA does before testing each item. Since pesticide contamination varies by crop, it is important to understand which items are most or least contaminated. Additionally, fresh items that are most contaminated, such as spinach, strawberries and other Dirty Dozen fruits and vegetables, still have high levels of pesticides in their frozen form."[5]

Nobody's perfect and everyone has different budgets, priorities, time constraints, and access to healthy foods, so the best advice I can offer is to prioritize the areas where you can make improvements. Whether it's switching to 100 percent organic fruits and vegetables, or replacing some of the non-organic and highly contaminated items (such as spinach and strawberries) with less contaminated ones, there are always ways to make improvements.

Keeping in mind that the body is constantly replacing old, ineffective, and dead cells and tissues with new ones, it might be helpful to provide your physiology with the optimal building blocks (vitamins, minerals, and other nutrients) for creating healthy cells and tissues. If you combine healthy eating with other strategies for reducing your toxic load (switching from vinyl to organic cotton shower curtains, replacing highly toxic cleaning supplies with vinegar and water, using body products that contain fewer human-made chemicals), you'll be rewarded with more energy, clarity, and vitality.

Take a look at the Dirty Dozen and Clean Fifteen from 2022.[6]

Dirty Dozen (beginning with the most contaminated)	Clean Fifteen (beginning with the least contaminated)
Strawberries	Avocados
Spinach	Sweet corn
Kale, collard greens, and mustard greens	Pineapple
Nectarines	Onions
Apples	Papaya
Grapes	Sweet peas (frozen)
Bell peppers and hot peppers	Asparagus
Cherries	Honeydew melon
Peaches	Kiwi
Pears	Cabbage
Celery	Mushrooms
Tomatoes	Cantaloupe
	Mangoes
	Watermelon
	Sweet potatoes

HOW MANY ORANGES

How many oranges would you have to consume today to enjoy the same nutritional value as someone consuming the same variety of orange in the 1950s? Some researchers say eight, others say 21.[7, 8] What's more concerning to me is the continued trend in the wrong direction. Modern intensive agriculture has depleted our soil by progressively reducing the volume of nutrients contained in it.[9]

In 2004 Donald Davis and his colleagues from the University of Texas published a paper that showed "reliable declines" from 1950 to 1999 in the amount of protein, calcium, iron, phosphorus, riboflavin (vitamin B2), and vitamin C found in 43 different fruits and vegetables.[10] They noted that there had likely been a decline in other nutrients as well (such as magnesium and zinc), but these nutrients weren't studied in the 1950s.

According to the authors, "Efforts to breed new varieties of crops that provide greater yield, pest resistance and climate adaptability have allowed crops to grow bigger and more rapidly... but their ability to manufacture or uptake nutrients has not kept pace with their rapid growth."[11]

Putting farming practices aside, as that is far too large a topic to discuss here, at an individual level you should invest in high-quality supplements and opt for food produced by local organic farmers. I worry that, because of today's agricultural practices, even with a healthy and balanced diet you may still be malnourished in terms of certain vitamins and minerals.

To Meat or Not to Meat?

After watching the eye-opening documentary *Forks Over Knives*[12] in 2012, I decided to try a vegan lifestyle for six months. I had the motivation, information, and enthusiasm to make a plant-based diet work for me. Although the word "vegan" is often associated with good health, some vegans eat unhealthy, processed foods all day long. I wanted to do it right.

Doing it "right" meant considerable food prep (such as soaking beans overnight), recipe research, and a lot of planning. I expected a surge in energy, maybe not on day one but certainly within a few weeks. I kept waiting and waiting . . . but it never came. I saw my naturopath regularly, took all the recommended supplements, and maintained an active and healthy lifestyle, but my energy level was lower than before the diet change. After the six months, I reintroduced organic salmon and immediately noticed an energy boost. I maintained that diet for a while and then added organic chicken and eventually beef.

You may be as confused as I was regarding my lack of energy while on a healthy, plant-based diet. Here's what I've learned since then: not every diet works for everyone. Our ancestry plays a major role in how our physiology responds to certain foods, regarding both the addition and omission of food groups.[13] But just as not all vegans are the same in terms of their food choices (and in terms of the quality and volume of food consumed), neither are meat-eaters.

By researching your heritage, you can determine where your ancestors came from and learn about the food they ate—which could provide you with valuable dietary information. For instance, if your ancestors lived near the sea, they likely consumed more seafood; if they lived inland, they probably ate more red meat. Learning about your family history doesn't mean you have to be strict about following a particular diet, but perhaps you should add more of what they consumed and less of what they didn't.

One thing all ancestral diets had in common was their reliance on nutrient-dense, natural, and whole foods free from the effects of industrialized processes. If you make this dietary alteration, you'll undoubtedly be much healthier.

As for me, I went from a good carnivorous diet to a good herbivorous diet and back to a good carnivorous diet. Most people in Western cultures (and in an increasing number of Eastern cultures) have an unhealthy carnivorous diet that includes too much poor-quality meat, too many processed foods, too little fiber, and too few vitamins and minerals. Even though ancestrally they may have come from a meat-eating culture, they would still benefit by cutting meat out completely. For these people, the vitamins, minerals, water (through the new foods they're consuming), and fiber that would be added to their diet would make up for the absence of meat.

A 2019 study on plant-based diets assessed data for 12,168 middle-aged adults from 1987 to 2016. The researchers found that "Diets higher in plant foods and lower in animal foods were associated with a lower risk of cardiovascular morbidity and mortality in a general population."[14] Another 2019 study, this one evaluating the effects of red-meat consumption on mortality rates, followed 53,553 women and 27,916 men over eight years. This study concluded that "Increases in red meat consumption, especially processed meat, were associated with higher overall mortality rates."[15]

These are just two of the many publications on the risks associated with a modern-day, meat-eating lifestyle. Although I believe that most people are far better off going completely plant-based, if you're seeking optimal you could study your heritage, go plant-based for a few months (perhaps indefinitely if you feel healthy), then add small amounts of organic, antibiotic-free, grass-fed, free-range meats that are associated with your ancestry.

ANTS IN YOUR SMOOTHIE?

Have you ever thought about eating ants? I certainly didn't until I learned about black ant powder and its potential for increasing energy, strength, memory, immunity, libido, and mental clarity,[16] as well as for reducing inflammation.[17] Think about an ant—its strength and stamina, the speed at which it moves. Ant extract has been referred to as the "Herb of the Kings"[18] and has been used in Chinese herbalism as an energy tonic for centuries. It contains beneficial vitamins and minerals—and is also rich in ecdysterone, the growth hormone of insects, which in humans impacts anabolism (the building phase of metabolism, where simple molecules combine and create new tissue, such as muscle).[19]

Before you rush outside to find ants for your morning smoothie, you should know that not all ants are created equal. The powdered ant extract you want is from an ant variety known as the polyrhachis. These ants live in the mountains and are often found around ginseng roots. Their proximity to ginseng roots may help to explain their ability to increase energy and enhance brain performance.

Not All Water Is Created Equal

As you can tell, I believe you should spend a lot more time thinking about what goes into your body, and that includes the water you drink. Most people likely know that "filtered" water is better than unfiltered. But why? Well, as great as it is that safe and clean drinking water is accessible to most people in the developed world, it still isn't perfect. Most city-supplied water contains the following:

- **Medications, such as mood stabilizers, antibiotics, and hormones.**[20] Do you really want the remnants of another person's medications? I'm guessing not.

- **Chlorine, to prevent bacteria from growing.**[21] The prevention of bacterial growth in your water is a good thing. According to researchers, however, "long term consumption of chlorinated drinking water is associated with bladder cancer, particularly in men."[22] Therefore, I'd advise that you opt for a water filter that removes chlorine. The chlorine will have already done its job of removing bacteria, so now you can filter it out and remove the associated risks.

- **Fluoride, added to drinking water in the mid-1900s to strengthen tooth enamel and reduce cavities.**[23] While fluoride has helped to reduce cavities, it's a known toxin that's linked to problems in the thyroid, gastrointestinal system, respiratory system, immune system, and liver.[24] It's also been linked to IQ deficits when there's an elevated fluoride intake during a child's early development.[25]

If you're interested in seeing what's in your city-supplied water (or in your well or other water source), you can order tests to determine exactly what's in it. However, even without a test, a water filter is a good start. What you need is a filtration system that removes the unwanted—viruses, harmful pathogenic bacteria, parasites, cysts, and any unhealthy chemical contaminates and impurities—but leaves the rest: beneficial minerals such as magnesium, calcium, potassium, and sodium. My favourite is the Berkey water filtration system, but everyone will have their preference. The point is filtered water is typically better than unfiltered water.

When my mom was diagnosed with cancer, I began to put a lot more thought into everything that was going into her body. Up until then, she had been using a reverse osmosis (RO) water system. RO may seem great because it removes just about everything from your water by using pressure to push water molecules through a semipermeable membrane, but this process also removes crucial minerals that leave your water devoid of everything, making it "dead."[26]

In fact, it has been proven that even short-term exposure to RO water can have deleterious effects. The Czech and Slovak populations began using RO water in home taps between 2000 and 2002, and within a few months there were various health complaints.[27] Thankfully in 2004 the World Health Organization (WHO) decreed that certain essential minerals were required in the drinking water in those countries and released a report proclaiming that RO water "has a definite adverse influence on the animal and human organism."[28] Even if you attempt to re-mineralize your RO water, it's extremely difficult to recreate natural water with all its minerals and trace elements.

You may think, then, that buying bottles of natural spring water is a good route to go. The problem with this is that plastic bottles will leach contaminants into your water.[29] Bisphenol-A (BPA) is an industrial chemical that's been used since the 1960s to make certain plastics and resins. Often referred to as the "everywhere chemical"[30] (along with phthalates, which are used to make plastic flexible), BPA is a toxic, endocrine-disrupting chemical that negatively impacts your hormonal system (because it mimics the chemistry of the hormone estrogen). It's also thought to be associated with certain cancers (breast and testicular), heart disease, obesity, diabetes, and impaired learning.[31]

There's also some research showing that BPA exposure can have negative health effects on the brain and the prostate gland of fetuses, infants, and toddlers.[32] BPA is commonly used in the production of baby bottles, sippy cups, pacifiers, and teethers[33]—and when children put their mouth on these products the BPA can leach into their bodies.

Plastics containing BPA are also used in food and beverage containers and in the epoxy resins used to coat the inside of metal products such as tin cans. As consumers become privy to the dangers of BPA and where this substance can be found, there are more plastic containers and cans with "BPA free" written on the label.

Again, it shouldn't have gotten to this point. I don't believe BPA should ever have been allowed to infiltrate our food and water supply. Again, responsibility has been placed on consumers to ensure they aren't ingesting harmful chemicals on a daily basis. There's no harm to you in avoiding this chemical, but lots of risk if you consume it, knowingly or unknowingly, on a regular basis. And . . . sorry to be the bearer of more bad news, but even if a company has removed BPA from their product, they may have replaced it with a less researched but still potentially harmful chemical like Bisphenol-S or Bisphenol-F.[34]

Even though the Food and Drug Administration (FDA) has said that the levels of these chemicals in consumer products are very low, if you're using them every day, what starts out as a small exposure will, if not properly eliminated from the body by its detoxification system, begin to accrue and will eventually reach a toxic level. The good news is that with simple changes you can reduce your BPA exposure. Consider adopting the following suggestions:

- **Use BPA-free products.** If the product is BPA-free, this will likely be advertised on the front of the bottle, can, or container.

- **Avoid heat.** Exposing polycarbonate plastics (which contain BPA) to heat via a microwave or dishwasher could cause them to break down and allow BPA to leach into your food.[35]

- **Find alternatives.** Substitute your plastics with glass, porcelain, or stainless steel.

So ask yourself, How good is my water?

Don't let *perfect* be the enemy of *good.* If you can't currently afford the water filtration system that you prefer or consider the best, you can start by making relatively inexpensive changes to the quality of your water.

To begin, eliminate soft plastic water bottles and opt for reusable glass or stainless steel. This small change will help not only you but also the environment (by reducing the volume of plastics that end up in landfills or bodies of water). Next, purchase a water filtration system that meets your budget—it may not filter all the unwanted elements, but you'll be lowering the toxic load on your body, and this will reduce the burden on your detoxification system.

Again, with small incremental changes you may begin to feel the positive effects on your physiology and, as a result, on your psychology. Taken a step farther, if you learn to recognize the early signs of physical or mental discomfort, you'll be able to act proactively and make sure you consistently feel your best. To do this, you must educate yourself in the language of the body, with significant attention to your GI system.

CHAPTER 9

Learning the Language
of the GI System

---

*"We cannot solve our problems with the same thinking
we used to create them."*—ALBERT EINSTEIN

GETTING TO THE root of your obstacle(s) requires some detecting skill on your part. You must be introspective about your habits and behaviors, and be able to pick up on the clues that something (such as an organ) isn't functioning as it should.

Your body is constantly sending you signs indicating what it needs. The problem for most of us is that we don't speak the body's language. Recognizing the difference between what your body and brain need and what they're craving, because of addiction or habit, is a skill you can (and must) master. Whether what you need is more sleep, hydration, minerals, connection, laughter, or exercise, there are bodily clues that you likely aren't aware of. Conversely, your body will warn you if you're having too much of something—such as sugar, alcohol, wheat, or exercise (yes, there's an upper limit for all of us).

We aren't sufficiently attuned to the deficiency, or the excess, and therefore we aren't able to properly remedy the situation. This section will focus solely on the GI system, given its relative importance to health and happiness and because GI issues are prevalent in both Eastern and Western cultures.[1, 2] But the human body is a vast landscape that's full of clues for those who are attuned to them. To learn more about the other areas (such as organs) of your body and how they communicate with you, scan the QR code on page 371.

DON'T SETTLE FOR BAND-AID SOLUTIONS

Unfortunately, we've come to rely on Band-Aid solutions for many of our health problems.

For instance, I've seen anti-inflammatory commercials where the actor has a sore knee but after taking the medication he's out jogging.

Is that really the best thing to do on a sore or injured knee? Perhaps we should figure out the root cause and resolve it first before risking more damage. Doesn't that make more sense?

Resolving the issue, however, hasn't been programmed into most of us, because solving the problem is difficult, and solving the problem may also reduce the financial gain of those who are making medications. Of course, certain medications are required by some people to live. These lifesaving medicines are an example of what the medical and scientific community do best, and we're eternally grateful for their work and for the availability of these medicines.

What concerns me is the overprescribing of medications,[3] and healthcare providers who don't work with their patients to dig a little deeper and attempt to resolve their issues. Remember, if your problems persist, you won't be able to live to your full potential.

It's time you became an active participant in protecting your health. If you take medication on a regular basis (prescription or over-the-counter), I recommend that you have a conversation with your healthcare provider(s) about whether you might be able to progressively reduce or eliminate your reliance on the drugs that you take.

Tell your doctors that optimal health is what you desire, that you want to work with them to reduce or eliminate your medications through proper diet and lifestyle. A good healthcare provider will be honest with you about the hard work ahead of you. And if you want to live optimally, you already know that the path will be difficult. The rewards, however, will be great.

Gastrointestinal Health

"All disease begins in the gut."–HIPPOCRATES

Gastrointestinal health is something that's been of interest to me for at least the last decade. Once I learned about the gut's role in immune function and happiness, I was sold. Also, as a child and teenager I was on antibiotics frequently, which eradicated the healthy bacteria that were there to serve me and resulted in a GI environment that had extreme dysbiosis. In my early years I was prescribed antibiotics for chronic ear infections; as a teenager it was for acne.

It wasn't until my twenties that I understood the deleterious effect that the acne medication had on the microbiome of my gut.[4] As an adult I wish I hadn't taken the medication, but to a teenager every zit is a very big deal, so I likely would have still taken it!

As children we're not typically taught about gut health. Even as a teenager I wasn't taught about happiness and immunity, and all the things impacting them. The habits formed early in life are likely to continue as you grow into adulthood. How your kids eat, their behaviors, and how they deal with emotions were likely influenced by you (their parents or guardian) when they were children.

We should be instilling habits that foster happiness, strength, personal growth, optimal immune function, emotional intelligence, and proper behaviors. Both in school and out of school, what is taught and modelled should reflect the life we desire for our children. Ignorance is not an option; their future is too important to leave to chance. Stack the odds in their favor. Do it every day.

Okay, rant done. Back to gut health.

There are many things you can do to support optimal GI health. This is good because, with the increasingly widespread education on gut health, more people are identifying an issue with this part of their physiology. Here's a list of some common GI issues and the symptoms associated with them. Look at the warning signs and get evaluated by a specialist if you suspect something might be wrong.

Remember, your behaviors may be leading you toward the cliff's edge—in this case, the GI cliff. If you stop (make changes) and turn around, you may never have to suffer the consequences of falling over the edge (which could result in chronic or irreversible disease).

Condition	General Info & Symptoms
Gastroesopha-geal Reflux Disease (GERD)	Occurs when stomach acid comes back into your esophagus (acid reflux) and you feel a burning sensation in the middle of your chest. This condition affects approximately 20 percent of people in the Western world.[5] Seek help if you experience pain in your chest or upper abdomen or if you have consistently bad breath, tooth erosion, persistent heartburn, or trouble breathing or swallowing.
Gallstones	As the name implies, they are hard stones that form in your gallbladder. According to the National Institute of Diabetes and Digestive and Kidney Diseases, gallstones affect 10 to 15 percent of the U.S. population, with nearly 1 million of those people requiring treatment, usually with surgery.[6] You may feel sharp pain in your abdomen (particularly in the upper right area).
Celiac Disease	People with this disease are very sensitive to gluten (a protein found in wheat, rye, and barley). When gluten is ingested, their immune system attacks the villi (the part of your small intestine that aids in nutrient absorption).[7] Symptoms include abdominal pain, diarrhea, constipation, bloating, vomiting, anemia, fatigue, depression, and even seizures. According to Beyond Celiac (formerly known as the National Foundation for Celiac Awareness), approximately 1 percent of Americans have celiac disease.[8] This statistic is likely low since it is estimated that more than 80 percent of people who have the disease don't know they have it or have been misdiagnosed with a different condition.[9]

The problem for most of us is that we don't speak the body's language.

Condition	General Info & Symptoms
Crohn's Disease	The exact cause is still unknown, but genetics likely plays a role.[10] It typically affects the part of the GI where the small intestine and the colon meet (the terminal ileum). The most common symptoms include abdominal pain, weight loss, diarrhea, fever, and rectal bleeding. According to the Crohn's and Colitis Foundation, it is estimated that approximately 780,000 Americans have Crohn's disease.[11]
Ulcerative Colitis	This inflammatory bowel disease causes the immune system to mistakenly associate certain foods with invaders; this results in sores and ulcers in the lining of the colon. The symptoms are similar to those of Crohn's disease but the affected area is just the large intestine. Frequent and sudden bowel movements, painful diarrhea, abdominal cramps, and blood in your stools are also symptoms to look for. According to the Crohn's and Colitis Foundation, approximately 907,000 Americans are affected.[12]
Irritable Bowel Syndrome (IBS)	The cause is unknown, but the symptoms to watch out for include bloating and large fluctuations in your stools (hard one day and watery the next). Diet is the main treatment for this syndrome.[13] The diet should not include anything that can trigger your symptoms—dairy, alcohol, caffeine, artificial sweeteners, and gas-producing foods are often culprits. Along with diet, stress is a contributor to IBS symptoms.[14] Following a low FODMAP diet is recommended to reduce symptoms.[15] It is estimated that 11 percent of the global population is impacted by irritable bowel syndrome.[16]

Condition	General Info & Symptoms
Hemorrhoids	Hemorrhoids are the result of an inflammation in the blood vessels toward the end of your digestive tract.
	Signs and symptoms include bloody stools and a painful/itchy anus.
	The cause is typically attributed to chronic constipation, bowel movements that require physical straining, diarrhea, and a diet that is low in fiber.
	Eating more fiber, drinking more water, and exercising more can help to treat the issue.
	It is estimated that 50 percent of Americans over the age of 50 experience symptomatic hemorrhoids.[17]
Diverticulitis	If there are weak spots along the lining of your digestive system, diverticula (small pouches) can form.
	Over 50 percent of people who are over the age of 60 have colonic diverticula.[18]
	According to research from 2020, the most common complaint is "left lower quadrant abdominal pain with symptoms of systemic unwellness including fever and malaise."[19]
	Obesity is a big risk factor for developing this condition.[20] Individuals should focus on a diet consisting of fruits, vegetables, whole grains, and plenty of fiber.[21]
Anal Fissures	Anal fissures result in tiny tears in the lining at the end of your digestive tract.
	Similar to those of hemorrhoids, symptoms often include pain and bleeding with bowel movements.
	A high-fiber diet can help to relieve symptoms.[22]

What is the current state of your gut health?

If you're struggling to determine the root of your GI-related symptoms, it's best to get checked out by your physician or alternative healthcare provider. But that doesn't mean you can't begin taking care of your gut today. Here are a few things you can do to improve your digestion and/or heal your gut.

- **Chew more.** I've certainly had my fair share of meals that were ingested way too quickly. You get caught up in what you're doing and aren't mindful of the quantity you're shoveling down, and the speed at which you're doing so. No judgment here—you should see me at Thanksgiving dinner!

  Chewing more not only forces you to be more mindful of what you're doing, but also begins the digestive process.[23] When you consume starches, ptyalin (an enzyme in your saliva) starts the digestive process in the mouth.

- **Avoid drinking liquids with your meals.** The additional fluid will dilute your stomach acid and therefore impede ideal digestion.

- **Drink bone broth.** Since bone broth contains the essential amino acids proline and glycine, it increases the collagen formation within your GI tract. Collagen is important in the healing of your stomach lining and intestinal wall.[24]

  Bone broth has also been shown to boost the immune function.[25] Additionally, it contains l-glutamine, which is beneficial in healing the gut lining, and therefore in repairing leaky gut syndrome (occurs when the tight junctions between cells start to "leak"—which can cause harmful substances to sneak into your circulation).

- **Eat fermented foods.** Foods such as sauerkraut, kimchi, and certain pickled vegetables contain live bacteria that serve to balance the microbiome of the gut. Also, fermented foods are typically easier to digest and aid in healthy motility (good bowel movement).

- **Eat blueberries.** Blueberries contain pectin, which has many positive uses but specific to the gut it can help to modulate the gut microbiota, therefore helping to properly balance the bacteria that reside within the GI tract.[26] They also contain resveratrol, a powerful antioxidant that can be used to neutralize free radicals. Additionally, the soluble fiber in blueberries aids in optimal motility within the GI tract.

- **Use peppermint oil.** Whether it's inhaled, taken by mouth, or applied topically, it can calm the GI tract muscles[27] and stimulate the movement of bile.[28]

- **Consume ginger.** Ginger can improve your gut health in numerous ways. It can reduce nausea and vomiting[29] (drinking canned ginger ale is a staple for most sick and nauseous kids), reduce indigestion,[30] aid in waste motility, and possibly reduce inflammation (which could help to heal leaky gut syndrome).[31]

  Additionally, ginger contains a lot of nutrients (fiber, vitamin B6, potassium, calcium, magnesium, and some trace minerals), antioxidants, and enzymes.

- **Consume apple cider vinegar (ACV).** Hypochlorhydria (low stomach acid) is a condition that typically causes indigestion. Including ACV in your diet (add 1 tablespoon to 1 cup of water before each meal) can help to replenish some of the acid needed to relieve certain stomach issues (such as stomach pain and gas). If you have a strong gag reflex, maybe start with half a tablespoon . . . trust me.

  An additional benefit of ACV is its ability to help combat unwanted GI fungus and bacteria. According to Yagnik and colleagues, "results demonstrate ACV has multiple antimicrobial potential with clinical therapeutic implications."[32]

- **Try rebounding.** I've never seen an upset adult jumping on a trampoline. I use the word "adult" because I've seen my kids jumping and crying multiple times—an odd sight indeed. As it relates to the gut, rebounding (bouncing on a trampoline, but not so high that your feet come off the trampoline) improves digestion[33] and bodily detoxification.[34]

  There are additional benefits that are widespread throughout the body. Rebounding just 10 minutes per day can increase lymphatic movement, bone density, balance, muscle mass, and circulation.[35] The benefits are numerous, so invest in yourself and get a quality mini trampoline. If nothing else, it may make you feel like a kid again!

- **Reduce your stress!** Your gut and your brain are in constant communication[36]—in fact, this is called the gut–brain axis. This bidirectional link ensures that signals can be sent from the gut to the brain and from the brain to the gut. If you irritate the GI system (via the foods you eat or any other irritant), it sends signals to your brain (via the central nervous system) that result in changes to your mood.[37] Also, changes to your mood (stress and anxiety, for example) send signals to your gut.

According to Dr. David Poppers, a gastroenterologist and clinical associate professor of medicine at NYU Langone Health, "There's a tremendous interaction between gut health, stress, and emotional health, and the arrow is bidirectional."[38] Dr. Poppers also explains what you likely already know: that high stress levels can make you feel hungrier or cause you to lose your appetite. With stress, the hormones ghrelin and leptin are produced by the gut, causing alterations to your hunger levels.

Some other things you can do to support your GI health are to make sure you're properly hydrated, getting adequate sleep, consuming enough fiber (both soluble and insoluble), taking a quality probiotic supplement, and reducing certain foods that contain FODMAPS.

FODMAPS

Don't feel bad if you've never heard the term "FODMAP" before. Unless you've suffered through chronic GI issues (such as irritable bowel syndrome), you likely haven't needed to be introduced to the term. FODMAP stands for fermentable oligosaccharides, disaccharides, monosaccharides, and polyols (all of which are carbohydrates). According to Kris Gunnars of Healthline, FODMAPS are "short chain carbs that are resistant to digestion. Instead of being absorbed into your bloodstream, they reach the far end of your intestine where most of your gut bacteria reside. Your gut bacteria then use these carbs for fuel, producing hydrogen gas and causing digestive symptoms in sensitive individuals. FODMAPS also draw liquid into your intestine, which may cause diarrhea."[39]

Here's a list of some common FODMAPS. Note that all of these can be found in whole foods and in packaged foods. If you're suffering from GI issues, it's a good idea to take a closer look at the ingredients of the food you're eating.

- **Fructose.** This can be found in table sugar and in many fruits (raisins, dates, and grapes, among others) and vegetables (broccoli, asparagus, and artichokes, among others).

- **Lactose.** This is a carbohydrate that can be found in many dairy products.

- **Fructans.** These are typically found in grains (such as wheat, spelt, barley, and rye). They are not absorbed in the small intestine, which leads to bloating and/or a laxative effect.

- **Galactans**. These are particularly abundant in legumes (such as pinto, navy, and kidney beans, as well as lentils).

- **Polyols**. These are sugar alcohols that are often used as sweeteners (such as sorbitol, xylitol, maltitol, and mannitol). They can also be found in certain foods, such as apples, peaches, plums, avocados, and apricots.

Personally, I'm sensitive to certain foods that contain FODMAPS. Getting to that realization has taken a lot of trial and error, and a lot of patience on the part of my wife (in dealing with certain—very unromantic—GI symptoms). My dietary do's and don'ts have taken years to narrow down. If you regularly suffer from GI discomfort and you aren't sure why, consult a registered dietitian to help you expedite the process. They might be able to analyze your symptoms to narrow down the foods, or food additives, that are the source of your problem. This could help you to avoid an enormous elimination diet that will take a long time to complete (typically it takes 2–6 weeks for the elimination phase and another month or so for the reintroduction phase).

Now that we've gracefully journeyed through the GI tract, I believe it's our *doody* to finish the job. (#DadJokes)

DID YOU KNOW . . .

Artificial sweeteners could be to blame for your GI bacterial imbalance.[40] According to Ariel Kushmaro, a professor in biotechnology engineering at Ben-Gurion University of the Negev, "the consumption of artificial sweeteners adversely affects gut microbial activity which can cause a wide range of health issues."[41]

Unfortunately, artificial sweeteners are so prevalent in our current food supply[42] that you likely don't even realize you're consuming them. And since new ones are being approved regularly, you have to remain diligent about reading labels. The best advice I can give you is this: when your craving for sweets kicks in, reach for some fruit that you know won't aggravate your digestive system.

Everybody Poops!

Now, don't get bashful. While it may not be appropriate dinnertime talk, it's important for us to have a little chat about it. Even though it provides very tangible (but don't touch!) clues to our health, I can't remember my family doctor ever asking me about my daily excrement. Conversely, every time I see my Chinese medicine acupuncturist, she asks—and she wants details!

When something is wrong with your gut you may not feel any pain, which allows the problem to linger and worsen with time. The issues may extend beyond the physical: you could experience unusual brain fog, mental health issues, or trouble focusing. By becoming a better bathroom detective, you may notice problems earlier and subsequently discover the root cause.

The etiology of gut dysfunction is multifactorial (immunity problems, chronic disease, blood sugar issues, etc.), so finding the exact cause may warrant a trip to your physician or specialist.

Before you make any bowel-related judgments, it's time you noticed trends. Although you might be too shy to admit it, I'm sure you already do it: you have a look before you flush. This habit that you've likely had since you were a kid is a good one, so keep it up!

Let's begin by examining why it's a good idea to peek into the toilet. Healthy poop can tell you the following:

- **Your core muscles are strong**—since core strength increases the pressure within your abdomen, which may assist in colorectal movement.

- **Your stress levels are good**—although stress is a necessary part of life since it helps you grow and adapt to the environmental demands that are placed on it, most people go well beyond their threshold and are therefore unable to properly recover. This isn't ideal for your daily bathroom trips since excessive mental stress and anxiety are known to cause bowel dysfunction.[43]

- **Your hormones are properly balanced**—since hormonal imbalance can impact the speed at which food moves through the intestines.[44, 45]

- **Your intestinal flora is plentiful and balanced**—since stool consistency has a close association with your gut microbiota.[46]

- **You've been ingesting the proper quantity of nutrients (such as fiber)**— since constipation is often linked to low dietary fiber.[47]

Interestingly, the coating on your tongue might provide clues as to the level of your dysbiosis (gut microbial imbalance) as well as the health of your digestive tract.[48, 49] In fact, it's one of the primary investigative tools that alternative clinicians (such as practitioners of Traditional Chinese Medicine) use in determining health.

Ideally the tongue is pink or light red (not pale), smooth (no cracks on the top or "teeth" marks along the side), with a very thin white coating of mucus.[50] Anything other than the ideal description could indicate an issue related to the health of your GI system.

Conversely, unhealthy poop may indicate the following:

- **You're dehydrated** (a very common issue[51])—which may be the source of your constipation.

- **You have increased stress and anxiety**—which affects hormone balance and stool consistency and regularity.[52]

- **You need more physical activity**—which will aid in bowel motility.[53] Conversely, too much exercise may lead to loose or watery stools.[54]

- **Your nutrition is lacking something**—such as fiber.

- **You have a food intolerance**—potential allergens such as gluten or dairy may negatively impact the ability of your gut to function optimally.[55]

Now that you understand how your excrement relates to your body, both physically and mentally, read the next table and reflect on what your poo quality is like most of the time.

You're looking for trends in your stools, not one-off issues. The information in the table is adapted from the Bristol Stool Scale,[56] which has been shown to be a valid and reliable tool.[57] This scale was developed at the University of Bristol to help patients discuss poo with their doctors with a little less bashfulness (my word, not theirs).

Type	Bristol Description	Joseph's Description
TYPE 1	Little hard lumps that are difficult to pass	*Ahk!*
TYPE 2	Sausage-shaped and lumpy	*Eek!*
TYPE 3	Sausage-shaped with cracks on the surface	*Decent*
TYPE 4	Shaped like a sausage or snake, and smooth/soft	*Awesome!*
TYPE 5	Soft clumps with clear edges	*Decent*
TYPE 6	Fluffy pieces with ragged edges (mushy stool)	*Eek!*
TYPE 7	Watery with no solid pieces	*Ahk!*

We're not done yet—there are a few other considerations to review before reaching any conclusions.

- **Frequency.** Ideally, you're going one to three times per day.

- **Color.** Healthy poo is light or medium brown (which is due to bile). The color may change based on what you've eaten (for instance, a reddish color could be the result of eating beets). Stools that are consistently pale brown, gray, yellow, black, or red indicate that there's an internal issue requiring immediate attention.

- **Smell.** It's never going to smell good, but poo that is very smelly could indicate an underlying issue such as a food intolerance or malabsorption (possibly caused by an infection or disease such as celiac disease or irritable bowel syndrome).

- **Ease of passing.** Bowel movements should be easy to pass. You shouldn't have to physically strain or run to the toilet when you feel the urge. In addition to ensuring that you're adequately hydrated, your defecation position plays a key role. Toilets are a relatively new concept, a luxury that our early ancestors didn't have. Humans used to squat (rather than sit) to relieve their bowels. Deep squatting helps to ensure that the puborectalis muscle is fully relaxed, which allows the colon to empty more in less time. No need to go running to your backyard to find an ideal poo corner; all you have to do is elevate your feet while on the toilet—that will mimic the squatting position. In our house we have a small step stool in each bathroom.

- **Sink or float?** Healthy poo might sink or float, but typically you want it to sink more often. This may provide insight as to the fat (float) to fiber (sink) ratio. If most of the time your poo is floating, it may indicate malabsorption of fat and other nutrients.

You should now have a better understanding of how healthy stools impact your overall health. So don't worry—it's okay to be disappointed the next time the automatic public toilet flushes your excrement before you can have a peek.

And if the information provided has revealed that you have a consistently less than ideal bathroom experience, don't fret! Improvements are possible with better nutrition and healthy habits that are more consistent. Part III will assist with your daily number two by helping you to rebuild your physiology and rewire your psychology.

BEFORE PROCEEDING TO Part III, please review the summary of Part II and reflect on your obstacles and the potential source, or root, of the issue. Having a clear understanding of what needs adjusting will allow you to narrow your focus and save time in your quest for optimal living.

Here are a few takeaways from Part II:

- Most people don't remember what it feels like to have a healthy body and a clear, focused mind. To (re)discover optimal energy, vitality, and enthusiasm, you will need to find the root of your issues.

- Getting to the root of your issues calls for some detective skill. You must be introspective about your habits and behaviors.

- Deeper roots will continuously form when you delay facing your fears. Use paradoxical intention to help overcome them.

- Twenty seconds of bravery may be all it takes to change your life.

- Worry is often emotional and very repetitive—and it plants scenarios into your subconscious of what you don't want to happen.

- Humans are designed to handle episodic stress, not continual stress.

- Something is negatively stressful only if you believe that it exceeds your ability to cope with it.

YOU ARE WHAT YOU ABSORB

Over the years I've spent thousands upon thousands of dollars on health supplements. Every time I pull out my credit card to pay the shockingly large bill, I think, "I sure hope these work." The truth is, I don't know where they've been stored (in a hot warehouse or in a warehouse that's temperature controlled, which could affect their efficacy), whether the ingredients listed are actually in them, or if I'm wasting my money. For those who've lived with GI issues, there's another layer of concern: Am I absorbing the ingredients?

Although the initial expense is greater, you may want to visit a naturopath and determine if intravenous (IV) supplementation is what you need until you've resolved your GI issues. If your medical doctor or naturopath deems it necessary, the first IV treatment would likely be a Myer's cocktail, which is a vitamin and mineral concoction that rapidly enters the bloodstream because it doesn't require absorption by the gut.

If you have a healthy lifestyle, a good diet, and take the recommended supplements, and still feel chronic fatigue, you might consider trying a vitamin IV drip. If you feel a noticeable difference in your energy levels, perhaps you need to explore possible GI issues to determine whether you aren't absorbing properly and are therefore wasting your money on expensive oral supplements.

- Your body, mind, and spirit are inextricably connected—the consequences of overworking one of these areas can be felt in the other areas.

- You're operating new software (modern stress) on an old operating system. By letting too many modern stressors impact your sympathetic nervous system you're not just exhausting your overall energy resources but also contributing to the excess weight in your midsection.

- Our conscious mind (which receives information from the outside world) *thinks* and our subconscious mind *executes*—it takes the information that it's given, then formulates a response and behavior that align with the operational paradigm that it's accustomed to.

- Limits and fears are created in your mind, and you might not even know they're there, comfortably rooted within your subconscious brain. Sustainable change requires you to develop a basic understanding of what it is you're trying to change.

- Consistency and clarity regarding your spiritual health will help to ensure you're aligned, focused, and purposeful in the decisions, conversations, and outcomes you aim to achieve for the day.

- Connectedness and fulfillment come from aligning yourself with something beyond just you.

- Your internal chemistry has likely been subjected to years, and perhaps decades, of improper treatment.

- Over 80,000 chemicals are used in everyday products—which makes it impossible to escape them. What starts out as a small exposure will, if not properly eliminated from the body through its detoxification system, begin to accrue and eventually reach a toxic level.

- The goal is to do whatever you can to get out of the body's way and let it do what it's intended to do, which is to keep your system (all your organs) working in flow.

- The body is constantly replacing old, ineffective, and dead cells and tissues with new ones—no matter where you currently are in your health journey you always have the option of providing your ever-changing body with the tools it needs to grow healthy, thriving cells.

- Modern intensive agriculture has caused soil depletion by progressively reducing its volume of nutrients—which is why you may need to supplement your diet.

- You need a water filtration system that removes the unwanted but leaves the rest.

- The ability to tell the difference between what your body and brain need versus what they're craving is a skill you can (and must) master.

- Optimal gut health contributes to your happiness, a well-functioning immune system, and an overall sense of well-being.

- Your stools provide valuable information about your health. Noticing trends in their frequency, color, consistency, smell, ease of passing, and whether they sink or float will help to determine the root of your physiological issues.

- You don't have to be a health expert. Simply noticing when something out of the ordinary is happening, and deciding to explore it, is a great first step toward optimal.

- Your body is wise—if you listen to it, it will reward you in spades.

PART III

Self-Optimization

"It is never too late to be what you might have been."
—MARY ANN EVANS

OUR DEFINITION OF "health" has changed a lot in the past 100 years. In the 1920s "health" was regarded as the absence of disease. In 1947 the World Health Organization updated its definition of health as "a state of complete physical, mental and social well-being and not merely the absence of disease or infirmity."[1] We now strive for optimal health, not just within the physical, mental, and social realms but also in other dimensions of health: occupational, spiritual, environmental, emotional, intellectual, and nutritional. While each has a distinct definition, they often overlap and influence each other. If one of these dimensions is severely mistreated or affected in some way, there's a ripple effect in the others.

This part of *Discovering Optimal* is about sharing with you the strategies and techniques revealed to us through science and ancient wisdom that can assist in optimal living. You'll be educated in the numerous ways you can effect sustainable change by changing your habits, both big and small. In Part IV, using these new habitual practices, I'll help you to make a plan for realistic self-experimentation and the development of sustainable habits and routines.

The initial adoption of healthy habits can be arduous, requiring a lot of willpower. With self-discipline, and the knowledge that you're actively making your life better, you will ensure that your habits eventually become a part of your daily routine. The day you get up and exercise without dreading it, the day you look forward to climbing into the cold plunge, the day you instinctively replace frustration with meditation and breath work, the day you realize that you haven't scrolled social media all day, the day you stop craving a cigarette, or any other vice, will be a glorious day, one that you've earned, and one that you deserve.

Your goal shouldn't be to adopt all the health and wellness strategies I present. Rather, you should examine your life situation (finances, time availability, desire, etc.) and try the methods that resonate most with you. Begin with those, examine their effectiveness, and then consider whether to cement them (through your work in Part IV of this book) into your lifestyle.

CHAPTER 10

Energy Management

"Energy and time are finite resources;
conserving them is very important."

—TWYLA THARP

ALTHOUGH MOST OF us associate the word "energy" with the vigor, vitality, and presence that we physically *feel*, there are other forms of energy that you need to acknowledge and respect. You're now aware that, in addition to the physical, energy exists within our mental, emotional, and spiritual selves. If you're overtaxed in one of these areas, the effects can be felt in the other areas. For instance, each day after I saw a therapist to help me properly grieve the loss of my mom, I was emotionally and *physically* exhausted. I eventually understood that I needed to conserve my energy and take it slow the day after an emotional psychology session. I knew that if I did that I would come out farther ahead.

To become better in any dimension of health we must push beyond our typical limits. Think about lifting weights: you'll get stronger only if you challenge yourself to lift more. But, as with anything, pushing too hard for too long will eventually lead to a breakdown of the entire system. For instance, if a weightlifter continues to push their body without the concomitant rest and recovery, they may develop a condition called rhabdomyolysis, which causes the breakdown of myoglobin from the muscles and its eventual expulsion through the urine.[1] If left untreated, rhabdomyolysis can lead to kidney failure and even death.

To build our mental, emotional, and spiritual capacity we must endure the same rigor that it takes to build physical muscle. You must expend energy in these areas, pushing beyond your current borders, and then take the recovery time necessary to come back stronger. Ideally, you'll be able to structure your life so you're growing in these areas without it seeming so daunting. To do so you must establish rituals. Before we get there, however, Part III will reveal strategies you can employ to help with your energy management.

Default Patterns

Good or bad, we all have a default emotion that we fall into. If your default emotion is anger, then you'll always find things to be angry about. If your default is gratitude, then you'll always find things to be grateful for. Every day we're faced with challenges and opportunities. It's when challenges arise that your default emotion presents itself most clearly.

You know yourself better than anyone. When something doesn't go as planned, when someone lets you down, when you get bad news, what happens? Of course, there are life events that warrant emotions that fall into the sad/angry/frustrated category. I'm not talking about those major events that occur periodically in your life. I'm more interested in the day-to-day emotion(s) that you regularly find yourself experiencing.

In 2017 Alan Cowen and Dacher Keltner conducted a study with 853 participants to determine the range of emotions that humans tend to exhibit.[2] They determined that there are 27 distinct varieties of an emotional experience. Here's a list of the 15 most common emotions.

Anger	Disappointment	Fear
Anxiety	Disgust	Guilt
Calmness	Envy	Joy
Confusion	Excitement	Sadness
Contempt	Frustration	Worry

 ## What Is Your Default Emotion?

Using the table as a guide, read the following scenarios and honestly choose the first emotion that you typically experience.

The only way this exercise works, and the way you'll get the most out of this book, is by conducting an honest and critical evaluation of yourself.

Read the scenarios and, as truthfully as you can, choose the first emotion that represents your typical response.

Scenario 1: You had a terrible night's sleep and woke up groggier and more tired than usual.

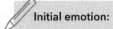 Initial emotion:

Scenario 2: You're stuck in traffic on your way to work or to an appointment.

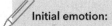 Initial emotion:

Scenario 3: Your kids are running around the house, not listening to you, screaming, and fighting with one another.

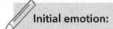 Initial emotion:

The objective, after a frustrating experience, is not to quash and negate your initial emotional reaction but to recognize it and quickly move toward a positive emotion. Negative emotions will quickly drain your store of energy resources. Remember, we want to preserve our most precious commodity: energy.

Do you find yourself lingering within an unwanted emotion?

The ability to quickly recognize an emotion that isn't serving you and make a rapid shift out of that state will help you tremendously in the long run. Now ask yourself if you actively work to quickly shift out of that negative state or if you let it propagate and subsequently steal your energy, joy, and happiness.

If you want to take this exercise a step farther, it's going to take some vulnerability. Try asking your significant other, or someone close to you, for their observation of your emotional state when difficult situations arise—and whether they believe you positively process and move through these situations.

Go ahead and ask them—you can return to this book when you're done.

By knowing your emotional habits, you can strategize the ways you might work to shift your dominant mental states and therefore help to preserve your energy (and make your day a little brighter as you move toward optimal living).

Take off the Mask and Change Your State

We all know people who seem a little too perky, a little too positive, and a little too optimistic. Our disdain is likely due to a tinge of jealousy. Admit it. The reality is if you know someone who fits this description, it's likely that they're really good at masking their unwanted emotions (this is not a good thing) or they move through sadness, worry, frustration, or anger more quickly than you might (and this is purposeful, practiced, and healthy).

The ability to move quickly from an emotion that isn't serving you to one that is serving you is a skill, and, like any skill, it can be developed. Soryu Forall is an ordained Buddhist monk and the founder of the Center for Mindful Learning in Lowell, Vermont. He says, "It's important to face the fact that there is suffering and there are real things to be afraid of. That alone gives us confidence to overcome them."[3]

You must complete the cycle of grief and sadness by recognizing their presence and processing their existence within you. Don't get stuck in an emotion that's no longer serving you—but also refrain from ignoring its existence within you (as I've done in the past).

Grief therapist and positive psychology coach Harriet Cabelly says, "You have to really let yourself feel—anxiety, grief, disappointment, sadness—and not run away. Whatever the feelings are, you have to go through them before you can get some reprieve."[4] This doesn't mean wallowing or obsessively ruminating on what's happened over and over. Remember, you know you better than anyone. If you know that your tendency is to get "stuck" in a swirling sea of "I wish I had . . . ," "If only this had happened . . . , " or any other thought pattern that isn't moving you forward, then you should seek the guidance of a trained professional or a family member/friend who can help you process what's happened and help you to move through it. The progress doesn't have to be at lightspeed, but you do need to progressively move forward so that healing can take place.

Remember, some life events warrant a certain amount of rumination and processing, but most people's day-to-day lives aren't filled with such events. As we've seen, it's important to properly work through those periodic situations. But it's equally important to recognize and quickly move through your negative day-to-day emotions. Your default patterns and behaviors will continuously knock at your door for you to let them in if you don't adopt a healthy emotional shift when you feel those old patterns creeping in. If you remain steadfast in your resolve to not let them occupy your home, you'll eventually change your patterns and the old unhelpful ones won't show up any more.

Easier said than done—believe me, I know. But to optimize requires courage. The most courage will emerge when you initially adopt your new strategies for emotional health and energy preservation. Eventually the new strategies won't take courage, because they will just be a part of who you are. You can get there; I know you can.

THE SPIRITUAL LAW of Relativity says that everything in the universe is neutral when seen in isolation. It's we who ascribe meaning and emotions to any experience. Accordingly, when something happens, there's no "good" and no "bad" until we provide meaning to the experience.

Remember, the objective isn't to deny a negative emotion or feeling but to recognize it and then work to quickly bring yourself back to a state that's more likely to serve you. It's hard, but, as with anything in life, the more you do it the more automatic it becomes.

In fact, I'd argue that the ability to change your state might be the most positive and life-altering skill you can learn. It's impossible to be happy, upbeat, positive, and motivated *all* the time, but that doesn't mean you can't live your life in a beautiful state *most* of the time. This is a crucial skill to master, since the quality of your life is determined by the state you spend most of your time in.

I know the challenges associated with trying to positively shift emotional states. Perhaps you need to discover why it's important for you to quickly get out of that state and into a healthier one. For me, the shift happened when I learned about the negative physiological effects of certain emotions on my overall energy levels. Because of my history with running myself into the ground, I'm now very conscientious about where I'm willing to let my energy go.

Ensuring that you have a variety of healthy ways to change your state will allow you to choose the best option for you, depending on the situation that is causing your unrest. Too often, people opt for unhealthy ways; although these ways may be temporarily effective, the long-term effect can be physiological and psychological disharmony.

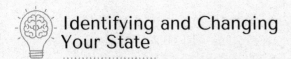

Identifying and Changing Your State

Here's a sampling of some common states that dominate people's lives. You'll see that not every state is a bad one. There are a few unicorns out there who are able to remain in a positive, happy, or grateful state most of the time, but they're the exception, not the rule. Circle the top two states you typically find yourself in; if they aren't listed, write them down.

Frustration	Anger	Envy	Worry
Fear	Shyness	Aggressiveness	Timidity
Sadness	Distress	Nervousness	Negativity
Gratitude	Happiness	Anxiety	Positivity

By now you're likely aware that engaging in unhealthy state changes (through alcohol, food, etc.) too often will make your situation worse. Here are a few examples of how people typically choose to alter their psychological state. Which of these do you employ most when you want a quick change to your emotional state?

Exercise	Caffeine	Alcohol	Drugs
Being in nature	Meditation	Listening to music	Prayer
Dancing	Sex	Sleep	Cold water immersion
Taking a sauna	A funny movie	Food	Yoga
Smoking	Deep breathing	Journaling	Positive affirmation
Therapy	Singing	Talking to a friend	Massage
Being around a positive person			

Be kind to yourself during this process. Developing sustainable change isn't easy, which is why so many people fail to succeed in the long run. We're searching for progress, not perfection.

If you're cognizant of the chronically unwanted emotional states you regularly find yourself in, refer to the list of techniques on the previous page (or brainstorm your own) and see if there are ways you can make a quick emotional change. For instance, if you find that anger or aggressiveness dominates when you're stuck in traffic, perhaps you could have a proactive strategy for when this happens—such as a few happy, upbeat songs that you sing along to, or a comedy routine from your favorite comedian.

A lot of people experience frustration (or some other low vibrational state) when their alarm goes off in the morning. In this scenario, perhaps you could commit to beginning your day by listing the things you're grateful for—followed by positive affirmations or incantations about yourself. It's very hard to feel frustrated and grateful at the same time, so *choose* gratitude.

Are there consistent scenarios in your life that cause a negative emotional state change? If so, list them, then brainstorm realistic strategies to cope with those changes and that you can commit to trying for at least a few weeks.

Scenario	State Change Strategy

WHEN MY WIFE and I first began dating, she told me that when she was feeling sad she would often go for a run and force herself to smile while running. She knew that it might look odd (I've seen it, and it does . . .) to people she ran past, but she said it was effective in changing her state from negative to positive. Although repressing or ignoring emotions isn't a goal you should work toward, when you're experiencing an emotion that isn't serving you, acting as if you're happy can accomplish two very important things:

1. It gives your subconscious the goal of being happy.

2. It causes your bodily cells to send signals to the brain that it's happy, and in turn the brain emits positive neurotransmitters such as dopamine and serotonin.

When something good happens to you, you feel happy. When your brain feels happy, endorphins are produced in your pituitary gland and signals are sent to your facial muscles to produce a smile. The contraction of the smiling facial muscles sends a signal back to your brain, which stimulates your reward system and produces more endorphins.[5] Therefore, faking a smile can help to trigger this feedback loop, which causes a positive shift in your level of happiness.

Another effective state-changing method is music and movie "therapy." What's unique about this approach is that you can determine your choice based on the mood you want to get into. Whether you want to feel inspired, happy, romantic, tense, motivated, melancholic (think about your high-school breakup blues), or even tearful, there's a song and a movie that can help you do so.

Let me show you my current music and movie choices based on the mood I want to shift into (or intensify even further). I want you to then brainstorm your choices and write them down. You might have multiple choices for each category, which is even better! I have several for each group, but to keep my word count manageable (and my editor happy) I painstakingly narrowed them down to two or three per mood. Following my examples is a blank table for you to write your selections.

Mood I Want to Elicit	Movie(s)	Song(s)
INSPIRED	*Rudy* *Invincible* *Coach Carter*	"Don't Give Up on Me" (Andy Grammar) "Eye of the Tiger" (Survivor) "Not Afraid" (Eminem)
HAPPY (LAUGHING)	*This Is 40* *Meet the Parents*	"The Power of Love" (Huey Lewis and the News) "Chicken Fried" (Zac Brown Band) "Diamond In the Sun" (Andy Grammar)
ROMANTIC	*The Family Man* *Crazy, Stupid, Love*	"For Sentimental Reasons" (Sam Cooke) "Lean on Me" (Bill Withers)
GOOFY	*Superbad* *Dumb and Dumber* *Zoolander*	"Funky Town" (Lipps Inc.) "Machine Gun" (Commodores)
PUMPED UP	*Remember the Titans* *Rocky* *I'm Not Your Guru*	"Can't Hold Us" (Macklemore & Ryan Lewis) "Thunderstruck" (AC/DC) "Sirius" (The Alan Parsons Project)
TENSE	*Free Solo* *Taken* *Green Street*	"Bulls on Parade" (Rage Against the Machine) "Way Down We Go" (KALEO)
MELANCHOLIC	*One Week* *The Pursuit of Happyness*	"A Long December" (Counting Crows) "Tuesday's Gone" (Lynyrd Skynyrd)
RETROSPECTIVE		"Last Time for Everything" (Brad Paisley) "See You Again" (Wiz Khalifa & Charlie Puth)
CURIOUS	*Forks Over Knives* *The Secret* *Heal*	

Mood I Want to Elicit	Movie(s)	Song(s)
INSPIRED		
HAPPY (LAUGHING)		
ROMANTIC		
GOOFY		
PUMPED UP		
TENSE		
MELANCHOLIC		
RETROSPECTIVE		
CURIOUS		

"That's Good"

A story I once heard that really stuck with me was about the CEO of a very large corporation who used the phrase "That's good" multiple times a day. I never did learn the name of the CEO or the corporation—or if the story is true. However, whether it's a fanciful tale or a true story, the lesson is important, and it's changed the way I approach difficult scenarios. The CEO in the story had so much responsibility and so many people reporting to them that they were regularly approached about company-related issues. Instead of focusing on the negative, the CEO routinely started their thought process about the issue with the simple phrase "That's good" to help their brain find a reason why the issue being raised wasn't a problem but was in fact a good thing. Doing this over and over helped to train the brain to do two things:

1. Discover quick solutions.

2. Look for the positive.

The CEO didn't waste precious time and energy on an emotion that wasn't serving them. They found a strategy that helped to quickly refocus their energy on problem-solving and find a benefit in the situation.

When the strategies I like to use for changing my physiology aren't immediately possible (going for a run or having a cold shower, for example), I employ this strategy. This simple phrase changes the amount of time I spend in a negative state. I've been using this strategy for years and have it taped up around my home and my office. This approach isn't always easy, but if you get your entire household on board with it you'll keep each other accountable and the habit will quickly become rooted in your everyday life. My wife and I are a testament to this.

When our kids are fighting and I feel my frustration level rising, I use "That's good" to find a way to turn their disagreement into a learning experience. At a very early age our boys were taught by my wife the meaning of the words "compromise" and "opportunity." If they want the same toy, they must come to a compromise or the toy will go away for the day—this makes them problem-solve and work together. Similarly, if one of them accidentally (or purposely) destroys something that was made by the other, we want them to verbally agree that this is an opportunity to make the destroyed object even better.

We also give our boys the space to be angry or sad about what's happened, and we ask them to consider their choice and to consider offering a genuine apology if necessary.

Try using this phrase the next time a situation arises that you'd normally view as problematic and see where thinking this way takes you. I'll bet you'll be pleasantly surprised. And if you're reading this and happen to be the CEO mentioned, thanks! (Email me!)

CHAPTER 11

Energy Fields and
Vibrational Frequency

*"The universe is not punishing you or blessing you.
The universe is responding to the vibrational attitude
that you are emitting."*–ABRAHAM HICKS

SEMYON KIRLIAN WAS a Russian photographer who perfected a way to photograph energy leaving the body (now referred to as "Kirlian photography"). It proves we're always emitting a vibrational frequency[1]—and since our emotions have an energetic frequency, the state you're in is often palpable to those around you.

For instance, when my wife walks in the door I can immediately tell whether her energetic frequency is positive or negative. This is good news for some people and bad for others. As we've seen, we all have a few emotions that we retreat to more than others. Whether it's guilt, joy, fear, jealousy, gratitude, or shame, the emotions that dominate your life emit a frequency.

Beyond humans, Kirlian discovered that all living things (plants, fruits, etc.) emit vivid, multicolored discharges[2]—which proves there's a vibrational energy surrounding all living things. Interestingly, even inanimate objects give off a coronal discharge, but the glow for them is more uniform.

Given that we all emit a vibrational frequency, you've likely noticed that the energy of the people around you is infectious, in both a positive and a negative way. It helps to explain why you connect with certain people and not others shortly after meeting them. They may not have said anything that creates or impedes a possible connection—you likely gravitate to them because you're vibrating symbiotically. This phenomenon may be hard to scientifically prove, but you certainly know when you feel it.

Do you want to know a secret? You have a superpower within you—and it's always accessible.

Your superpower is that you possess the ability to positively change someone's vibrational state, and in the process access the best parts of the individual's personality. You just have to learn how to "tap" into it.

If you train your mind to see in all people what they don't see in themselves, it can be shockingly simple to turn someone's day around, enhance their mood, and have them view you in a positive way. All you have to do is leave them with the feeling of "increase"—that is, leave them feeling better because of having seen you. Shockingly, this is easily done.

When you see (or feel) that someone's state is low, there are many ways you can change their frequency. You could look for what they do well and then tell them. This can be done with every person you interact with. For instance, if you see that the cashier is having a bad day, you can compliment them on something you notice, then watch how quickly their mood changes; the vibration they had is quickly transformed.

Of course, there are those stubborn cases who are determined to stay wedged in their vibrational state. But even then, I'm willing to bet that although they might not show it, they've had a shift on the inside.

With an acquaintance you may not be able to go very deep into their personality, but there's *always* something you can comment on and compliment them on. If you're trying to enhance the vibration and mood of friends and family, you can comment on superficial and/or deep personality characteristics or traits. Make sure your observations are sincere and you'll likely notice that while a negative mood or vibration can be triggered quickly, so can a shift to a positive mood or vibration.

Aside from the feeling that you've made someone's day a little brighter, there's another reason why you should be doing this on a consistent basis. According to Bob Proctor, when you leave someone with the impression of "increase" (make them feel good), you're putting yourself in harmony with the higher side of their personality.[3] People will notice this and realize that by associating with you they will enjoy an increase in themselves.

By practicing this technique on a regular basis, you're training your brain to see the good in everything, which will leave you in a positive vibration as well. Additionally, people will inevitably "return the favor" and begin to notice positive things about you. Have you noticed that the positive energy you project to the world tends to find its way back to you?

As stated in Luke 6:38 in the King James version of the Bible, "Give, and you will receive. Your gift will return to you in full—pressed down, shaken together to make room for more, running over, and poured into your lap. The amount you give will determine the amount you get back."[4]

Identifying Your Energy Field

"If you want to know the secrets of the universe, think in terms of energy, frequency and vibration."—NIKOLA TESLA

As a teenager, I took Tae Kwon Do for six years. At the end of every practice, we'd sit cross-legged with our back against a wall and our teacher would guide us in eyes-closed energy work. We'd do some calming breath work, then vigorously rub our hands together and hover them over various parts of our body. I was always amazed that I could feel the heat and energy between my hands and where I was hovering them.

If you want to become aware of your energy field, try the following exercise.

- Sit comfortably with your back straight, then spend a few minutes breathing deeply into your abdomen, allowing your mind to become quiet.

- Straighten your hands and rub them together rapidly for about 15 seconds.

- Hold your hands out in front of you with the palms facing each other— relax them so they are slightly curled.

- Slowly bring your hands together until they're about six inches apart.

- Make small circular movements with the palms facing each other—feel the variation in sensations. Then separate your hands with the palms still facing each other—move them closer to each other and apart.

- Repeat this process several times, slowly moving your hands toward each other and away.

- Pay close attention to your palms. You may experience a sense of pressure, similar to magnets repelling each other. You may also experience a feeling of warmth, tingling, or pulsing.

- Do this for five minutes and you may notice the sensations becoming stronger.

   Incredible, isn't it!

Global Resonance

Have you ever been to an event and felt that the energy was infectious?

One of the reasons why it's more exciting to attend a concert or sports event rather than watch it on television is because having a large group of people vibrate together creates an atmosphere that intensifies the feelings you have, positive or negative. If sports or concerts aren't your thing, you likely felt "unity" with others the last time you went through a major life event with a group of people. You probably felt more connected to them than ever before; this is because compassion and fear are two strong emotions that elicit interconnectedness between humans.

One of my favorite experiences with resonance is when I meditate with a group of people. Before I started doing mindfulness regularly, I wouldn't have predicted this—I'd have assumed it would be too distracting to have others around me. This all changed after I went to a meditation studio for the first time. I was able to get into a deep meditative state very quickly. I'd lose track of time and feel mentally refreshed afterwards.

I can achieve a meditative state on my own, but I've found it takes more focus and more time to do so, and I never seem to get quite as "deep." The reason why it's such an effective experience is the combined consciousness of everyone in the room—our frequencies align and the experience is intensified.

Human resonance like this can actually be measured. In 1998 Princeton University began something called The Global Consciousness Project where they use multiple random number generator (RNG) machines to collect data. According to the university, the project is "an international, multidisciplinary collaboration of scientists and engineers . . . [who] collect data continuously from a global network of physical random number generators located in up to 70 host sites around the world at any given time . . . Our purpose is to examine subtle correlations that may reflect the presence and activity of consciousness in the world. We hypothesize that there will be structure in what should be random data, associated with major global events that engage our minds and hearts."[5]

With many years of data, researchers have been able to monitor over 500 major world events such as the nuclear accident in Japan, the grand jury regarding President Clinton's alleged affair, Hurricane Katrina, Obama's presidential acceptance speech, the COVID-19 crisis, George Floyd's death and the subsequent demonstrations, multiple bombings, earthquakes, U.S. elections, Olympic Games, Christmas Eves, and the list goes on. The major events and the associated fluctuations in the generators (which the scientists attribute to consciousness changes) were not due to chance. The researchers conclude that "The probability that the effect could be just a chance fluctuation is less than 1 in a trillion."[6]

So what does this tell us? Not only do you have the ability to positively (or negatively) alter someone's vibrational state but in doing so you're creating something very powerful—you're creating *connection*. And the more people you have symbiotically vibrating together, the stronger the bond or the more united the purpose.

Harnessing Flow and Becoming Decisive

Remember the last time you had a day that seemed to flow perfectly? The conversations, the activities, the events, the people—they all blended so well. You felt connected, present, and calm—sensations that likely went away as soon as you were hit with something that caused you to stop, overthink, and worry.

The word "flow" in this sense was made popular by psychologist Mihaly Csikszentmihalyi. When in complete flow (a.k.a. optimal experience), you're in a peak performance state (mentally and/or physically), singularly focused with your conscious mind remaining "quiet." Csikszentmihalyi describes this moment as "being completely involved in an activity for its own sake. The ego falls away. Time flies. Every action, movement, and thought flows inevitably from the previous one, like playing jazz. Your whole being is involved, and you're using your skills to the utmost."[7]

I like to call this being "in the zone," and there's no better way for me to get there than by playing a sport. It's like moving meditation. When this happens, my conscious brain is quiet, which allows my subconscious mind to execute the task before me. It has been discovered that there's

THE LAW OF ATTRACTION

Call it chemistry, call it serendipity, or call it a spark—whatever it is, the law of attraction is likely the matchmaker. Whether it's meeting someone new and feeling as though you've been friends for years, or finding the love of your life, we'll always gravitate to those who vibrate symbiotically with us. The law of attraction helps to govern the circumstances that we find ourselves in. As Napoleon Hill states in his iconic book from 1937, *Think and Grow Rich*, "Every human brain is both a broadcasting and receiving station for the vibration of thought."[8]

If you're skeptical, then ask yourself: What's the worst that can happen by thinking positively, shifting your emotions from negative to positive, and opening yourself up to the possibility of attracting the situations, circumstances, and people that make you happy? To me, it sounds pretty darn good—I highly recommend you give it a try.

Some of you may still have limiting beliefs about what is possible, or what you think you deserve, but if you want to work on breaking that glass ceiling and soaring to heights you hadn't even dreamed of (yep, that sounded cheesy in my head as I typed it, but it's too true not to be included!), then you must continue to challenge your old way of living.

One of the ways people lose time, energy, and special moments is by living a life of disconnect and hurry. To combat this tendency, you must design your days, and the situations within those days, so that they flow gracefully.

a temporary decrease in activity in the frontal area of the brain when an individual is in flow—this results in the neurons of the basal ganglia (primarily responsible for motor control) to activate more efficiently.

What if you don't play a sport (or music, as in Csikszentmihalyi's example)? Can you not obtain the benefits of a flow-like experience? Yes, you can!

Think about anything you do that causes you to be fully in the moment, devoid of conscious thought and interruption. According to Arne Dietrich in the article "Neurocognitive Mechanisms Underlying the Experience of Flow," when you experience flow the analytical aspect of your brain is halted so the creative sensorimotor area can flourish.[9]

Here's a list of activities that can, under the right circumstances, cause a flow-like experience in me. Following my list, I've left space for you to list the activities that inspire flow in you. Once you've identified your activities, I encourage you to find ways to include these in your regular schedule to enhance your overall well-being.

Watching a captivating movie	Playing with my kids
Sports	Journaling or writing
Sex	Teaching
Meditation (especially group meditation)	A great conversation

You find yourself lacking flow when you feel as though you're stutter-stepping through your day, which makes it hard to progress in any area. You end up feeling as if you're moving a millimeter in every direction, never getting anything substantial accomplished. For instance, imagine you wake up feeling good and decide to go for a jog. On your run there's a lot of traffic so you keep having to stop and let the cars go by before you can continue running. The cars forcing you to stop are like the moments you have each day that interrupt your flow.

Some common flow-jackers are those times when we must learn something new, when we experience ambivalence (the co-existence in one person of opposing feelings toward the same objective), or when we're indecisive or experience decision fatigue.

Think about the last time you tried a new activity. You spent a lot of time in your head, ruminating over all the things that were required to do it well. And since you were constantly thinking about what to do next, or whether you were doing it correctly, you likely never obtained any flow.

In contrast, consider the efficiency of professional athletes: they have trained their bodies and minds to use intuition and instinct in the decision-making process. This allows them to stay in the moment and move forward without getting stuck for too long. In sports, as in life, if you remain ambivalent for too long the play and the players move on without you; to keep up you must make quick decisions when the moment arises.

Decisions are necessary from the moment you wake up in the morning. My advice regarding decisions is that you aim to become like the captain of a professional sports team. Good captains set the pace for the game. You can become the captain for those around you.

If you are direct, decisive, and confident, others will trust your leadership. This doesn't mean you'll always be right, because making a wrong decision is part of life. What's worse than making the wrong decision? Wasting precious time before you make that wrong decision. As author and motivational speaker Tom Peters puts it, "Test fast, fail fast, adjust fast."[10] Remember, even if you're wrong, being decisive allows you to find out sooner—which allows you to correct the course of action and move forward appropriately.

For people who regularly struggle to make decisions, decision fatigue can cause physiological turmoil in their body. For some, they fear making the wrong decision, especially if they believe it will affect other people. They tend to spend an inordinate amount of time mulling over their options, often stuck on the scary notion that the incorrect choice will affect the other person involved and therefore reflect poorly on them.

Where to eat? What to watch? What to do? These might seem trivial and easy decisions for you, but for others they can cost precious time and energy as they weigh all options until decision fatigue sets in and they finally decide.

We all have a wall that we hit when it comes to decision-making: that point at which your brain is so fatigued that it chooses the easiest and most gratifying option. Roy F. Baumeister and John Tierney, authors of *Willpower: Rediscovering the Greatest Human Strength*, say, "Decision fatigue leaves you vulnerable to marketers who know how to time their sales . . . And this isn't the only reason that sweet snacks are featured prominently at the cash register, just when shoppers are depleted after all their decisions in the aisles. With their willpower reduced, they're more likely to yield to any kind of temptation, but they're especially vulnerable to candy and soda and anything else offering a quick hit of sugar."[11]

Also located at the cash register are gossip magazines. Undoubtedly, you've stood in the grocery line while blankly staring at the magazine covers. If your willpower was low, you might have given in to the temptation and opened one. Your exhausted brain was surely enlightened to find out which celebrity cheated on whom, where they got their coffee, the quickest ways to lose 10 pounds, or, my personal favorite from back in the day, the latest sighting of Bigfoot or the Loch Ness Monster published in the *National Enquirer*. We've all been there, so don't feel bad about spending the $7.99 on nonsense.

But, with practice and dedication, you can improve the speed of your decision-making and the number of decisions you can handle in a day before decision fatigue sets in. Think about running. The fitter you are the farther and faster you can go before you get tired (or before you "hit the wall"). The same can be said of making decisions.

Become the captain for those around you!

As you've likely experienced (perhaps daily), your emotions have an impact on the decisions you make. According to Naqvi and colleagues, various emotions cause physical feelings that can affect your decision-making in favor of choices that bring you a "reward."[12] For instance, if you're sad you might choose a sugary snack because you know it will make you (temporarily) happy.

Think about the life motto carpe diem (to live in the moment while giving little thought to the future), which some people choose to live by. People who have this life philosophy are more likely to make decisions based on their emotional state. Conversely, people who focus on the past or the future are more likely to base their decisions on previously experienced emotions.

It's certainly difficult to take emotions out of decision-making, but the next time you reach for a gratifying treat, whatever it might be, pause and consider your options. Are you making that decision because you're avoiding dealing with the emotional state you find yourself in? If the answer is yes, there's likely a better, more holistic way to acknowledge your emotional state and then, when you're ready, move out of it and into an emotional state that will serve you better. If, after that, you still want the treat, go for it!

Outsourcing Your Decision-Making

My wife prefers that I do all the grocery shopping. And you know what? So do I. She says that the constant decision-making needed when walking down the aisles is draining and not how she wants to spend her energy. Conversely, I love it. I've always loved roaming the grocery aisles. They're well lit and full of fresh produce, and I get to see if my favorite foods or supplements are on sale. However, it must be *my* grocery store! I must go to the same one every time, or the extra time and energy spent trying to find my usual items is annoying and sometimes frustrating.

In this way, Lauren has done a great job of outsourcing the decisions that she dislikes most. Having a partner, a roommate, or other family members balance the decision-making load can help ensure that your home is operating in flow.

Consider ways that you might reduce your decision-making. Can you split some of it up among the people in your home or your workspace?

When you're regularly tasked with more decisions than your brain is effectively able to handle, you should aim to reduce those that don't move the needle regarding your health, career, or well-being.

Everyone is different in terms of the amount of time they spend making decisions—but some people devise strategies to reduce the time spent finding an answer. Quick or automated decisions will ensure that you have more time for the questions or decisions that will bring real growth.

For instance, Mark Zuckerberg, the founder of Facebook, is famous for wearing plain gray T-shirts. He chooses to wear the same thing repeatedly because this reduces his decision-making. Similarly, in a 2012 *Vanity Fair* article former U.S. president Barack Obama says, "You'll see I wear only gray or blue suits . . . I'm trying to pare down decisions. I don't want to make decisions about what I'm eating or wearing. Because I have too many other decisions to make. You need to focus your decision-making energy. You need to routinize yourself. You can't be going through the day distracted by trivia."[13]

For me, keeping up with the latest fashion trends has never been of interest; paring down my wardrobe and opting to wear only a few items repeatedly was an easy decision to make. Most days you'll find me in a white V-neck T-shirt and a pair of jeans. As I sit on a train and write this sentence, that's exactly what I'm wearing.

If decision fatigue is a problem you encounter, consider using this table. Beside each day of the week write down the outfit you'd like to wear. Of course you don't have to be so militant as to wear the same thing every day—but having an outfit for each day of the week, and then putting the list on your dresser, might do wonders for your tired morning brain.

Day	Outfit
Monday	
Tuesday	
Wednesday	
Thursday	
Friday	
Saturday	
Sunday	

As with the seven-day outfit list, I highly recommend you try a seven-day list for your food intake. Most people are very habitual when it comes to their breakfast and lunch while dinner tends to be the meal that uses up the most mental energy. Instead of spending precious time every night wondering what you'll eat, and whether you have the ingredients to make it, you should make a list of seven dinners and which day of the week you'll have each of them. My wife and I love this plan, and so do our kids. Of course it fluctuates a tad some weeks, but having a list on the fridge ensures that we get all the necessary ingredients at the grocery store, and my weekly shopping run ensures that we have dinners for the entire week.

Let me share a fairly standard week of dinners at the Gibbons house during the winter months. After the list, I've left a blank table for you to fill in with your week of dinners. Ideally you'd write it out on a larger piece of paper and stick it on your fridge as a reminder. This strategy may also end up saving you money. Buying exactly what you need, rather than arbitrarily choosing items in the grocery store, will likely lead to less food spoilage.

Day	Meal
Monday	Salmon, Brussels sprouts, and sweet potatoes
Tuesday	Spaghetti with organic red meat and konjac noodles
Wednesday	Taco Tuuuuesdaaaay! (Yes, I know it's Wednesday . . . and yes, that's how my kids yell it)
Thursday	Tofu salad
Friday	Homemade pizza night (my favorite)
Saturday	All-star salad (quinoa base with a crazy number of toppings)
Sunday	Steak and sweet potato fries

Day	Meal	Ingredients
Monday		
Tuesday		
Wednesday		
Thursday		
Friday		
Saturday		
Sunday		

A modern decision-making dilemma comes at the end of the day: What should we (or I) watch? Before streaming came along, we weren't faced with this issue—you knew what shows were on TV each night of the week. Of course, you still had the Friday-night dilemma of roaming the Blockbuster aisles—is it weird that I miss that?

This is another task that my wife has outsourced to me. It doesn't matter what I choose; she says, "Sure," because at this point in the day she wants to turn off all decision-making responsibilities. If this is a nightly battle for you, here's my suggestion: On your phone, make a list of shows, movies, and documentaries. Whenever someone highly recommends something (which people love to do), jot it down. This may seem trivial, but it's important.

If you approach each day as though you have a certain number of *quality* decisions in you (let's say 20), then you don't want to waste them on issues that don't appreciably enhance your relationships, career, health, or well-being.

CHAPTER 12

Happiness

"Happiness is when what you think, what you say, and what you do are in harmony."—MAHATMA GANDHI

PEOPLE CONSTANTLY SEEK out circumstances, opportunities, and relationships that they believe will make them happy. From what I've surmised, fame, fortune, and power aren't likely to positively shift your daily happiness baseline. Actor Jim Carrey says, "I think everybody should get rich and famous and do everything they ever dreamed of so they can see that it's not the answer [for happiness]."[1]

Before I had kids, I lived way too much for work, because I believed that if I accomplished this or that the end product would be happiness and fulfillment. Once I achieved something I was usually happy for a time, but when my level of happiness returned to its baseline I'd set my sights on other projects, certifications, or achievements. This is known as the hedonic treadmill.

According to an article in *Psychology Today*, the hedonic treadmill is "the idea that an individual's level of happiness, after rising or falling in response to positive or negative life events, ultimately tends to move back toward where it was prior to these experiences . . . Starting a new romance or being promoted at work may cause a brief burst of extra joy, but these events will not necessarily change people's everyday levels of happiness in the long run. Instead, people often adjust their expectation to the new status quo and find themselves desiring even more to maintain the same level of happiness."[2]

I believe that having ambition and career aspirations is good and healthy. I certainly want more for me and my family in this life, but I'm now careful about my reasoning for the *more* and the way I pursue it. I've accepted the fact that having a healthy life balance requires me to be okay with achieving things within a larger time frame than my old self would have liked. This life shift was a huge breakthrough for me!

Our collective desire to constantly be in pursuit for *more* reminds me of "The Story of the Mexican Fisherman." The story was originally written by German author Heinrich Böll, but has been adapted by many people since. The essence of the story remains true. Here's a summary of the version I remember most:

An American investment banker was on holiday in a small coastal Mexican village. He noticed a small boat with just one fisherman. In the boat were several large yellowfin tunas. The American was impressed with the quality of the fish and asked how long it took to catch them all.

"Only a little while," the Mexican replied.

"Why don't you stay out longer and catch more fish?" the American asked.

"I have enough to support my family's immediate needs," the Mexican replied.

"But how do you spend the rest of your time?" the American asked.

The Mexican fisherman said, "I sleep late, fish a little, play with my children, take siestas with my wife, Maria, stroll in the village each evening where I sip wine, and play guitar with my amigos. I have a full and busy life."

The American scoffed, "I have a Harvard MBA and could help you. You should spend more time fishing—you can use the proceeds to buy a bigger boat. With the profits from the bigger boat, you could buy several boats and eventually have a fleet of fishing boats. And instead of selling your catch to a middleman you would sell directly to the processor, eventually opening your own cannery. You would control the product, processing, and distribution. You would need to leave this fishing village and move to Mexico City, then LA, and eventually New York City, where you will run your expanding enterprise."

The Mexican fisherman asked, "But how long will this take?"

To which the American replied, "15 to 20 years."

"But what then?" asked the Mexican.

The American laughed and said, "That's the best part. When the time is right you would announce an IPO and sell your company stock to the public and become very rich; you would make millions!"

"Millions—then what?"

The American said. "Then you would retire. Move to a small coastal fishing village where you would sleep late, fish a little, play with your kids, take siestas with your wife, stroll to the village in the evenings where you could sip wine and play your guitar with your amigos . . . "

This is one of my favorite parables of all time. In fact, I have it framed in my house. It's a daily reminder of what's really important in life: the simple things. For too many, this remains true in their heart, but since society encourages more stuff, bigger houses, faster cars, and so on, we inadvertently push the envelope just as the American banker advised the Mexican fisherman to do.

We're programmed to believe that the accumulation of *more* will lead to what we all desire: happiness. Like a kid chasing the pot of gold at the end of the rainbow, you'll always be chasing happiness if you tie it to things outside of yourself. So be careful. Be careful how often you use the words (aloud or in your head) "as soon as."

"As Soon As . . . "

You've likely uttered the phrase "as soon as . . . " on many occasions in your life. "As soon as I get X (a degree, a partner, a promotion) I'll be able to relax and be happy." But how long does that happiness last after you've achieved what it is you want? For most, their happiness begins diminishing (and returning to baseline) shortly after their "as soon as" is realized.

Rick Hanson, author of *Hardwiring Happiness*, says that if you employ the right strategy, positive short-term experiences can elevate your baseline mood. He recommends a three-step routine to help with this process:[3]

1. When you feel happy, grateful, or appreciated, you should sit with that feeling (for at least a few slow breaths) rather than let it quickly pass by. Hold on to the positive emotion and soak it in.

2. Try to feel the happiness throughout your entire body.

3. Focus on what's enjoyable about the experience you just had.

Hanson expands on this idea: "Each step elevates the way your brain converts passing experiences into lasting changes in your mind and mood."[4] This practice will also bring you back to appreciating the simple things. Achievement and goal-setting are healthy and encouraged, but you must stop tying your happiness to them. It's time to reprogram your mind to be happy with what you have and where you are—recognize your blessings and maintain a realistic balance as you proceed with your life. If you tie your perceived happiness to an outcome, then you'll always want to expedite the process. In doing so, you'll be missing out on life.

Countless people say that it's the little moments in life that bring them the most joy: playing with their children, feeling the warm sun on their skin, laughing with a friend. But since our brains are wired to seek out trouble, and due to modern society telling you (consciously and subconsciously) what it takes to make you happy, you're stuck in the perpetual cycle of seeking happiness.

Bronnie Ware, an Australian palliative-care nurse, works with people in the last months of their lives. She's been privy to the regrets of people as they're dying. Ware's list of the regrets of dying people went viral online and was picked up by *The Guardian*.[5] It reveals some common themes, two of which stand out for me:

1. I wish I hadn't worked so hard.

2. I wish that I had let myself be happier.

When I think of the first regret, "I wish I hadn't worked so hard," I deduce that to work "hard" means to work for too long and for too many hours. I value hard work, and I'll instill that work ethic into my children. However, as you've read, my tendency is to work hard *and* for too long.

I've had to learn the hard way what happens when you spend an inordinate amount of time working. Not only do you miss out on life but you also put your health at risk because too often our work is associated with high levels of stress—and too much stress will wreak havoc on your mind, your body, and even your spirit.

When it comes to your career, what is the pinnacle for you?

Often, people don't define their ultimate work-related goal and therefore just keep striving for career advancement. This is akin to someone who lifts weights to build muscle but neglects the other types of exercise (aerobic, flexibility, balance, etc.). When it comes to resistance training, some people become fixated on the numbers, on how much they can bench press, dead lift, squat, et cetera. But if you don't have an end goal, you'll be perpetually aiming to achieve more in this area while neglecting other areas. For people with this mindset, I have them write down the weight they would be happy with for each exercise; once that goal is achieved, they can maintain the weight (maintaining is much easier than gaining) and then work to improve the other dimensions of their fitness routine.

The same principle applies to people who devote a disproportionate amount of time and energy to work. Determining the income, job title, or responsibilities you desire will give you an end goal that, once achieved, will allow you to prioritize the other, neglected, areas of your life. Additionally, this will provide your subconscious with a much clearer picture of what you want to attain and allow it to help you realize your goal.

Although I like this strategy, I'd still caution any self-described workaholic not to wait until they reach their career pinnacle before implementing any other strategies necessary to achieve a degree of balance.

 ## Identifying Your Work-Related Pinnacle

I want you to give some thought to what your work-related pinnacle is. Place it at the top of a pyramid and then work backwards, down the slope, indicating all the steps required to achieve your goal. The example I provide is a very broad-strokes outline that can be expanded upon, perhaps with the help of a career counselor.

CAREER TITLE: Senior Manager
COMPENSATION: $150,000 per year
RESPONSIBILITIES: Oversee the operation of my entire division

Become assistant manager

Learn a new skill that improves
my value within the company

Attend night school
to complete my trade
certification

Find a mentor within
a similar industry

Hire a performance coach to
enhance my sales skills

Request an informational
interview to determine
everything required

YOU ARE HERE

CONCERNING THE OTHER regret, "I wish that I had let myself be happier," it took me a while to understand just what this means.

So what does it mean to let yourself be happier? Nurse Bronnie Ware expanded: "Many did not realize until the end that happiness is a choice. They had stayed stuck in old patterns and habits. The so-called 'comfort' and familiarity overflowed into their emotions, as well as their physical lives. Fear of change had them pretending to others, and to their selves, that they were content. When deep within, they longed to laugh properly and have silliness in their life again."[6]

In the ground-breaking 1996 article "Happiness Is a Stochastic Phenomenon," researchers David Lykken and Auke Tellegen describe a study in which they determined (after studying more than 2,000 twins from the Minnesota Twin Registry) that approximately 50 percent of life satisfaction is attributed to genetics.[7] This suggests that the other 50 percent is variable, which means you have a great deal of control over it!

When your body is functioning optimally and your mind is clear, what is typically elevated? That's right—it's your happiness. After all, it's hard to feel happy when you're tired and weak. That said, having abundant energy and vitality isn't an automatic precursor to happiness. Your level of happiness is distinctly tied to you and the habits you foster.

HAPPINESS SCHOOL?

"When there are no enemies within, the enemies outside cannot hurt you."
—ANCIENT AFRICAN PROVERB

At my high school and university there were a few practical courses but nothing as outwardly obvious as a happiness class. I think most people were under the impression that the courses you took, and what you would gain from them and from your degree, would eventually lead you to the unicorn they call happiness.

"Keep striving for X, and then happiness will come." "Now do X, and happiness is just around the corner." On and on you go until you're decades older and you realize that perhaps the most important life skill of all hadn't been taught to you—at least not in a direct way.

Martin Seligman, a professor at the University of Pennsylvania and the director of its Positive Psychology Center, has said that "Psychology had only been about mitigating what was wrong. That will [only] take you to zero."[8] Much like the earlier definition of "health," the old approach to psychology just got you back to the status quo.

But what about those who want more out of life, those who want to live in a state that allows for more opportunities to experience joy, laughter, balance, and contentment?

In 2006 Harvard University ran a course called "Positive Psychology 1504." It was taught by Tal Ben-Shahar and 1,400 students were enrolled—making it the most popular course in Harvard's history.[9] In 2018 Yale University offered a course called "Psychology and the Good Life," taught by Laurie Santos (who's also the host of *The Happiness Lab* podcast), with approximately 1,200 undergraduate students enrolled. This course, the most popular course at Yale to date,[10] sought to answer two questions: What actually makes us happy? What can we do to achieve the good life?

Of course, if there were a magic recipe for happiness, that wisdom would be worth billions to whoever held it. Although there isn't a one-size-fits-all approach, courses like those at Harvard and Yale can teach students about life approaches that have been proven to increase your contentment and happiness. After all, success leaves clues (as well as a road map to help you navigate).

Remember Joy?

My kids don't keep their emotions close to their chest. They don't subdue their joy or hide their anger—in fact, they don't temper any of their feelings. For a parent this can be very challenging at times, but their emotional swings are still something to marvel at. In particular, I love watching them when they're immersed in something that's bringing them joy—joy in every sense of the word: their smile couldn't be any bigger, their laugh couldn't be more genuine, and their little bodies are so happy they're almost buzzing. I often think to myself, when was the last time I felt that level of unbridled enthusiasm? And honestly, I usually draw a blank.

As adults we're taught to be tempered, to act a certain way, to stay within societal boundaries. I understand that tempering emotions in certain circumstances is appropriate, but too often that becomes the dominant outcome—which leads to a subdued life where we don't dare explore the boundaries of happiness. We settle for mediocre contentment and the occasional grin or chuckle.

Remember belly laughs?
Remember not caring what others think of you?
Remember pure joy?

Let's explore the concept of joy a little further. Let's see if we can move your barometer of happiness to the right just a little.

What is joy? To put it simply, joy is the surge in dopamine experienced from the systematic neural firing of the amygdala to induce stimulation of the olfactory bulb, the orbitofrontal cortex, and the cingulate gyrus . . . just kidding! You can't break joy down into a physiological sequence that works with absolute certainly. There can be no universal definition of joy— that would kind of defeat the purpose and authenticity of it. At least that's what I believe.

Remember belly laughs?

However, if it were necessary to provide an explanation for it, I'd say you should close your eyes and think of an event, a moment, an action, or anything that has taken you out of your "head." A moment that takes you out of the need for societal appropriateness, away from the wet blanket that we've cloaked ourselves in. A time when you laughed so hard that

- your drink came out of your nose

- your abs hurt

- you struggled to catch your breath

- your cheeks became painful because of the massive grin plastered on your face

If it's been so long since you had any of these experiences, think of something that fills your body with happy vibes—like the feeling you get when riding a roller coaster, the happiness of hearing a baby giggle, the excitement of tobogganing down a steep hill. Those are the moments that take you out of your head and into the moment. I dare you not to smile while tobogganing, jumping on a trampoline, or tickling a baby while they belly laugh. Go on, I dare you!

Now, to be fair, I'm coming from a Western view of joy. What this word means for me may not be the same as what it means for people in other cultures. For instance, certain Asian cultures view joy as a sense of calm, peace, and serenity.

Joy vs. Happiness

In the Merriam-Webster dictionary, "happiness" is defined as "a state of well-being and contentment,"[11] whereas "joy" is defined as "the emotion evoked by well-being, success, or good fortune or by the prospect of possessing what one desires."[12] How different are the two? People have been trying to distinguish between the two emotions for a long time. A panel discussion with four academics from the Yale Center for Faith and Culture didn't reach a consensus on the difference between them. One suggestion was that joy is a more intense feeling, one that can overwhelm you, while happiness is a more consistent emotion.

Now, does it really matter that we make a distinction between the two? Probably not. According to some, they are intertwined in a human being's overall well-being and general sense of satisfaction. Dan Harris, author of *10% Happier*, says that "People confuse happiness with excitement."[13] If we work to shift our notion of what it means to be happy, then perhaps we can include contentment and calm in the definition. Psychologist Rick Hanson says that "Bad stuff happens to everyone . . . When it does, it's normal to feel sad, irritated or rattled. Being a happy person means having an underlying sense of well-being that lets you return to your baseline more quickly."[14]

It's time you approached the enhancement of your happiness in a different way. You should strive for a consistent and sustainable boost to your baseline level of happiness.

At this point in your life, you've likely noticed that things such as a promotion, a trip, material stuff, and so on won't lead to a fundamental change in your deep-rooted sense of happiness. While you may have felt temporarily happy, you've always returned to the level of contentment and happiness that you had before those things were attained. An authentic shift must be derived from your psychology and your physiology.

From a psychological standpoint you must alter your subconscious programming. This may be the most difficult self-improvement step you ever endure. It will require consistent action and belief in the process to ensure its permanent adoption. But if you commit to it, you'll be amply rewarded. Refer to Part II if you need a refresher on how this can be accomplished.

From a physiological standpoint you must optimize the functioning of your body. You want your organs to be working at their best—while having healthy communication with one another. This, combined with a reduction in toxins, a healthy diet (that's tailored for you), and positive lifestyle choices (exercise, quality sleep, appropriate supplementation, etc.), will result in a boost to your energy levels. Enhanced energy (Qi/life force) typically makes people feel happier, which in turn helps them to make more positive lifestyle decisions.

Later in Part III we'll discuss how certain hormetic stresses (hot and cold therapy) can result in a positive shift in your day-to-day baseline level of happiness.

Is Laughter Really the Best Medicine?

You've heard the saying a thousand times: "Laughter is the best medicine." But is it true? Even if it is, I'm not expecting hospitals to start hiring comedians to join their daily medical rounds, but wouldn't it be great if they did! Since 1988 Lee S. Berk, Associate Dean of Research Affairs for Loma Linda University School of Allied Health Professions, has been studying the effect that laughter has on the body. Research results have concluded that after exposure to humor there's an increased level of activity in the immune system.[15] Berk's research has demonstrated the following immune-system improvements:

- An increase in the number and activity level of natural killer cells that attack viral-infected cells and some types of cancer and tumor cells

- An increase in activated T cells (T lymphocytes)

- An increase in gamma interferon, which tells various aspects of the immune system to "turn on"

- An increase in the antibody immunoglobulin A (IgA), which helps to fight upper respiratory tract infections

According to the *Time* magazine article "Smiling through Trying Times," laughter "prompts muscle relaxation, increases blood flow and reduces arterial-wall stiffness associated with cardiovascular disease."[16] And although it may be impossible to determine whether laughter is the best medicine, it certainly seems that adding more of it to your life will have distinct benefits.

Here's another interesting thing about laughter. When my wife and I had to make frequent visits to the Fetal Medical Unit at Mount Sinai Hospital in Toronto, we sometimes acted in a way that we thought was inappropriate. We had one or two appointments per week, which required us to be there for five to six hours. We'd sit in the waiting room until we were called to go into the ultrasound room, where the nurse would check our babies' vital signs, do measurements, and take pictures before the doctor came in to let us know how they were doing. Both before and after Lauren's laser ablation surgery, we were terrified during those appointments, because we knew that at any moment the babies' environment could worsen and they might not make it—especially since the odds weren't in their favor.

The oddest thing would happen when we were left alone in the waiting rooms—we'd have laughing fits, the kind that you can't stop even if you want to, and if you try to it will only make it worse. We didn't understand it at the time—how we could be so terrified and spend hours upon hours praying, but then be in hysterics while waiting for the specialist to come in and talk to us. Well, it makes a lot more sense now.

According to Naomi Bagdonas, a Stanford University lecturer and co-author of *Humor, Seriously*, "When we laugh, our brains release a happy cocktail of hormones . . . It primes us for resilience, human connection and being more open to joy."[17]

Harriet Cabelly, an expert in positive psychology and the author of *Living Well despite Adversity*, explains that "We can be sad and happy—we can hold grief, pain and joy together. Even through our darkest moments, it's possible to let tiny bits of sunshine peek through . . . If you don't incorporate some joys and pleasures into the hard times, then you're basically signing yourself up for a life of misery, darkness and victimhood."[18]

Humor was definitely our crutch during those excruciating appointments—it helped us to cope with the uncertainty of the news awaiting us after each ultrasound. According to Bagdonas, "When we're primed for something . . . we are more likely to find it, faster and more often. The simple act of looking for joy will lead to people reporting more of it serendipitously appearing in their lives."[19] Of course, the inverse is also true. If you're stuck in a negative frame of mind or if you believe you have "bad luck," then you'll likely attract more of those thoughts and more of those people/circumstances.

Stacking All the Chips in Favor of Happiness

For most of us, our brains tend to focus on the negative rather than the positive. Working toward seeing the positive and expressing regular gratitude should be one of your ongoing goals. Building a routine into your everyday that helps to ensure that your mind sees the glass as half full will lead you to become happier over time.

Here are some things you can do in your everyday life that will lead to more happiness, and possibly begin to change the expression of your DNA for the better:

- **Begin mindfulness practice**. The scientific benefits of incorporating a regular mindfulness routine are not up for debate. In addition to the numerous studies demonstrating positive structural changes to the human brain (creation of new neurons, generation of new nerve cells, and a reversal in the brain's natural tendency to thin),[20, 21, 22] there are many studies that prove the effectiveness of mindfulness in enhancing an individual's level of happiness.[23, 24, 25]

- **Express gratitude regularly**. When you express gratitude, it's important that you take the time to feel it in your body. Feel the emotion and the happiness that it brings. This will help to improve your baseline level of happiness because you'll be engaging your subconscious.[26]

  Many experts believe that gratitude and appreciation are among the highest vibrational emotions we can have.[27] Spending more time in this state will provide positive benefits for your body, brain, and sense of well-being and happiness. Conversely, on the lower end of the vibrational spectrum are emotions such as guilt, shame, apathy, grief, and fear.[28]

· **Display "happy" body language**. Picture yourself standing with your head up and shoulders back with a big smile on your face versus sitting slouched with your head down. Your posture and facial expressions contribute to your mood. This isn't hyperbole; there's science to back it up.

A genuine smile over your entire face can trigger the release of endorphins into your bloodstream,[29] and power-posing (as in the Superman pose) may help to reduce cortisol levels (in addition to raising testosterone levels) while simultaneously increasing our "happy" hormones.[30]

Also, you should avoid "body blocking" (closing your body with crossed arms and legs) when you're nervous or afraid. You can avoid this universal sign of discomfort by making yourself larger with your arms and legs. Not only will this convey confidence to those around you, but it will also send signals to your subconscious that you're confident.

· **Socialize**. Positive social connections can fuel happiness. Quality over quantity is the key. Having a few people who you can rely on, be yourself around, and have fun with will help you feel connected and happier. *New York Times* best-selling author Daniel Gilbert, author of *Stumbling on Happiness*, writes: "If I wanted to predict your happiness and I could only know one thing about you, I wouldn't want to know about your gender, religion, health, or income. I'd want to know about the strength of your relationships with your friends and family."[31]

· **Speak positively**. If you replace your typical vernacular with words that you want to be associated with, your subconscious will have the goal of achieving that state. For instance, when I take my dog for a walk, I go slowly, talk to God, and give thanks for all the blessings in my life. I notice the beauty of the world around me, and if I see a neighbor who asks, "How are you?" I usually reply, "I'm great, thanks! How are you?"

Simple changes implemented over time end up having a big impact. As with exercise, you mightn't notice the changes right away, but there'll come a day when you wake up and notice that you look and feel different. Consistency is the key!

- **Exercise**. It's likely no surprise to you at this point that exercising makes you feel good. The rush of endorphins that you get, as well as the release of dopamine, norepinephrine, and serotonin, gives you a boost of energy and happiness. Many people prefer to work out in the morning because it helps to set the tone they want for their day.

  Exercising first thing in the morning will also help reduce the mental negotiating you may encounter later in the day. If you wait to do your workout, you may find reasons (too many emails, a long to-do list, "too hungry") and put it off until tomorrow.

- **Pray**. There are many possible benefits of regular prayer, such as a positive shift in your happiness level. One of the ways that prayer reaps this benefit is by reducing stress. A study published in the *British Journal of Health Psychology* notes that praying can reduce your risk of developing depression and anxiety—and the benefits are enhanced when you choose to pray in a place of worship.[32]

  According to Dr. Andrew Newberg from the Department of Psychiatry at the University of Pennsylvania, you can boost your levels of dopamine by praying.[33] Additionally, Dr. Newberg's study noticed a reduction in an individual's ego (since praying affects that area of the brain) with regular prayer—therefore, you're more likely to be humble and to be less focused on material desires.

These are just a few examples of what you can do to improve your happiness. How many of these practices do you engage in regularly?

You have a lot of control over whether today will be filled with happiness or will be another frustrating, worry-filled, and stressful day. And by stacking good, or even great, days together, not only will you attract more positive people and situations into your life, but also, as we've seen, you may experience epigenetic changes that help to solidify the new behavior and its positive outcome (happiness).

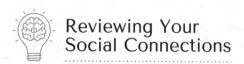

Reviewing Your Social Connections

Feelings of loneliness can contribute to depression, low self-esteem, anxiety, and stress.[34, 35, 36] Conversely, socializing positively impacts happiness, well-being, and cognitive skills, and may even help you live longer.[37, 38]

Within the blue zone (where there's a disproportionate number of centenarians) of Okinawa, Japan, infants are placed in social groups called *moai* (a group of people who meet for a common purpose).[39] Typically, they are in groups of about five young children, and they share a lifelong commitment to jointly work and play and to pool their resources.

According to Klazuko Manna, an Okinawan woman who belongs to a moai, the social groups are about support and respect for one another: "Each member knows that her friends count on her as much as she counts on her friends. If you get sick or a spouse dies or if you run out of money, we know someone will step in and help. It's much easier going through life with a safety net."[40]

Ask yourself, How strong are my social connections? Have they weakened over the years as you've become increasingly busy with work and family commitments?

If you want to give your social circle a boost, complete the activity on the next page. Begin by listing some of your closest friends from over the years—the ones you want to reconnect with. Next, decide when, and how (text, email, call), you'll connect with them.

The last category is your *purpose* for getting in touch. That may seem odd, but there's value in this exercise. It can be as simple as reaching out to say thank you ("Hey, Larissa, I was reminiscing about the old days and wanted to reach out to say thank you for being a great friend back in college. I hope the family is well!"). If nothing else, it's sure to make their day a little brighter—and perhaps that's all you're hoping to gain from the exchange. Or maybe you want to get together in the hope of inserting a former friend back into your life. Whatever your purpose, reconnecting opens the door to possibility.

I think about the *purpose* before most of my encounters with people—this helps me stay mindful of why I'm with them. The purpose could be

Person	How	When	Purpose

strictly to have fun and to laugh; it could be to problem-solve; it could be to help them through a difficult time. Whatever the purpose is, it helps me to be mindful and fully present.

If you want to expand your social circle and human connection even more, join a club, try a new hobby, or just strike up a conversation with people in your community.

Two Types of Happiness

Rick Hanson explains in *Hardwiring Happiness* that there are two broad categories of happiness, hedonic and eudaemonic.[41] Both types are essential for our overall happiness. Here's the difference between the two:

Hedonic happiness is what you feel when something makes you happy. Whether it's a hug from your grandmother, a raise at work, a great golf shot, or an invigorating workout, hedonic happiness is achieved through experiences of pleasure and enjoyment.

Eudaemonic happiness is the feeling you get when you live in accordance with your spirit. Derived from the word "eudaimonia" based on the Greek words *eu* (good) and *daimon* (spirit), this type of happiness is experienced when you get up in the middle of the night to comfort your child, when you've spent a weekend volunteering at an old age home, or when you complete a fundraising campaign to support your favorite charity. Eudaemonic happiness is achieved through experiences with meaning and purpose.

You've heard the expression "It's better to give than to receive." This is true for several reasons. If you give your time, energy, and enthusiasm to a cause you believe in, eudaemonic happiness resonates deep within your soul.

For most people there isn't an appropriate balance between the two forms of happiness. Hedonic happiness is typically what dominates. For a more fulfilled life you must discover (and implement) ways to boost your eudaemonic happiness. Think of things that align with your spirit, with the deepest sense of who you are or who you want to become.

Here are some examples of what boosts my eudaemonic happiness. I've included a space for you to write down the activities that bring you eudaemonic happiness.

- Serving food with my home church group

- Doing an activity that my kids want to do (which usually means chasing them around the house pretending to be a "monster")

- Helping my family with their health

- Helping my family with their errands or important tasks

- Sleeping with my kids when they're sick and want me close

- Sending money and supplies to children in unfortunate situations

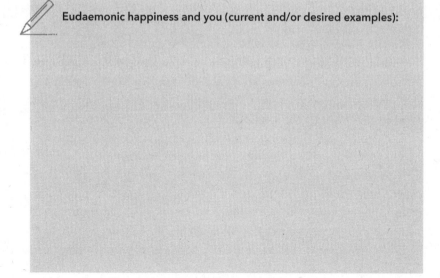

Eudaemonic happiness and you (current and/or desired examples):

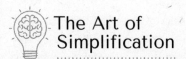

The Art of Simplification

"Wealth consists not in having great possessions, but in having few wants." —EPICTETUS

If you've been stuck in the "rat race" long enough, you've likely uttered the words "I need to slow down" more than a few times. Maybe you're looking at it the wrong way. Instead of "slowing down," perhaps you should work to *simplify* your life. The tasks you're doing right now (working, raising kids, household chores, social engagements) likely aren't being done at a faster pace than they were generations ago; the problem is that you've stacked too many things together, so your brain is stressed because you always feel a step behind and your body is stressed because you've built in so little time for rest and recuperation.

The number of responsibilities and commitments we face today makes it hard for us to appreciate the small things, because we're always moving on to the next commitment, the next meeting, the next activity. Let's work on that. Let's see if we can start simplifying.

Believe it or not, my life was busier before I had children. When my wife gave birth to our boys, I took parental leave so I could be home. While caring for kids may not be the most relaxing thing you'll ever do (understatement of the century!), for some parents it does allow them to learn about simplification. There's certainly a ton to do, and the lack of sleep that often accompanies caring for a newborn makes every task infinitely more challenging, but your focus is more unilateral in those first few months of your children's lives. It's all about them.

I'm one of the many people who've repeatedly said, "I need to slow down." But it's not just about slowing down. I've learned that I need to eliminate unnecessary commitments and keep only those that I value. Essentially, I've needed to "cut the fat"—whether it be unnecessary commitments, toxic people, or anything that's robbing me of time, and, more importantly, energy. What little time and energy I do have, I need to reserve for my family.

It's time to start simplifying!

In this exercise, ask yourself what (or who) you can eliminate in order to simplify your life. Are there things that have unnecessarily robbed you of time (social media, TV, poor decision-making, etc.) or created life-related complexity (people causing drama or gossip, etc.)? List all the elements you can think of and beside each one write a strategy for how you'll eliminate it from your life.

To Be Eliminated	Strategy for Elimination

NOW IT'S TIME to bridge the gap between the mental and physical to ensure a holistic approach to wellness. After all, health optimization is possible only when you learn to marry your body and your mind.

Eudaemonic happiness is the feeling you get when you live in accordance with your spirit.

CHAPTER 13

Bridging Mind and Body

"Take care of your mind, your body will thank you.
Take care of your body, your mind will thank you."
—DEBBIE HAMPTON

IN WESTERN SOCIETY we've been programmed to believe that to heal from disease, aches and pains, and mental health issues we need pharmaceutical intervention.

To be perfectly clear, modern medicines are entirely appropriate and necessary for our optimal health. Science and technology have done a great service in enabling us to live longer and more healthfully. However, I believe we've lost touch with the natural ways derived from ancient cross-cultural traditions and wisdom that can create more internal harmony and healing within our bodies and minds.

Throughout this chapter I'll explore methods and techniques derived from ancient wisdom and cultures that you can use to connect your mind and body.

Vagus, Baby!

Have you ever heard of tickle therapy? I first heard about tickle therapy when I came across an internet video of a man being "tickled to sleep" (technically, he fainted). After watching the video, I quickly investigated what caused him to pass out. Due to the tickling, there was an immense amount of stimulation in the vagus nerve (a.k.a. the "wandering nerve" because of its wide distribution throughout the body). Since the vagus nerve connects the brain and the digestive system, one of its jobs is to manage blood flow to the gut (as in the case of digesting the food we eat).

If there's a lot of stimulation in this nerve it can pull too much blood away from the brain and result in fainting (but the bodily response of fainting is quite rare).

Tickle therapy, or, as it's referred to scientifically, "transcutaneous vagus nerve stimulation," is an emerging therapy that uses a small and painless electric current to the ear. Stimulation in this region will cause controlled stimulation of the nervous system through the vagus nerve. Dr. Beatrice Bretherton from the School of Biomedical Sciences at the University of Leeds explains that "The ear is like a gateway though which we can tinker with the body's metabolic balance, without the need for medication or invasive procedures."[1] Dr. Bretherton is optimistic about this therapy: "We are excited to investigate further into the effects and potential long-term benefits of daily ear stimulation, as we have seen a great response to the treatment so far."[2]

Let me tell you something else about the vagus nerve. Traditional Chinese Medicine (TCM) practitioners have known about the vagus nerve and its influence for thousands of years! The Huangdi Neijing text from 500 BCE describing yang and yin meridians points to the centrality of the vagus nerve and its ability to influence the body.[3]

Strengthening your vagal tone helps in the conservation of energy while also enhancing your sense of calm, relaxation, and connectedness within your body. Living too much of your life in a sympathetic state (fight or flight) will drain bodily resources, leaving you exhausted and, most likely, frustrated.

In addition, you must learn to recognize emotional states that are cutting into your vitality and serenity; otherwise you'll be perpetually taking two steps forward and two back, never coming out ahead.

If your emotions too often reside in the realms of frustrated, angry, worried, sad, and guilty, then you have an energy leak that must be addressed. It's fine to be filling your cup with good nutrition, mindfulness, exercise, and any of the other things that your mind and body love, but if you're pouring those positive habits into a cup that has holes in it, you'll always struggle to come out ahead.

Here are some strategies you can use to enhance your physiology, stimulate your vagus nerve, and reap the benefits of a body that's operating in harmony:

- **Traditional Chinese Acupuncture.** A TCM practitioner will place acupuncture needles at various sites (called meridians) around the body to enhance your Qi. My TCM practitioner determines her needle placement based on the evaluation of my sleep patterns, bowel movement quality and consistency, pulse strength, tongue color and shape, and my subjective well-being.

   It's been proven that auricular (relating to the ear) acupuncture can directly impact vagal regulation. In their study, Wei He and colleagues found that "auricular acupuncture plays a role in vagal activity of autonomic functions of cardiovascular, respiratory, and gastrointestinal systems."[4] Further, they suggest that this type of acupuncture may "prevent neurodegenerative diseases via vagal regulation."[5]

- **Tapping.** Also referred to as "EFT (emotional freedom technique)," this therapy involves the stimulation of meridians and energy flow by tapping on them. It's said to work in the same manner as acupuncture but without the invasiveness of needles. Studies have found a positive correlation between EFT and anxiety,[6] post-traumatic stress disorder,[7] and stress.[8]

To perform the EFT tapping method, follow these five steps:

1. Identify the issue. Think about the problem you'd like to have resolved (do just one at a time).

2. Determine how intense the issue is currently, perhaps using a 0–10 scale: is it a 10/10 (meaning it's the worst it's ever been), or is it less intense than that? This will give you a reference point as to how much the tapping has helped.

3. Come up with a phrase to repeat aloud while you're tapping the Karate Chop point (KC, located on the outside of the hand—the fleshy part beneath your little finger). This will tell your system what you're trying to address.

   For me, I repeat "Even though I'm experiencing symptoms of depersonalization, I deeply and completely accept myself." This helps to alleviate the anxiety that typically accompanies such symptoms.

4. Next, cycle through the tapping points while repeating your chosen phrase. Make sure to use two or more fingers and tap each point five times.

Here's the sequence:

- top of the head (TOH): in the center of the top of your head

- beginning of the eyebrow (EB): at the start of the eyebrow (just above and to the side of the nose)

- side of the eye (SE): outside corner of the eye, on the bone

- under the eye (UE): about one inch below the pupil, on the bone that's under the eye

- under the nose (UN): between the nose and the upper lip

- chin point (CH): halfway between the lower lip and the bottom of the chin

- beginning of the collarbone (CB): where the sternum (breastbone), collarbone, and first rib intersect

- under the arm (UA): about four inches below the armpit, on the side of the body

5. Finally, you need to test the intensity again on your 0–10 scale and then repeat the steps if necessary.

The bulk of EFT research is for people dealing with anxiety. A 2016 systematic review that included 14 studies ("Emotional Freedom Techniques for Anxiety") by Morgan Clond determined that people who used tapping saw a significant reduction in anxiety.[9] Remember, if you're reducing anxiety, you're also preserving energy—a win–win.

- **Mindfulness meditation.** I often call exercise the wonder drug because of its ability to provide numerous physiological and psychological benefits. The same can be said of mindfulness. The concept and execution of mindfulness meditation is so simple that it should be taught to every child and reinforced in the school system to help children develop a life skill that's capable of so many positive things.

I certainly don't remember any calculus from high school, but I'd have remembered group meditation and the associated stress reduction. Taken a step farther, imagine if schools were to teach collective consciousness and meditation on global events that require humanitarian efforts to provide relief—think of the compassion that students would learn to develop!

Here are some of the proven benefits of mindfulness, along with scientific backing for it:

1. Reduction in anxiety and depression[10]

2. Improved immune function[11]

3. Better brain health[12]

4. Enhanced mental clarity and focus[13]

5. Reduced cellular aging[14]

6. Better sleep[15]

- **Visualization (or guided imagery).** *Think and Grow Rich* by Napoleon Hill contains some of the most famous quotes of all time, but to me there's one that really stands out: "Whatever the mind can conceive and believe, it can achieve."[16] The key, however, is the belief that you can achieve it—that you have the skills, resourcefulness, determination, and persistence to see it through.

    Later, we're going to go much deeper into the "how" of visualization, and, when it's done correctly and repeatedly, the deep-rooted and lasting impact it has on your subconscious mind. But if you can't wait, try this:

    - Find a comfortable place (your bed, couch, backyard, or anywhere you feel relaxed). Make sure it's quiet and calm.

    - Take some slow, mindful breaths to calm your sympathetic nervous system. Repeat as often as needed until you feel a shift in your breathing rate and mental clarity.

    - With your eyes closed, imagine yourself in a peaceful and tranquil setting. But don't just see the image—place yourself in the midst of it. Feel the air on your skin, hear the birds softly singing, notice the warm sun embracing your skin like a comforting hug, recognize your emotions and the gentle smile that begins to form. Whatever relaxed and peaceful means to you, envision and embody it.

- Stay in this place for 5 to 10 minutes and notice how you become more and more relaxed. Enjoy it to the fullest.

This can be done to help you relax, to improve your athletic performance, to make you a better public speaker, to enhance your social skills . . . the possibilities are endless!

- **Slow, rhythmic, diaphragmatic breathing.** Since the vagus nerve passes through the opening in the diaphragm, if you take deep, mindful breaths, you're causing your diaphragm to move and the concomitant stimulation of that nerve.

- **Singing or humming.** Since your vagus nerve is connected to your vocal cords, by singing or humming, or just repeating the "ommm" sound, you'll stimulate the nerve. When you combine this technique with another relaxation method, such as mindfulness, you're stacking the benefits and enhancing the vagal response.

- **Washing your face with cold water.** Cold water on the face stimulates the vagus nerve, because whenever your body is asked to adjust and acclimate to the cold it causes a decrease in sympathetic nervous system activity and an increase in parasympathetic nervous system activity.[17] According to researchers, "cold habituation lowers sympathetic activation and causes a shift toward increased parasympathetic activity."[18]

- **Balancing your gut microbiome.** If you have a diet rich in fermented foods (kimchi, sauerkraut, kefir, etc.) or take probiotic supplements, you're enriching your gut microbiome. This helps to create a positive "feedback loop" through your vagus nerve and therefore will help to increase its tone.[19]

The therapeutic techniques described all have a positive influence on the vagus nerve, which positively influences the relaxation response of your parasympathetic nervous system. There are other ways to enhance the parasympathetic nervous system. One of the simplest and most effective is deep breathing.

The Power of Deep Breathing

"If I had to limit my advice on healthier living to just one tip, it would be simply to learn how to breathe correctly. There is no single more powerful— or more simple—daily practice to further your health and wellbeing than breathwork."[20] —ANDREW WEIL, M.D.

Have you ever wondered why taking deep breaths can be beneficial when you're frustrated, angry, or anxious? From a physiological standpoint, when you take deep breaths (called diaphragmatic breathing) you move your diaphragm up and down a lot more than with normal breathing (called tidal breathing). During the process, you're stimulating the vagus nerve. This is beneficial, because when you're in a negative mindset you have much higher stimulation in your sympathetic nervous system. Living in this state for too long will deplete important resources such as adrenaline and cortisol, and over time will contribute to excessive daily fatigue.

Stimulating your parasympathetic nervous system via your vagus nerve doesn't have to be part of a formal meditation or mindfulness session. Similar to a regular exercise routine, a regular mindfulness routine is extremely beneficial. However, you don't need to limit it to just the time you've set aside. When you feel a negative emotion coming on, take a few deep, mindful breaths. This will help to stimulate your parasympathetic nervous system and reduce the amount of sympathetic energy loss you would have experienced.

Think of doing a formal mindfulness practice as "exercise," and think of taking some mindful breaths throughout your day as "physical activity." "Exercise" typically refers to a planned activity that you schedule into your day, whereas "physical activity" is the daily physical movements that you've incorporated into your life. Both are important.

If you were to wake up, sit in your car to get to work, sit at work all day long, go to the gym for your scheduled exercise session, go home and sit for dinner, sit to watch television, and then go to bed, you'd have spent a lot of your day stationary. Although going to the gym regularly is very beneficial, you'll see even more benefits if you also incorporate daily physical activity (walking to work, taking the stairs, etc.) into your day, outside of the planned exercise session. The same is true of mindfulness.

While it's very important to set aside time to practice mindfulness in an undisturbed setting, you'll reap even more benefits if you also use deep breathing and mental refocusing whenever you feel stress, anxiety, or frustration coming on. In some instances, just a couple of deep, intentional breaths can help to calm your sympathetic response and pull you back to a more relaxed physiological and psychological state.

Give it a try right now.

Wherever you're reading this book, I want you to relax, close your eyes, and slowly take five deep breaths while focusing only on the feeling of air coming into your nose and going out of your mouth. As the air is going out of your mouth, try pursing your lips (as if you were about to whistle)—this will ensure that your slow, deep inhalation isn't followed by a quick exhalation.

Go ahead . . .

I'm willing to bet that some of you didn't make it through the five breaths without opening your eyes. If this was you, that's a pretty good indication that slowing down and relaxing is a foreign concept for you. If this is where you are, that's okay—but it's time for a change.

Although you may not be able to close your eyes in every situation, you'll still see the benefits by taking deep, intentional breaths with your eyes open.

Breathing in through your nose and out through your mouth might not seem natural at first. Typically, when you formally meditate it's recommended that you allow your breathing to occur in whatever way is most comfortable for you. However, what I tell my students is that you'll see some additional benefits of the formal meditation if you begin the process (the first 1–2 minutes) with some breaths that enter via your nose and exit via your mouth, with pursed lips. This is because it takes longer to fill your lungs with air when you breathe in through your nose. So taking full, deep breaths will result in the slowing down of your breaths per minute and therefore let the relaxation response begin. This process will get you primed for the meditation to follow.

Think of the warm-up you do before you begin physical exercise. A proper warm-up can enhance the benefits, especially in the early moments of the exercise or the sport. In mindfulness, you'll still see the benefits without some priming breaths, but doing them for a minute or two at the beginning helps to signal your body and mind to relax.

If you'd like to learn about a variety of breathing techniques, and see which resonate most with you, scan the QR code at the end of this book—there are a variety of techniques outlined on the *Discovering Optimal* website.

One of the ways that deep, intentional breaths can return your body (and mind) to a more harmonious state is by enhancing the internal resonance between organs. This helps your body to operate in flow. And just as you love it when your days flow smoothly from one task, conversation, or event to another, your organs covet the same harmony.

Heart Rate Variability and Harnessing Your Internal Resonance

Heart rate variability (HRV) is an index of autonomic balance (the harmonious equity within your nervous system); it refers to the beat-to-beat changes in your heart rate, specifically the variation in time between each heartbeat. It was once believed that a healthy heart was one that beat regularly (think of the consistency of a metronome) and thus that having a low HRV was a good thing. It is now understood that the opposite is true. The healthier you are, the higher your HRV is. This means that the time between each beat is very irregular.

Studies have shown that HRV decreases with illness, age, and stress.[21, 22, 23] However, it's been proven that moderate-intensity exercise is sufficient for increasing absolute vagal-related HRV indexes.[24] Additionally, you can improve your HRV by implementing stress-management strategies.[25] In doing so you'll help to create an internal environment that's calmer, more efficient, and better prepared to handle the episodic stress it will inevitably encounter.

If you want to induce a quick boost in your parasympathetic nervous system, and therefore improve your HRV, you can implement breath work. The optimal breathing rate for achieving the highest HRV is five breaths per minute—therefore each inhalation lasts six seconds and each exhalation lasts six seconds.[26]

Try it.

Practice breathing in gently for a count of six and then breathe out smoothly for a count of six. Don't force it. If this is too difficult, begin with four in, four out and then advance to five in, five out. When you're comfortable you can try six in, six out. The goal is to balance your sympathetic nervous system with your parasympathetic nervous system. Initially you can count aloud or use a visual cue, but eventually you'll want to just go based on feel (because counting or watching a clock could mildly activate your sympathetic nervous system).

Do this for at least five minutes and see how you feel. I'm guessing that you'll be calmer, more relaxed, and have an increased sense of presence.

Do you want proof that this works? With the advanced technology we have access to today (such as smartwatches), you can monitor your HRV at home. And knowing your HRV (which fluctuates from day to day) can help determine what your body needs. For instance, if your smartwatch indicates a low HRV, because your heart is beating with more regularity, it may signify that your body is overtired—possibly resulting from poor sleep, alcohol the night before, or an infection.

The data I get about my HRV allows me to plan my energy output for the day—especially as it relates to my workouts. If my readings are showing that my body is tired, I don't want to strain my already exhausted internal physiology, so instead of working out I choose activities that support bodily recuperation (such as a light jog, meditation, or stretching).

Since many people carry their stresses with them all day, and into the bedroom at night, you should try the resonance breathing exercise when you get into bed. This will help to bring your body into a harmonious state before you drift off to sleep, which in turn will increase the likelihood of a restful and recharging night. After all, have you ever gone to bed stressed and woken up feeling great? Likely not.

Conversely, think about the sleep you get when you're on vacation. I'm guessing you wake up a lot more rested and refreshed when you're on holiday—and one of the reasons for this could be your mental and emotional state when you fall asleep.

To create even more connection between your body, mind, and soul, you can (re)connect with nature.

The Healing Power of Nature

Have you ever noticed how you feel after spending some time immersed in nature? There's something about engaging with the natural elements that leaves you feeling more grounded, relaxed, and connected. One of the reasons why my wife and I chose the location of our first house was that it was on a dead-end street close to a river and a beautiful walking trail. Just about every day we'd go for a walk, even a short walk, to the water and along its bank. While we may have been stressed before leaving the house (thinking of bills, our messy house, or our current to-do list), there was always a calm we'd feel just a few minutes after arriving at the river's edge.

According to Lisa Nisbet, an associate professor of psychology at Trent University in Peterborough, Ontario, "A body of research demonstrates that being in natural environments reduces the human stress response." [27] Feelings of well-being and overall life satisfaction can also be increased if you spend just two hours per week in nature. [28]

Have you ever heard of *grounding* (also known as *earthing*)?

I hadn't heard of grounding until my family and I were about to head off on a trip to England and the UAE (by the way, taking four seven-hour flights with one-year-old twins is not advised . . .) and my naturopath recommended it. She told us to walk outside barefoot when we got to our destinations. Now, before you roll your eyes, hear me out.

The Earth has natural magnetic frequencies (approximately 8 hertz)[29]— when you place your bare feet on the ground you expose yourself to the Earth's negative ions. This is beneficial because your body likely has a buildup of positive ions (resulting from cellular metabolism). This accumulation unfavorably affects the natural electrochemical gradient that exists across your cell membranes. When this gradient is disrupted (such as when positive ions have accumulated), it has an adverse effect on cellular metabolism and results in bodily inflammation.

Exposing yourself to negative ions (such as being barefoot on the ground) allows your body to release some of the accumulated positive ions.[30]

You can take advantage of this phenomenon by walking barefoot whenever possible, wearing grounding shoes (or sandals), using a grounding wristband, placing your feet on a grounding mat, or even sleeping on a grounding device (placed under your fitted sheet).

It's clear that nature provides many benefits, but what about its downsides? Are you going to have those same feelings of connectedness when the weather is less than ideal (too many mosquitoes, high winds, you wore the wrong shoes and now have wet feet, etc.)? Mark Coleman, author of *Awake in the Wild*, believes that these moments are perfect opportunities to practice observation without judgment. He says that with mindfulness you must "First, acknowledge your discomfort. But then ask yourself, 'What else is happening?' The sky is beautiful. The leaves on the trees glisten after the rain. You have the power to choose your response and shift your attention."[31]

We all have chaos in our everyday lives. Using this technique regularly can help to train your brain to find the joy despite the chaos.

"Most people live from the outside in. True leaders live from the inside out."

—BOB PROCTOR

CHAPTER 14

Sleep

"Sleep is the best medicine."—DALAI LAMA

WE'VE ALL EXPERIENCED sleepless nights and exhausted days. I would be remiss if I wrote a book about discovering your optimal self and didn't include a chapter on sleep. Maximizing your sleep quality might be the silver bullet that unlocks your true potential—because without it you're destined to sleepwalk through life no matter how great your other health dimensions are.

For some, lack of sleep is their own fault (for instance, staying up too late even though they must get up early), but for others it's an issue they just can't seem to remedy despite following all the best sleep practices they come across.

If this section is of no interest to you, then you're one of the lucky few! Unfortunately, most people either have a sleep-related issue currently or have had one in the past (and will likely have another in the future). To give you an idea of the scope of the problem, the National Sleep Foundation found that among American adults[1]

- 75 percent have at least one symptom of a sleep problem (such as frequent night waking or snoring)

- 54 percent have at least one symptom of insomnia

- 30-40 percent suffer from occasional insomnia—10-15 percent have chronic insomnia

- 40 percent snore

- 2-4 percent suffer from obstructive sleep apnea

- 5-10 percent have restless leg syndrome

- Americans average about 6.9 hours of sleep per night

- Americans spend approximately $2 billion on sleep medications

According to Lawrence J. Epstein, M.D., past president of the American Academy of Sleep Medicine, "Sleep deprivation and sleep disorders are estimated to cost Americans over $100 billion annually in lost productivity, medical expenses, sick leave, and property and environmental damage."[2] Consistent sleep deprivation has even caused some of the worst catastrophes in recent memory—such as the Exxon *Valdez* oil spill,[3] the space shuttle *Challenger* disaster,[4] and the nuclear accident at Three Mile Island.[5]

It's undeniable that quality sleep is not only a life-improver but also a lifesaver. A 2017 systematic review and meta-analysis, which included over 5 million participants, concluded that there's a "statistically significant increase in mortality" when people average less than six hours of sleep per night.[6]

Sleepwalking through Life?

Less than 3 percent of Americans with sleep problems get treatment.[7] This is partly because many people believe that poor sleep is inevitable and therefore don't broach the subject with their doctor. Also, many primary care doctors who were educated in the 1990s or early 2000s tend not to see sleep as a health issue. Dr. Epstein reports that, as recently as 1998, "the average amount of sleep education averaged a little more than two hours during the four years of medical school."[8] This has changed over the past two decades and sleep medicine is now recognized as a medical subspecialty. But even with physicians having more training in this area, many people still chronically suffer from poor sleep—and although medications are necessary for some, too many people resort to medications to try and remedy the persistently poor sleep and constant exhaustion.[9]

My dad was one of the 97 percent whose poor sleep went untreated. He would be tired most of the day despite sleeping the recommended number of hours each night. He had brain fog, felt exhausted, and trudged through his days. He attributed his low energy levels and poor sleep quality to age and years of working the night shift.

He accepted this reality even though a better life was possible. It wasn't until my wife urged him to spend a night at a sleep clinic that things got better. During his one-night stay, he woke up 283 times! Yes, you read that correctly. When the doctor called my father to review his results, they determined that he stopped breathing an average of 42 times per hour, which meant that he had a severe form of sleep apnea. I'm thankful that he finally resolved this serious issue but I couldn't help but think about how many memories he'd missed over the years, how many laughs, how many experiences, how many connections.

The deleterious effects of chronic sleep deprivation are many. According to the article "The Effects of Sleep Deprivation on Your Body," the negative effects of sleep deprivation are widespread throughout the body.[10] They include (but aren't limited to)

- memory issues
- mood changes
- trouble thinking and concentrating
- high blood pressure
- weakened immunity
- risk for diabetes
- weight gain
- low sex drive
- risk of heart disease
- poor balance

On top of this disturbing list, there are two other dangerous phenomena arising from sleep deprivation that substantially increase your risk of injury (to yourself or others):

- **Microsleep (or "nodding off")**. This is characterized by having very brief moments (2–15 seconds) of stage 1 sleep. The brain doesn't respond to sensory input and therefore the risk of an adverse event goes way up.

- **Automatic behavior**. This is when you're awake and performing typical daily tasks or routines but aren't cognizant of your surroundings (for instance, when time passes while you're driving but you don't remember).

A better life for my dad was always possible, but it was delayed because he accepted his suboptimal life. My advice to you: if you're suffering from poor sleep, the time to act is now! Sometimes the key to unlocking your potential is closer than you think. Whether you require a medical intervention to help with your sleep, or you just need to develop better sleep habits, getting a better night's sleep is crucial to allowing things like growth, repair, immunity, and memory retention.

Interestingly, it wasn't until 1929 that scientists discovered that our brains do more than simply "shut down" when we sleep.[11] Using electrodes placed on a person's scalp (this is called an electroencephalogram, or EEG), scientists determined that the brain is very active at night. The level of brain activity is correlated with the associated brain wave that the brain is in.

Scientists have separated sleep into two different types:

1. Rapid eye movement (REM) sleep, also known as dreaming sleep

2. Non-REM sleep, or quiet sleep

Quiet sleep is represented by alpha (stage 1), theta (stage 2), and delta (stages 3 and 4) brain waves. After you've cycled through these stages, you'll enter REM sleep, which, as the name suggests, causes your eyes to dart back and forth. Although you're typically dreaming in this phase of sleep, your body is in a "paralyzed" state known as atonia; therefore you do not act out your dreams. There've been a few rare instances where people have acted out their dreams because their body wasn't in a state of paralysis; this usually leads to severe injury.[12]

Both types of sleep are required for optimal health. Dr. Epstein summarizes the characteristics and benefits of the different phases of sleep (refer to the following chart).[13] It's important for you to understand these so you can prioritize quality of sleep over quantity. You want to maximize the time spent in stages 3 and 4 because of the regenerative benefits they provide.

Chronobiology and Your Internal Clock

Another bodily process that is heavily intertwined with sleep is our circadian rhythm. This rhythm is part of our chronobiology—our body's natural cycles (mental, physical, and emotional) that are affected by solar

Sleep Cycle	Approx. Time	Characteristics and Benefits
STAGE 1	5 minutes	· Body temperature drops. · Muscles become relaxed. · Eyes move slowly from side to side.
STAGE 2	10-25 minutes The time spent in stage 2 increases throughout the night.	· Eyes are typically still. · Heart rate and breathing slow down. · The brain's electrical activity is irregular.
STAGES 3 AND 4	20-40 minutes These stages get shorter as the night progresses, which is why you dream more in the morning (because you move into REM sleep more quickly).	· Breathing slows and becomes more regular. · Blood pressure and heart rate fall to about 20 percent to 30 percent below their waking rates. · There is less blood flow to your brain, which causes it to cool. · Your brain becomes less responsive to external stimuli, which makes it more difficult for you wake up. · This is when your body renews and repairs itself by releasing growth hormone (which stimulates tissue growth and muscle repair from the pituitary gland). · Blood levels of interleukin are increased (which activates your immune system and helps your body to defend itself against infection).
REM SLEEP	Lasts only a few minutes in the early part of your sleep but can be as long as an hour in the later stages. Represents about 25 percent of your total sleep.	· Body temperature, blood pressure, heart rate, and breathing rate all increase to daytime levels. · Helps to restore your mind by clearing it of irrelevant information and facilitating learning and memory by processing and consolidating memories.

and lunar rhythms, also known as biological rhythms.[14] Interestingly, this process occurs in all living organisms.

In your brain there's a small but very important region called the hypothalamus. Among its other functions (regulating body temperature, controlling appetite, managing sexual desire, and regulating emotional responses), the hypothalamus is responsible for the release of hormones and the maintenance of daily physiological cycles. More specifically, the suprachiasmatic nucleus (SCN) region of the hypothalamus is our internal clock.[15] Keeping this region healthy (through exercise, adequate sleep, and a healthy diet) is crucial to your overall health and wellness.

It would be amazing if we had the financial and responsibility-related freedom to schedule our life around our circadian rhythm, but unfortunately this isn't a reality for 99 percent of the population; that said, there are likely some ways you can adjust your lifestyle to parallel your body's natural rhythms more closely and therefore act more harmoniously with them.

Even though you might not have the time to schedule your day to mimic the exact desires of your circadian rhythm, this doesn't mean you need to actively fight it, day after day. Most people battle with their natural rhythms, and over time the result is more and more internal fatigue—which results in the body and mind not getting what they need, when they need it.

Here's an example provided by chronobiology.com of a typical circadian rhythm for someone who wakes up early in the morning, eats lunch around noon, and goes to bed around 11 p.m.[16] As we've seen, there are many factors that affect the body's timing, but this will give you a rough idea of timeline—it's kind of like your body's to-do list:

6 a.m.   The body's systems awaken

7–9 a.m.   Hormones are at their peak

8–9 a.m.   Highest pain threshold

10 a.m.–
12 p.m.   Fully fit and wide awake—brain is at its most efficient

12 p.m.   Time to eat—digestion in top gear

1–2 p.m.   Afternoon low—time for a nap

3–4 p.m.	New upswing—phase of learning and long-term memory
5–6 p.m.	Second peak—best time for manual work (body temperature and grip strength peak)
6–9 p.m.	Regeneration and relaxation, optimal sense of smell and taste
9 p.m.	Stomach rests—time to stop eating
11 p.m.	Time for bed
4:30 a.m.	Lowest body temperature

As you probably know, not everyone has the same ideal sleep and wake schedule—but the variation in ideal sleep and wake times isn't as great as you might think. According to Dr. Michael Breus, who's often referred to as "America's Sleep Doctor," genetics plays a role in determining your internal clock.[17] Your chronotype is largely determined by a gene called the Period Circadian Regulator 3 (PER3). It's a circadian gene that determines your ideal sleep and wake schedule based on its length. If your PER3 gene is longer, you're more likely to be an early riser; if it's shorter, you're more likely to prefer rising late.[18]

Dr. Breus has developed an in-depth questionnaire that places people into one of four chronotypes (Dolphin, Lion, Bear, and Wolf). Here's a brief depiction, as well as the ideal wake-up time, for each of the four chronotypes. To find out your chronotype, I recommend that you head to his website (thesleepdoctor.com) and take the quiz.[19]

- **Lion**. These people typically wake up early with lots of energy (you know the type . . . cue the slightly envious eye roll) and are exhausted by early evening; ideal wake-up is 5:30 a.m.; represents about 15–20 percent of the population.

- **Dolphin**. These folks tend to be light sleepers and are more likely to be diagnosed with insomnia; ideal wake-up is 6:30 a.m.; represents about 10 percent of the population.

- **Bear**. These individuals have a circadian rhythm that follows the rising and setting of the sun and usually require a full eight hours of sleep; ideal wake-up is 7 a.m.; represents about 50 percent of the population.

- **Wolf**. These people have a hard time waking up early and are most energetic in the evenings; ideal wake-up is 7:00–7:30 a.m.; represents about 15–20 percent of the population.

Although Dr. Breus provides the ideal sleep time for each chronotype, I believe there's more variation in this due to people's wildly different lifestyles. Those who are busier and get regular physical activity will have undoubtedly accumulated more adenosine in their brains throughout the day—this will drive their desire to sleep (so that proper recovery can take place).

Also, the "ideal" times based on your chronotype can be shifted. While you're unlikely to turn a Wolf into a Lion, through lifestyle choices (when you consume caffeine, meal timing, exercise schedule) you can move it a bit closer to your ideal (for instance, you really want to be a morning person) or your reality (you must get up early for work).

Consider this: You call yourself a "night person" (as many falsely people do), yet you feel tired most days even though you're getting the "recommended" amount of sleep. Perhaps your ancestral biology would rather you woke up earlier, but you've fought it for years and therefore believe that you're a Wolf. So, if you've been living with chronic exhaustion perhaps it's time to make some adjustments and try something new. It will take a few weeks to adjust (both mentally and physically), but you may feel that you're more energetic and happier with an earlier bedtime and wake-up schedule. If this represents you, there are many ways you can adjust your biology to induce sleepiness at the time you desire.

Improving Your Sleep

It's no secret to you at this point that there's a lot you can do to help with sleep quality and quantity. Here are some ways you can promote better sleep.

You may have heard of some of these recommendations before; that's why I've qualified my advice with a brief justification. I'm hoping that, with a little more information, you'll decide to adopt these measures in your nightly routine.

Better Sleep through Your Physiology and Psychology

- **Regular exercise.** Research has repeatedly shown that exercise provides three key benefits in relation to sleep: you'll fall asleep faster, attain a higher percentage of deep sleep, and wake up less often throughout the night.[20, 21] These benefits may even be increased with age. A systematic review determined that exercise positively affects sleep in middle-aged and older adults—and could be "an alternative or complimentary approach to existing therapies for sleep problems."[22]

  Another study found that older men and women have more deep sleep if they're aerobically active.[23] This finding is not surprising given the body's desire to repair and regenerate itself while in a deep sleep.

  Note: Don't exercise too close to your bedtime if you can help it. For some individuals, doing so may impede their ability to fall asleep. Finishing your exercise session at least three hours before you go to bed will ensure that it doesn't negatively impact sleep latency (the time it takes to fall asleep).

- **Maintaining a healthy diet.** This is another obvious pro when it comes to overall health and wellness. The type of food you consume, as well as the timing of your food intake, will play a role in determining the quality of sleep you'll be able to get. At this point you're likely aware of the foods that make you feel good and the ones that make you feel tired, bloated, and sluggish. Whether it's avoiding known food allergens, or eliminating the foods that make you feel bad, you should take measures to improve your eating patterns.

  This can be challenging, I know. However, with diligence and fortitude you may improve your sleep (and therefore your energy levels) so much that sustaining the dietary change is easy. Here are a few obvious, and not so obvious, examples of dietary choices that negatively affect sleep quality and/or sleep latency:

  - Acidic foods may cause acid reflux.[24]

  - Alcohol inhibits deep sleep.[25]

  - Caffeine may affect sleep quality and latency.[26]

  - Late-night snacking requires your body to digest while you're asleep, thus affecting sleep quality; also, foods with a high fat content take longer to digest.[27]

- Consuming too much fluid close to bedtime may cause frequent bathroom trips and therefore sleep disturbances.[28]

- Nicotine is a stimulant that may affect sleep quality and latency.[29]

- Certain medications negatively impact sleep quality or latency;[30, 31] do some research and determine the optimal time for you to take the medication.

- **Increasing your core temperature.** You can increase the amount of deep sleep you get by warming up your body (warm shower, sauna, bath, etc.) within an hour before going to bed. According to Dr. Greg Potter, co-founder of Resilient Nutrition, you want to raise your skin temperature by a couple of degrees shortly before sleep—this will create a temperature gradient between your core and your skin, which will help to radiate heat out from your core.[32] Doing this will help to improve sleep latency and the amount of deep sleep you achieve. This can be accomplished by having a warm shower (about 104°F/40°C) for about 10 minutes within an hour of your scheduled sleep time.[33]

- **Promoting adenosine.** "Somnogens" are sleep-promoting chemicals in the brain (the term encompasses any agent that induces sleep). Part of its function is to act as a barometer for how long you've been awake. The main somnogen is adenosine, which progressively accumulates during your waking hours. As explained in Part I (see page 5), adenosine binds to receptors within your brain, which causes you to feel relaxed and sleepy.[34] As you sleep, the adenosine is metabolized, which helps you wake up feeling refreshed. Unfortunately for all the late-night coffee drinkers out there, adenosine and caffeine are competitors.[35] By having caffeine in your system, you're potentially inhibiting the binding of adenosine, and therefore reducing the percentage of deep, restful sleep you get.

- **Going to bed happy.** When you wake up in the morning and when you go to bed at night you naturally go through the alpha and theta states. Worry, anger, fear, and frustration are very powerful emotions. If you're in a negative state as you enter these brain-wave frequencies, then whatever you're upset or worried about is more likely to have a lasting impression on your subconscious mind—and could potentially impact your memory.[36] If you're consistently going to bed in a negative state, then whatever you're ruminating over is likely to begin growing roots. The longer you continue this trend, the harder it will be to reverse that psychological damage.

- **Expressing gratitude**. Expressing gratitude, especially at bedtime, can produce powerful shifts and transformations in your life. Appreciation and gratitude elicit very high vibrations.[37] When you go to bed in this vibrational state, you're more likely to have a peaceful and restful sleep.[38] Remember, though, simply using your conscious brain to think about the things you're grateful for isn't utilizing the full potential of that power. To get the most out of the positive vibrations of gratitude, try to conjure up emotions that reflect whatever it is you're grateful for. For instance, if what you're grateful for today is your children, then before you sleep use imagery to bring yourself to a moment you had with them that evoked joy. Put yourself back in that situation. Try to envision the feeling in the room, what you felt in your heart when you were there—anything that pulls you back to that moment. Once you're able to do that, stay there as long as you can. Your body will feel the positive effects of gratitude on a deeper level when emotions accompany the thoughts.

- **Investing in sleep-aiding supplements**. Magnesium citrate or magnesium glycinate can act as a stress reliever and mild sedative.[39] It's believed that nearly half of Americans are magnesium deficient[40]—and since magnesium is involved in more than 300 biochemical reactions, ensuring optimal levels is vital to your well-being. If you're wary of magnesium supplementation because of previously experienced GI issues (namely, diarrhea), you can opt for a magnesium spray that's applied to your skin.

    Other supplements that have been linked with a better night's sleep include zinc, lavender, l-theanine, tryptophan, valerian root, and melatonin.[41, 42] Even certain adaptogens (such as ashwagandha and reishi mushroom) can enhance sleep quality.[43] Consult with a dietitian or naturopath to determine whether your current diet or supplement regime is optimal for the promotion of sleep quality.

- **Reducing light exposure.** Since the retina of our eye is what connects to the part of the brain called the suprachiasmatic nucleus (an area of the brain that contains receptors for melatonin), light is the most influential zeitgeber we have.[44] A zeitgeber is a circadian rhythm time clue that impacts our levels of fatigue—other clues are eating patterns, temperature, and social interaction. Therefore, it's crucial to expose yourself to light when you want to be alert and to darkness when you want your body to begin releasing hormones that help in the transition to sleep.[45]

  At least an hour before going to bed, you should begin dimming the lights in your home and avoid blue-light emitters (such as the computer, phone, or TV). Blue light has shorter wavelengths that cause increased suppression of melatonin production.[46] If blue light can't be avoided, invest in blue-light filtering glasses or computer screen covers.

- **Listening to binaural beats.** You're now aware of the importance of sleep cycles and brain-wave frequencies in achieving a deep and restful night's sleep. If you have a hard time slowing down your high-frequency beta brain waves, you may want to try listening to binaural beats.

  Binaural beats use two tones, each at a different frequency, one for each ear. Your brain will create an additional tone that is the frequency difference between the two tones.[47] So, if you want to induce a deep, delta brain-wave frequency (0.5–4 hertz), the difference in tones should be in that range. The resulting tone can help to reduce your brain-wave frequency.

- **Maintaining regular sleep schedules.** I know how challenging this can be. You have a social life, an erratic work schedule, a show you're binge-watching that you "just can't" turn off. But maintaining consistency in your circadian rhythm is paramount for your energy and vitality—it's one of the reasons why you must go to bed and wake up at roughly the same times every day. According to Dr. Epstein, "If you must deviate from this schedule on weekends, try to limit the change in wake-up time to a maximum of an hour."[48]

  Consistency shouldn't be reserved for your bedtime and wake-up time; you should "aim to do other significant activities—such as meals and exercise sessions—at consistent times. If you have dinner at six on Monday, at nine on Tuesday, and at eight on Wednesday, you send your body conflicting messages about when it should expect sleep to begin," explains Epstein.[49]

Better Sleep through Your Environment

- **Reserve the bedroom for sleep and intimacy.** Train your mind to know that the association between you and your bed is sleep. Avoid watching TV, scrolling on your phone, or doing work while in your bedroom.

- **Can't sleep? Get out of bed.** We've all been there: lying awake and getting increasingly frustrated knowing that the time from now until your alarm clock goes off is getting shorter and shorter. I can always tell by my eyes. I'll periodically open them to determine how tired I am. If they open wide and there's no heaviness at all to my eyelids, I know sleep isn't right around the corner. You don't want to perceive the bed as a battleground. If sleep is evading you, get up and do some reading, make some herbal tea, or do something else relaxing.

- **Control bedroom noise.** White noise is very popular for helping people to stay asleep. If the room is too quiet, then any atypical sound will likely jolt you awake. Increasingly more people are opting for pink noise, which is designed to have louder, lower frequencies and more diminished higher frequencies. Pink noise has been shown to improve sleep quality by having a significant effect on reducing brain-wave complexity.[50]

- **Block out light.** Keep your room as dark as possible to signal your brain that it's nighttime. Use blackout curtains or eye shades to help keep it dark. And if you're someone who uses an eye mask, it's still necessary to keep your room as dark as possible—this is important because it's been discovered that we also have photoreceptors outside of the eyes (mainly on the skin).[51] The visual cells that detect light use a group of proteins called opsins. When exposed to light, the opsin will change its shape and turn on signaling pathways in photoreceptor cells; this will send a message to the brain that light has been detected.

- **Keep the room cool and well ventilated.** While the temperature of your room is a personal preference, having it cool (especially at the beginning of the night) is more beneficial for sleep promotion. However, since your body temperature typically drops as the night progresses, keep an extra blanket handy. The best bedroom temperature for sleep is approximately 65°F (18°C).[52]

- **Hide the clock.** For many, knowing the time can increase frustration. Cover the clock up or turn it off. You don't need to be doing that sleep math every 10 minutes (determining the hours remaining until you wake up).

- **Upgrade your bed and bedding.** If what you sleep on every night doesn't properly breathe, it could induce allergies. Consider switching to materials that promote better thermoregulation (such as organic cotton or silk) and that aren't produced with polyurethane foam and chemicals that may be an allergen for you.

- **Have plants in your bedroom.** Plants can help turn carbon dioxide into oxygen, increase the humidity level (most people prefer 30–50 percent humidity), and release negative ions into the air (which help to clear certain airborne allergens like pollen, mold spores, viruses, and bacteria). It's been determined that some of the best plants, in terms of improving indoor air quality, include the snake plant, peace lily, philodendron, Barberton daisy, English ivy, and chrysanthemum.[53]

- **Filter your air.** A proper air filter or purifier (such as HEPA or carbon filtering) can ensure that the air you're breathing is clean and fresh. This is important because when pollutants impact air quality it affects sleep efficiency.[54]

DID YOU KNOW . . .

According to some ancient traditions, such as *vastu shastra* (an Indian system of architecture), the most ideal position to sleep is when your head is pointed toward the south, and therefore your feet are pointed north.[55] The concept stems from Hindu beliefs that the human body has its own north and south poles, similar to the Earth—therefore, this sleeping position will align your magnetic energy with that of the Earth.

According to the Sleep Foundation, "Your 'north pole,' or your head, is oriented towards the Earth's south pole, so opposite poles can attract. When you lie the other way, you have two similar poles facing each other, which practitioners believe may contribute to headaches and high blood pressure."[56]

Also, according to the principles of feng shui your bed should be "directly against a wall, but not underneath any windows. Ideally, it should be placed on the wall opposite to your bedroom door, in a spot where you can see the door clearly but are not directly in line with it."[57]

Develop a Pre-Sleep Routine

At this point in your life you've gone to bed and woken up thousands of times. You are your best research study. The trial and error you've experienced is enough to create an ideal pre-sleep regimen. You know the challenges of falling asleep, as well as how you feel the next day when you eat late at night, drink too much alcohol, go to bed too late, stare at your phone before bed, or go to sleep angry or worried.

If you spend some time brainstorming what works and what doesn't, and you consider the knowledge and tips from this chapter, you'll quickly develop the ideal routine for you. Let's give it a try.

To begin, list all the things you've found that inhibit your sleep (either falling asleep, staying asleep, or overall sleep quality).

-
-
-
-
-
-
-
-
-
-

Next, list the things you've found that enhance your sleep (either falling asleep, staying asleep, or overall sleep quality).

-
-
-
-
-
-
-
-

Now that you've written down what works and what doesn't, develop an ideal routine. I understand that you'll waiver from time to time—but start with your ideal and do what you can to stick to it. Here's an example of my ideal bedtime routine.

Joseph's Ideal Routine

5:30 p.m.	Dinner with the family
7:00 p.m.	Optional snack (then no more eating until 11 a.m.)
7:15 p.m.	Turn all the lights in the house down (or off) (to stimulate melatonin production) and have quiet time with the family/put kids to bed
8 p.m.	Watch a TV program, light a fire, play a game with my wife, et cetera
9 p.m.	Get ready for bed and take nighttime supplements (magnesium and ashwagandha)
9:15 p.m.	Read something that doesn't stimulate thinking too much
9:40 p.m.	Write in our gratitude journal
9:45 p.m.	Pray
9:50 p.m.	Meditate
10:00 p.m.	Sleep

Your Ideal Routine:

-
-
-
-
-
-
-
-
-
-

Wake Up More Refreshed

It's time to come full circle and be reminded that your goal should be to wake up refreshed without the "need" for morning stimulants. Starting the day groggy, sluggish, and exhausted is something too many people experience daily and accept as an inevitability. Don't worry, there's a better way!

Here are some ways to make waking up naturally and with more energy a much more frequent occurrence.

- **Invest in a wake-up light**. Waking up to light mimics how our ancestors arose each morning. The light creates a cascading flow of hormones that slowly begins to release adrenaline into your bloodstream, which leaves you waking up more alert.

- **Have a glass of water**. Drink 10-14 oz. (300-400 mL) of water upon waking. During sleep, your body loses water. Replacing it first thing helps to ensure that your bodily processes are getting what they require. It can be especially beneficial if you add some lemon juice for gastric acid balancing (unless you're intermittent fasting, in which case save the lemon juice until before your first meal) and some Himalayan salt (half a teaspoon) for your adrenal glands.

The salt is beneficial because when you wake up in the morning your blood pressure rises to awaken your physiology—it accomplishes this via cortisol and adrenaline from the adrenal glands. To spare the already exhausted adrenals, the morning salt will temporarily raise blood pressure and therefore take some of the load. Also, if you already have adrenal fatigue, then you likely have trouble retaining salt (because the adrenals aren't producing enough aldosterone to maintain bodily sodium levels). Adding Himalayan salt to your diet helps to restore 84 trace minerals necessary for normal physiological functioning.

Note: If you currently have high blood pressure, the sodium may exacerbate the issue. Speak with your healthcare provider before proceeding. If you do adopt this strategy, I recommend using Himalayan salt, not regular table salt.

- **Begin your day with movement**. It doesn't have to be a formal exercise session; start by performing some jumping jacks, rebounding, or anything that gets your blood and lymphatic fluid moving.

- **Try the Nordic Cycle**. A warm shower followed by a cold shower can energize you and make you feel more alert. Subjecting yourself to low temperatures results in a dramatic increase in norepinephrine within the brain,[58] which causes you to feel more energized. Additionally, low temperatures have been shown to "relieve depressive symptoms rather effectively."[59] There'll be more on the benefits of cold therapy in Chapter 16 (see page 227).

- **Invest in a sleep app**. You know the feeling of waking up from a deep sleep versus a light one. The sleep cycle you wake up from can make a substantial difference in how you start your day. There are sleep apps and technologies that determine which stage of sleep you're in and then initiate your alarm when you're no longer in a deep sleep. Since you don't know exactly when you'll be in a light stage of sleep, you set sleep windows (such as between 6:15 and 6:45 a.m.) so your alarm can wake you any time between those times.

Another beneficial way to begin your day is with sunlight. Most people are prone to the overexposure risk that excessive ultraviolent (UV) light brings (increased chances of sunburn, skin aging, and skin cancer). Between 10 a.m. and 3 p.m. UV indexes are typically higher,[60] which means you must be extra careful to protect your skin from its damaging effects. That said, the light of the sun is very beneficial for your mental and physical health[61, 62]—but it's important that you time your exposure to maximize the benefits while limiting the downsides.

It's advisable for you to expose yourself to early-morning sunlight (before 10 a.m.) to receive the wonderful benefits it can provide. Here are some of the benefits of early-morning light.

1. **Helps to wake you up.** When light enters our photoreceptors (particularly the ones located within the eyes) it sends signals to our pituitary gland to release cortisol (which increases blood sugar, blood pressure, and heart rate) and downregulate melatonin.

2. **Increases feeling of happiness.** Sunlight boosts serotonin levels by triggering certain areas within the retina.[63] Serotonin is known to positively affect areas of the brain associated with mood.

3. **Ensures that our circadian rhythm is synchronized with the sun and moon.** Since humans are diurnal, we thrive best when our sleep and wake cycles are similar to the rising and setting of the sun. Early morning sunlight helps with the synchronization of biological rhythms.[64]

4. **Increased immunity.** Sunlight has been shown to increase white blood cell production, which plays an active role in fighting the infections we may encounter.[65]

5. **Enhances the production of vitamin D.** Sunlight on our skin helps to produce vitamin D (which, among other benefits, promotes immunity, bone health, and dental health).[66] In fact, unless you supplement your diet with exogenous vitamin D, approximately 90 percent of its production happens in this way.[67]

NOW THAT YOU'VE read about the many strategies that can be used to improve your sleep habits, are there any that you want to try?

As with any change in your routine, it's important to be realistic about the addition of something new in your life. You need to know that you can commit to sustaining the behavior long enough to evaluate the results. If necessary, take small steps and gradually build on those habits. Perhaps choose one or two a month that you can commit to.

If you have a partner who you sleep with every night, come up with strategies together. My wife and I do this and it makes a big difference to have someone who motivates and encourages the good behavior(s) on days when your resolve may be low. Eventually, with determination, you won't require willpower to continue—that's the point at which you can add a few more positive habits to your nightly routine.

So, then, what are some actionable steps you're willing to add immediately? List them here.

The positive effects of sleeping well consistently can be felt in just about every aspect of your life. For me, one of the primary benefits is the boost in immune-system functioning. Since a priority for me is feeling energized and present every day, having a strong and robust immune system is necessary for maintaining internal harmony.

CHAPTER 15

Immunity

"The best and most efficient pharmacy is within your own system."
—ROBERT C. PEARLE

IN ONE WAY or another, much of this book is about promoting habits and routines that will have a positive impact on your immune system. Your immune system is a network of organs, white blood cells, antibodies, and various chemicals, all living and working together in your body. It protects you from infection, illness, and disease by quickly recognizing invaders and swiftly executing a broad and efficient response to the threat.

We all know people who rarely get sick and when they do the illness doesn't last long. Unfortunately, they're the exception rather than the rule. In some ways, medicine has gone too far. At the first sign of illness too many people rush to ingest pain relievers and fever reducers. In most Western cultures the healing power of a fever has been forgotten.

A fever is a cell-mediated immune response that amps up the body's resources to coordinate a strategic attack on foreign invaders—but this physiological response is blunted by our world of over-prescription and self-medicating. Additionally, drug companies devalue rest in the recovery process by advertising their medication's ability to get you out of bed (despite being sick) and carrying on business as usual.

Sometimes medication is necessary and sometimes it isn't. The ability to determine when it's appropriate versus when you should focus on rest, proper hydration, and healthy food is an important life skill.

Before we explore the ways you can enhance your immunity, you must first have a basic understanding of what makes up this self-protection network.

- **The lymphatic system.** This is responsible for transporting lymph fluid (which contains white blood cells that fight infections).

- **The skin.** This is often the first line of defense from our external environment. This permeable layer of connective tissue is estimated to host more than 20 billion T cells (which is a type of white blood cell).[1]

- **The respiratory system.** This is a complementary set of organs (mouth, pharynx, larynx, trachea, and lungs) that inspire oxygen and expel carbon dioxide. Your respiratory system's defense mechanism includes a thin layer of mucus over the airways that is designed to trap particles and pathogens before they reach the lungs.

- **Lymphocytes.** These are white blood cells that identify and eliminate pathogens. There are two types of lymphocytes:

  - B cells make antibodies that are designed to attack bacteria and certain toxins.

  - T cells work to dispose of infected and cancerous cells.

- **The gut microbiome.** Our gastrointestinal tract has a tremendous amount of contact with the outside environment (particularly through our consumption of food, drinks, and medications). Residing within the gut are beneficial bacteria that help to mitigate the harmful effects of the bad bacteria we encounter.

  Maintaining a healthy microbiome (through diet, probiotic supplements, stress management, etc.) is critical, since it has been estimated that up to 70 percent of our immune system is found within our gut-associated lymphoid tissue (GALT; located on the outside of our intestinal lining).[2] The GALT is responsible for determining whether what we eat or drink is safe; if it deems that it isn't safe, it will prompt your immune system to respond.

- **The spleen.** The main job of the spleen is to act as a filter for your blood by recognizing and removing old and damaged red blood cells (RBCs). If the spleen detects an issue with certain RBCs, it will deploy macrophages (large white blood cells) to break them down.

Perhaps the best way to enhance your immune system is by making sure that your lymphatic system is circulating efficiently—which will in turn ensure that immune cells are being properly transported and unwanted cellular debris is taken to where it can be eliminated or recycled. Keeping this system moving is vital to your overall well-being.

Unlike the cardiovascular system, which uses the heart to pump blood throughout your body, the lymphatic system doesn't have a natural pump, so it needs bodily movement to reduce built-up congestion (dead blood cells, pathogens, toxins, cancer cells, etc.) and deliver important compounds (such as white blood cells and certain vitamins). Remaining stagnant (due to sitting or lying down too long) isn't natural for our physiology.

Your body wants to move, which is why it was designed to do so. Improving your detoxification system may be one of most important things you do in your life, so it's time to prioritize it. Given the sheer volume of toxins that you encounter every day, and the risk associated with their progressive accumulation, ensuring that your system is recognizing and eliminating them should be a top priority.

Your body wants to move!

Below are some ways you can enhance the functioning of your detox system and therefore improve your immunity. Most of these strategies are designed to aid the movement and functioning of your lymphatic system; keeping this system healthy is possible with very simple changes to your daily routine.

- **Physical activity and exercise.** This is perhaps the easiest and most accessible way of improving lymphatic flow.[3] Along with structured exercise routines, make sure you implement additional ways of moving your body such as parking farther away from your destination, taking the stairs instead of the escalator, taking the dog out for an extra walk, or setting a timer to get up from your desk and move at regular intervals. There are many ways to add movement to your day. Be creative!

Bodily movement also improves the efficiency of the lungs, kidneys, immune system, circulatory system, and intestines—this results in enhanced capability to detoxify unwanted substances.

- **Rebounding.** This has been proven to aid in the movement of your lymphatic system by stimulating numerous one-way valves.[4] Just a few minutes of rebounding correlates to a significant improvement in blood circulation and oxygen uptake.[5]

  Also, it is theorized that the up-and-down mechanics of rebounding causes the compression, and subsequent decompression, of bodily tissues and organs due to the added G-force on your body at the lowest point of the bounce.[6] This may result in toxins being expelled from tissues (which would allow the lymph system to carry away and eliminate waste) and blood to be cycled within organs.

  Additional benefits of rebounding include improvements in body composition, blood pressure, glucose and lipid profiles, pain severity and tolerance, and aerobic capacity.[7]

- **Dry skin brushing.** Since the lymphatic system doesn't have a central pump to effectively move lymphatic fluid, dry brushing helps to exfoliate and unclog pores by shedding dead skin cells.[8] It also helps with blood circulation and lymphatic flow/drainage.[9]

  To skin brush effectively, you need to purchase a brush that is designed to do so. Start at your feet and brush the skin in an upward motion toward the heart. I use circular motions as I travel up the body.

- **Massage therapy and foam rolling.** Through deep tissue physical stimulation you may be able to remove toxins that have built up within the tissues. The toxins would then be released into the bloodstream and eliminated from the body. This is one of the reasons why therapists will tell you to drink plenty of water after deep tissue massage (since an underhydrated lymphatic system will struggle to mobilize the toxins within your body). Also, cupping therapy may aid in "releasing of toxins and removal of wastes and heavy metals."[10]

- **Apple cider vinegar (ACV).** In addition to being great for your gut health, ACV can help to reduce body fat and therefore aid in the removal of toxins that have built up within the fat cell. Kondo and colleagues report that "vinegar intake reduced body weight, visceral and subcutaneous mass, and serum TG (triglyceride) levels without causing adverse effects in our obese Japanese study subjects. Intake of 15ml of vinegar per day was sufficient to achieve these effects."[11]

Another way that ACV aids in the removal of internal toxins is by relieving constipation. According to researchers, "Chronic constipation is a prevalent, burdensome gastrointestinal disorder whose aetiology and pathophysiology remains poorly understood and is most likely multifactorial."[12] Since ACV can beneficially alter the microbiota of the GI system, it helps with detoxification because "the altered intestinal microbiota may play an essential role in the pathogenesis of chronic constipation."[13]

Additionally, the pectin (a fiber) found in ACV helps to reduce inflammation and stomach cramping.[14] It's also been shown to treat diarrhea in people suffering from irritable bowel syndrome (IBS). A 2015 study concluded that "Pectin acts as a prebiotic by specifically stimulating gut bifidobacteria in IBS-D patients and is effective in alleviating clinical symptoms, balancing colonic microflora and relieving systemic inflammation."[15] [translated from the Chinese]

- **Proper hydration**. This will help to flush your body of toxins via the skin, urine, and feces. Symptoms that suggest that your hydration is too low include dizziness, dry eyes, dry mouth, inability to sweat, feeling of sluggishness, weakness, heart palpitations, confusion, increased thirst, and a decreased urine output.

   Dehydration by as little as 2 percent of our body mass is enough to have harmful effects on the body (such as trouble concentrating, diminished alertness, and decreased motor skills).[16, 17] The amount of fluid you should consume per day depends on several factors (heat and humidity level, how much exercise you do, the type of food you eat, body size, etc.). However, it's estimated that women consume approximately 2.5 quarts/liters, men 3.5 quarts/liters.[18]

   Another way to boost your hydration is to eat water-rich foods like cucumbers, tomatoes, blueberries, broccoli, strawberries, and celery. These foods aid in bodily cleansing for a variety of reasons: they elevate your internal water content, they're often from the earth (which means they aren't processed with ingredients and fillers that burden our physiology, especially if they're organic), and they typically contain a high percentage of vitamins and minerals.

- **Supplementation.** Certain nutrients have been linked to a positive immune response—as well as the growth and function of immune cells. Zinc, folate, iron, copper, selenium, and vitamins C, D, E, B6, and B12 all play an important role. The micronutrients that have shown the strongest evidence include vitamins C and D as well as zinc.[19]

  According to Wessels and colleagues, "Zinc ions are involved in regulating intracellular signalling pathways in innate and adaptive immune cells."[20] Therefore, if you want to enhance your immune system you should consider zinc supplements. This is especially important as you age since zinc deficiency has been proven to be prevalent among the elderly.[21] Additionally, zinc deficiency has been linked to depression, cerebral aging, Parkinson's disease, and Alzheimer's disease.[22, 23, 24]

- **Increased fiber intake.** Increasing fiber will enhance your body's ability to remove waste through your GI tract. Eating organic fruits and vegetables will ensure that your body has the necessary fiber without the unwanted pesticides.

- **Sauna.** The increased sweating and blood flow that using a sauna causes can assist in toxin elimination. Especially effective are infrared saunas, because they deliver deep infrared energy into the body (as opposed to a traditional sauna, which heats up the air inside the sauna).[25] The wavelength of infrared rays that are emitted from the panels is set at a level that causes them to be absorbed by the body. Other items that you bring into this type of sauna, like your towel, do not heat up like you do (because these items do not absorb the rays). Additionally, according to Chun-Chih and colleagues, an infrared sauna reduces oxidative stress in the body.[26]

- **Wear loose clothing.** Tight clothing prevents optimal fluid movement— underwire bras and waistbands tend to be the most restrictive. There's a high concentration of lymph nodes in the upper torso, so a tight bra will impede the ability of fluid to move and drain from this area. The unforgiving waistband of most underwear will reduce fluid movement as well. So perhaps it's time to convince your partner to sleep naked . . . you know, strictly for health reasons.

It's pretty easy to see that boosting your immune system is a simple matter—move your body, promote sweating, stay hydrated, eat a healthy diet containing lots of fiber, prioritize certain supplements, and limit restrictive clothing. These are strategies that don't require a lot of time or money, so there's no excuse for not beginning immediately. In Part IV you'll create your new life blueprint that will include the addition of most of the techniques mentioned.

Once you've committed to these simple and cost-effective strategies, perhaps you'll be ready to level up your health routine. An uncomplicated, but uncomfortable, way to do so is to add temperature-related hormetic stresses. Hot and cold therapies aren't new, but they're becoming more mainstream as people become privy to their numerous benefits. Enhanced energy, clarity, and happiness, as well as improved physiological repair and growth, become a reality when you regularly expand your comfort zone this way.

CHAPTER 16

Temperature Therapies and You

"Champions aren't made when the game is easy."

—JAMIE KERN LIMA

THE MAJORITY OF people—dare I say everyone?—would like to be happier. So here's a thought. Did you know that certain types of hormetic stress (pushing your body to the limit so it can adapt and thus become more resilient) can make your body more sensitized toward feelings of happiness? Exercise is a form of hormetic stress, but so too are heat and cold therapies.

You'll likely have to endure some discomfort to reap the rewards, but a new happiness baseline is out there. Also, temperature-related hormetic stresses enhance internal cleansing, which positively impacts the level of vigor and vitality you feel each day.

During a discussion at the Biohacker Summit in Finland, Dr. Rhonda Patrick, founder of *Found My Fitness*, discussed the benefits of heat as a form of hormetic stress. She summarized some of the benefits of regular sauna exposure (we'll expand on these benefits later):[1]

- Sensitizes brain to endorphins
- Improves cardiovascular health
- Improves overall longevity
- Increases heat shock proteins (HSP)
- Activates Foxo3 gene
- Increases growth hormone

Imagine, all that goodness from something so simple as sitting in a hot box!

Saunas and Happiness

What does Dr. Patrick mean when she says the use of saunas "sensitizes" our brain to endorphins? The science behind it is interesting. When you're exposed to excessive heat and your internal body temperature rises above the normal 96.8°F–98.6°F (36°C–37°C), dynorphins are released from presynaptic neurons, which then bind to kappa opioid receptors to prompt an uncomfortable (or dysphoric) feeling within you[2]—this causes you to remove yourself from the situation. You may be asking yourself, Why is this a good thing?

Endorphins (our feel-good hormones) bind to receptors called mu opioid receptors. When our body releases dynorphins, it causes the creation of more opioid receptors. More receptors equals more endorphin binding—which in turn equals greater feelings of happiness when endorphins are released. Also, with regular exposure to dynorphins, the receptors may become more sensitized, which means they will bind more easily with endorphins.[3] Don't you just love physiology?!

Another neat feature that heat can induce in us is activation of the Foxo3 gene and heat shock proteins (HSP). Foxo3 is associated with the process of autophagy. Autophagy (Greek for "self-eating") is a natural cleansing process within the body that allows cells to "eat" themselves—this detox process helps to clean out damaged cells and toxins, which ultimately helps the body create new, healthy cells.

Cell damage is a normal part of our physiology. However, as damage to a cell accumulates, the cell can eventually become senescent (cells that aren't alive but also aren't dead). These cells reside in tissues and organs and secrete pro-inflammatory molecules and cytokines that damage nearby cells (and may cause them to become senescent as well), accelerating the aging process.[4] Thankfully, Foxo3 and autophagy help to clean up our systems.

The upregulation of Foxo3 is beneficial for other reasons as well:[5]

- It activates genes that are involved in DNA repair—which prevents cell mutations.

- It activates genes that are involved in cell death—this is important because if a gene does get a mutation, the cell will sacrifice itself and die.

- It activates genes that are involved with stem cell function—which is important because stem cells can make white blood cells.

In addition to Foxo3, Dr. Patrick explains, heat shock proteins play an important role within your cells: "Their role is to make sure that proteins maintain their three-dimensional structure. And that's really important because every protein inside your cell has a certain three-dimensional structure in space, and that three-dimensional structure is essential for that protein's normal function. And if you disrupt that three-dimensional structure then the protein can't function optimally."[6]

The three-dimensional structure of protein is being damaged all the time—this is a completely normal part of our physiology. However, what you want to avoid is excessive and continuous accumulation of protein aggregates. HSPs can repair damaged proteins and return them to their original three-dimensional shape, which then reduces the number of aggregates that are formed.

Here are some additional biochemical functions of HSPs:[7, 8]

- Prevent the accumulation of free radicals and cellular damage
- Help to promote the body's cellular antioxidant capacity
- Help with autophagy and cellular turnover

Remember, whenever possible you want to stack healthy habits together; this can supercharge your ability to achieve optimal health. In the article "Heat Alteration: Health Benefits of Traditional Sauna & Infrared Heat Room," Olli Sovijärvi outlines the additional benefits that are possible if heat stress is combined with intermittent fasting and cold exposure: "Greater benefits come from heat stress with elevated autophagy (for example while fasting) while including heat alteration through cold exposure."[9] Sovijärvi explains that the best way to activate HSPs and take advantage of autophagy is to fast for 16 hours and then exercise for 20-30 minutes before completing a heat alteration session of three 15-minute periods with 2 minutes of cold exposure in between.

Cold-Water Therapy

"Successful people do what unsuccessful people are not willing to do."
—JIM ROHN

Intentionally subjecting yourself to cold isn't something that most people do. Most humans prefer consistent comfort—they like to stay "coooozy" (that's how my kids say it when they climb into their beds at night). I'm the same, *except* when there's a discomfort that could increase my energy and immunity; then I'll happily oblige.

Exposing yourself to cold via an ice bath, cryotherapy, or a cold shower is another hormetic stress. One of the most robust responses to cold stress is the large increase in norepinephrine in the brain.[10] This is important because of norepinephrine's ability to assist with focus, attention, and mood—which is why it's targeted to help individuals with depression and attention deficit hyperactivity disorder (ADHD).[11]

Submerging yourself in 40°F (4.4°C) water for just 20 seconds can result in a 200–300 percent increase in norepinephrine.[12]

Cold stress can also result in mitochondria biogenesis (which means more mitochondria are produced).[13] Mitochondria are responsible for generating most of your chemical energy that powers cellular activity. This adaptation to cold exposure makes sense because one of the byproducts of your body producing energy is heat. More mitochondria = more energy capability = more heat production. So, in addition to your body being more capable of warming itself when encountering very low temperatures, the increase in mitochondria enhances your ability to use oxygen to produce and use more energy. This helps you lose weight, because the biogenesis happens within fat cells—and it makes you more aerobically fit, because the increase in muscle mitochondria gives you the ability to use more oxygen to create energy.

I know that the adoption of a cold-water immersion routine is uncomfortable, so I'm going to add some more credence to its addition to your life.

- **Decrease in inflammation.** It's been proven that cold water immersion helps your body to reduce muscle inflammation by decreasing damage to the affected tissue.[14, 15]

- **Increase in adiponectin.**[16] This is a protein that helps with blood sugar regulation, fat metabolism, the immune response, and energy regulation.

- **Activates brown adipose tissue.** This helps to improve mitochondrial functioning, resting metabolic rate (by increasing it), and thermoregulation. According to researchers, with regular cold-water immersion brown adipose tissue is activated in the back of the neck and the upper back—this helps to generate more heat, because brown adipose tissue (which gets its color from higher iron levels) burns conventional white adipose tissue.[17] So, the more you engage in cold-water immersion, the more tolerant you become to the cold (which is great news for those of us living in colder climates!).

    It's not just cold water that activates the thermogenesis; a cold environment can do the same. When your body is exposed to the cold it must work harder to maintain homeostasis and regulate core temperature, which stimulates more brown adipose tissue.[18]

- **Heal the Blood Brain Barrier (BBB).**[19] Keeping this very thin layer of protection intact is important in ensuring that destructive toxins and infectious pathogens don't enter the brain. You want osmosis into the brain reserved for substances the brain wants, such as glucose, amino acids, certain nutrients, and ketones.

- **Immune system activation.** Buijze and colleagues found that, in healthy adults, a daily hot-to-cold shower resulted in a 29 percent decrease in self-reported absence from work due to sickness.[20] This may be explained by the increase in white blood cell count, decrease in inflammation, and stimulation of norepinephrine release with cold thermogenesis.

- **Enhanced feelings of alertness and energy.** Immersion in 14°C (57°F) water for one hour results in a 350 percent increase in metabolic rate, a 530 percent increase in norepinephrine, and a 250 percent increase in dopamine.[21]

    One hour is a long time, so it's a good thing you experience benefits in as little as 20 seconds.[22] The length of time you expose yourself to the cold is directly related to the temperature of the water. Typically, you want the water to be below 59°F (15°C), and you want to build tolerance slowly by incrementally staying in longer or reducing the temperature as the weeks progress.

Remember to always listen to your body. Hypothermia, which usually occurs when the body temperature falls below 95°F (35°C), is nothing to brag about! Notice dangerous symptoms such as a distinct rise in breathing rate, confusion, and drowsiness. And if you're living with a chronic disease, it's best to consult with your physician before adopting this therapy.

When I first read about the positive effects of cold-water immersion, I gave it a try by having cold showers. I'd keep turning the tap lower and lower while focusing on using my breath to regulate my body. Eventually I wanted to take my cold-water experience to the next level. I wanted to know the exact temperature of the water so I could tailor a suitable time frame for immersion. I bought a large chest freezer (14.8 cu ft./ 0.42 cu m) and converted it to a cold plunge. I followed the advice of John Richter in his book *The Ultimate Chest Freezer Cold Plunge DIY Guide*[23] on the proper way to convert it. It's far more complicated than just adding water—but worth the investment!

ACCLIMATIZE

I'm not a monster, so I can appreciate the difficulty of giving up your warm and comforting shower every day. Even though the evidence is very clear that routine cold-water exposure is great for the body and mind, I know this might not be enough to make you want to jump in. Slowly acclimatizing yourself to this form of hormetic stress may ensure that you continue doing it day after day. I'm willing to bet you'll begin to crave it! Once you feel the positive effects, and it becomes a daily habit, you'll miss it if you can't do it for a day or two.

Below are some tips from the *Biohacker's Handbook* on building up your tolerance and cold-water practice.[24] Remain at each step for as long as it takes for you to feel comfortable moving on to the next one.

1. Put your hands in cold water for 20-30 seconds.

2. Put your face in cold water–40°F–50°F (5°C–10°C)–for 20–30 seconds. This is beneficial because the highest concentration of cold thermoreceptors can be found in the face and ears. It has the bonus of activating the trigeminal nerve, which will then activate the vagus nerve.

    Before submerging your face (or your entire head, if you can), breathe in until your lungs are about 80 percent full (so you can still relax your body). Perform three repetitions while doing at least a minute of slow breathing (to ensure that the stored carbon dioxide effectively leaves your lungs) between attempts.

3. Finish your warm shower with a cold shower. Aim to increase the length of cold exposure each day.

4. While showering, try alternating from warm (30 seconds) to cold (30 seconds), going back and forth for a few minutes.

5. Start having strictly cold showers.

6. Immerse yourself in a cold plunge or a cold-water swim. Increase your time and frequency as you progress. Submerge your head periodically during the immersion.

Also, try adding some visualizations to your pre-exposure routine. Envision yourself as a cold-water animal such as a seal or a penguin–they are impervious to the cold, so it doesn't faze them (which is your goal). Ideally, you'll be able to use your breathing and visualization technique to enter a cold plunge and not hyperventilate and tense up as most people would. This will take time, but each day you do it you'll be building your mental and nervous system resilience.

Cold Therapy 2.0–The Mammalian Dive Reflex

First studied in the 1930s, the mammalian dive reflex (DR) is a phenomenon found in all mammals. This incredible physiological response causes breathing cessation (which inhibits humans from inhaling water) as well as a slowing of the heart rate and an increase in peripheral vasoconstriction when the face is submerged in water.[25] Also, as a survival mechanism your body conserves oxygen for the brain and heart.[26]

Total-body cold-water exposure (including the face) is important because when the cold water fills the nostrils it triggers sensory receptors in the nasal cavity (as well as other areas of the face) to send information to the brain that induces the DR.[27] This hormetic stress can be used to enhance the tone of your vagus nerve and therefore the overall functioning of your parasympathetic nervous system.[28] Additionally, due to the hydrostatic pressure of the water (at deeper levels in particular, especially for people who practice free diving) and the lower levels of oxygen and higher levels of carbon dioxide, there is splenic contraction that results in red blood cells being released into the circulatory system.[29, 30] More red blood cells means that there is more oxygen available to your system.

To induce the added benefits of the mammalian DR reflex, submerge your face five or six times while in your cold plunge. Does it feel great when you do it? No. Do the benefits outweigh the cost? That's for you to decide.

Cold Exposure and Physical Training

I'm willing to bet that most of the people reading this book have the goal of increasing their endurance and/or muscle mass. The question, then, is, Should you cold-shock the body after either endurance-based exercise or resistance-based exercise? The answer is yes and no, respectively.

There's evidence suggesting that, after endurance-based exercise, cold-shocking the body provides additional benefits (immediate mitochondrial biogenesis and a reduction in inflammation).[31] Conversely, if your goal is to increase muscle mass, cold-water immersion immediately after might inhibit muscle adaptation.[32, 33]

According to Dr. Patrick, "Immediately after strength training there's inflammation that occurs, and that inflammation is very important as a hormetic response to activate all these anti-inflammatory pathways. And also, it's important to activate some immune cells that play a role in producing IGF 1 [insulin-like growth factor] in muscle tissue, which helps you make your muscle grow."[34] She suggests waiting at least an hour after resistance-based training before you do your cold plunge. Perhaps while you wait you could spend some time in an infrared sauna, as this has been demonstrated to speed up recovery from exercise.[35]

Personally, I don't like to cold plunge directly after endurance-based exercise either. I wait about an hour after the endurance exercise so my body can normalize (return enzymes, hormones, and heart rate closer to resting levels) by itself. During the hour before a cold plunge (if time and my daily schedule permit), I'll stretch for 10–15 minutes, rebound for 10–15 minutes, and then go into my infrared sauna for 20–30 minutes.

DID YOU KNOW . . .

According to researchers, if you fail to maintain adequate hydration levels and dehydration occurs, it impairs the production of testosterone after strength training.[36] This outcome (diminished testosterone) has also been found after endurance-based activity when dehydration was present.[37] The bottom line: stay hydrated!

Transferable Benefits

By adopting a consistent cold-water immersion routine you'll likely gain an additional benefit, and it's not something that can be measured quantifiably. Pushing the boundaries of your comfort zone via cold therapy will be very difficult at first, but with repeated exposure and the expansion of your comfort zone your brain will develop a transferable strength that may be useful in other areas of your life.

There's a bubble around you. You can't see it, but it's there. If you take one step outside of that bubble your body and brain will coerce you back to safety, back to your comfort zone. Leaders and risk-takers regularly challenge the borders of this zone. They feel the fear just as you or I would but decide to push on anyway. In doing so they're able to achieve things that the average person can't.

Challenge the borders of your bubble!

As time goes on and their comfort zone becomes larger, their subconscious mind grows increasingly confident in their ability to accomplish what's within their zone—but it also gains confidence in accomplishing what's outside their zone. Since they regularly push their limits their subconscious mind grows assured that even though they haven't done something before, because they've had success in pushing their boundaries they know they'll find a way—that's true confidence.

The Comfort Zone

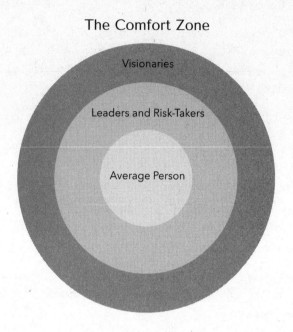

Visionaries

Leaders and Risk-Takers

Average Person

Although adopting a cold-plunge routine may seem an extreme step to get you accustomed to the discomfort of venturing out of your comfort zone, it's helped me in a variety of ways. It's helped me with the difficult task of ending relationships that were toxic, to push through adversity with a sense of calm, and even to write this book. In striving toward an optimal life, you are routinely going to be challenged. The physiological and psychological priming that must be done to endure the discomfort of a cold plunge has helped to expand my comfort zone.

Additionally, you may opt to try the Nordic Cycle of exposing yourself to heat, then cold, followed by a period of relaxation. Nordic countries have been using the hot, cold, relax cycle for generations. It may seem counterintuitive to follow your hot sauna, and the zen-like relaxation that occurs, with the brutal shock of a cold plunge or shower. Why would you want to create tension immediately after you've spent time letting tension melt away? Here are a few reasons.

- **Immunity boost.** Lymphatic circulation is improved via the contraction of your lymphatic vessels. This enhances the detoxifying power of your body.

- **Quick pore closing.** This will ensure that germs and bacteria have a tougher time entering your body.

- **Improved circulation.** When you're hot, circulation is directed to your skin in order to release heat. The cold shock will quickly send blood back to the organs, giving them the additional oxygen and nutrients they need to thrive.

- **Decreased inflammation.** This is especially noticeable in the joints, where inflammation is felt most.

- **Skin appearance.** The closing of the pores and the enhanced circulation contributes to the skin appearing rejuvenated.

- **Increased happiness.** The hot-to-cold experience will raise your heart rate, release adrenaline, and release endorphins.[38] For most, this will lead to an enhanced mood.

Disclaimer: If you have heart-related issues, the immediate vaso-constriction of the cold shock may be contraindicated. Discuss possible issues with your physician.

To summarize, you can boost your mental and physical health by adopting routines that require some psychological fortitude. I don't recommend implementing every hormetic approach mentioned on the first day of your transformational journey. Start slowly and notice the changes in your health and wellness as the months progress. Who knows—you may wake up one day and find yourself craving a cold plunge. Stranger things have happened.

Another hormetic stress that's attracted a lot of attention in recent years is intermittent fasting (alternatively called time-restricted eating). Similar to the strategies we've discussed, this lifestyle approach requires you to persevere through an uncomfortable adjustment phase. Your physiology, and particularly your psychology, must remain steadfast so intermittent fasting can eventually transition into a sustained habit.

CHAPTER 17

Intermittent Fasting

---

*"Discipline is the bridge between goals
and accomplishments."*—JIM ROHN

IT SEEMS THERE'S a new fad diet, superfood, or eating strategy every couple of years. Something I want to caution you about is the adoption of a dietary protocol that restricts certain food groups. A lot of people get hooked on these novel eating strategies because they initially make you feel fantastic. For some this can lead to it becoming a dogma—they stop listening to their body and to science because they've tied their belief structure to it. This is dangerous as both a dietary choice and a lifestyle strategy.

For me, the food dogma I had to address was my long-standing belief that eating in the morning was necessary for optimal health. Like many, I'd been told that breakfast was the most important meal of the day. My belief in breaking the fast upon waking up was so ingrained in me that I sought (consciously or subconsciously) to support that belief—but due to extreme fatigue and exhaustion it became clear that I needed to challenge my assumptions. Not breaking the fast—or intermittent fasting—had been on my radar for quite some time due to the many accounts I'd heard of it boosting energy levels and enhancing focus. So, armed with research, I decided to try a new way.

Intermittent Fasting: My Experience

I don't typically ease into things, so when I make a decision regarding a certain path I want to go down, I follow it to the letter. There are a variety of styles of intermittent fasting, and each has its benefits and challenges.

Here are some common methods.

- 16-hour fast (black coffee/tea allowed) followed by an 8-hour eating window

- 18-hour fast (fatty coffee allowed) followed by a 6-hour eating window (a.k.a. Bulletproof Intermittent Fasting)

- 20-hour fast with a 4-hour eating window (a.k.a. The Warrior Diet)

- 24-hour fast 1 to 2 days per week (a.k.a. Eat Stop Eat)

- 36-hour fast followed by a 12-hour eating window (a.k.a. The Alternate Day Fast)

I began with the 16-hour daily fast for a variety of reasons, chief among them was that it seemed the simplest to begin with; if I liked the results, I could try the more extreme versions.

The first task was choosing my 8-hour eating window, and I picked 11 a.m. to 7 p.m. I won't lie: the first week was very tough. My body (and mind) woke up craving food; making it to 11 a.m. was a challenge. On the flip side, my belly would fiercely rumble after 10 p.m. I knew there'd be an adjustment phase—I just didn't know how long it would last. Fortunately, it lasted only about a week.

Following this adjustment phase, things got easier—once I made it through the first hour of the day my hunger subsided and getting to 11 a.m. wasn't too difficult. The hardest mornings were the ones when I would be at home. The physical sensations of hunger weren't any worse, but the psychological craving for food was high.

Part of my strategy in curbing my hunger pangs at the start of the day became morning exercise. Over the course of my intermittent fasting journey, I've found that if I'm hungry and have a strong desire to eat but decide to exercise instead, my hunger sensations are reduced for another few hours. This knowledge about my personal biology motivates me to exercise when I wake up—and it helps in the achievement of my 16-hour fasting window. It's a win-win!

Here are some of the firsthand benefits that I've experienced with my 16/8 fasting strategy.

- **Better workouts.** I typically exercise in the morning. In the past I'd make sure I ate something at least an hour before I began exercising (especially if it was going to be a resistance-based workout). To my surprise, exercising before breakfast made my body feel more present and better able to respond to what I was asking of it. No longer did I have to time my pre-workout eating and make sure I had the right balance of macronutrients for quick gastric emptying. I could just get up and begin. What freedom!

- **Increased energy.** This was enough for me to make this fasting strategy a staple in my life. I'm fixated on creating more "clean energy"—this is what I call energy that's derived from within rather than from an outside source (such as coffee and other stimulants).

- **More focus.** Since my career requires me to research, write, and present information, being able to focus and execute efficiently is very important. I noticed that my brain fog diminished the longer I continued with the 16/8 intermittent fasting diet. Sometimes you don't know how foggy your brain and thoughts are until they become clearer.

My experience has been excellent, and at this point I'm a lifer, but before I get into some of the general benefits you might experience with a similar regime, I will say that this lifestyle adjustment isn't necessarily beneficial for everyone. Whether it's because you have a chronic disease that makes it contraindicated to go too long without eating (perhaps because of its relation to your medication, blood sugar levels, etc.), or for some other reason, it's important to find the best eating strategy for you. Consult with a trained professional on the potential benefits and drawbacks of this lifestyle. For instance, people who are pregnant, breastfeeding, living with chronic fatigue syndrome, or under 18 years of age should avoid intermittent fasting unless otherwise recommended by their primary care physician.

Intermittent Fasting—What the Literature Tells Us

Before I get into some of the other benefits of intermittent fasting, I want to remind you of something: our bodies are incredibly adept organisms capable of executing countless tasks at the same time without you having to consciously control any of them. Logically, then, it makes sense that if we get out of the body's way it stands a good chance of cleaning up the internal "mess" and restoring health.

If our body is busy digesting and absorbing food every hour that we're awake, and even a few hours while we're sleeping (if you eat right before bedtime), then it doesn't have a chance to get back to a baseline it's happy with. What follows is a slow but steady accumulation of toxins that begin to interfere with the proper functioning of our organs—and can contribute to chronic disease, daily exhaustion, and poor concentration.

Aside from the benefits I experienced, there are a lot of other proven perks of this lifestyle. Here are some of the additional benefits of intermittent fasting:

- **Human growth hormone (HGH) elevation.** Blood levels of growth hormone may increase as much as fivefold with a two-day fast.[1] Although fasting for two days might be too extreme, it's been demonstrated that the 16/8 method provides ample return on your investment.[2] It was concluded that "an intermittent fasting program in which all calories are consumed in an 8-h window each day, in conjunction with resistance training, could improve some health-related biomarkers, decrease fat mass, and maintain muscle mass in resistance-trained males."[3]

- **Faster stem cell regenerative capacity.** A 2018 study found that a 24-hour fast significantly improved the regeneration of intestinal stem cells in mice.[4] Since human aging results in reduced ability of intestinal stem cells to regenerate (which makes it more difficult to repair and regenerate tissues and recover from GI infections or other intestinal issues),[5] periodic 24-hour fasts may boost stem cell regeneration and therefore aid in the functioning of the gut.

- **Improved cellular repair.** Removing waste from cells is crucial for the overall health and well-being of your body and mind. Alirezaei and colleagues found that fasting led to an upregulation of autophagy.[6]

- **Increased longevity.** Research has found beneficial changes in various genes and molecules that relate to longevity and disease protection.

According to researchers, "results suggest that alternate fasting could exert a beneficial antioxidant effect and a modulation of the oxidative stress associated with aging."[7]

- **Less oxidative stress.** Researchers Mark Mattson and Ruiqian Wan report that intermittent fasting leads to a reduction in the levels of oxidative stress, which is indicated by "decreased oxidative damage to proteins, lipids and DNA."[8]

- **Weight loss.** Intermittent fasting enhances hormones (such as insulin, HGH, and norepinephrine) that aid in weight loss. A study from 2000 concluded that "Resting energy expenditure increases early in starvation, accompanied by an increase in plasma norepinephrine."[9]

- **Reduced inflammation.** A 2007 study concluded that prolonged intermittent fasting has "some positive effects on the inflammatory status of the body and the risk factors for cardiovascular diseases."[10] With so many people experiencing heart-related issues, as well as persistent bodily inflammation, doing what you can to minimize these issues should be prioritized.

- **Beneficial for heart health.** According to the World Health Organization, heart disease remains the leading cause of death globally.[11] In 2009 Varady and colleagues evaluated modified alternate day fasting (ADF; you consume 25 percent of typical energy needs on the fast day and eat as usual on the other days) and its relation to coronary artery disease (CAD) for obese individuals. They found that "ADF is a viable diet option to help obese individuals lose weight and decrease CAD risk."[12]

- **Possible cancer prevention.** There has been a lot of promising evidence from animal studies showing that intermittent fasting can help to prevent cancer.[13, 14, 15] Tiwari and colleagues determined that "Emerging evidence suggests that fasting could play a key role in cancer treatment by fostering conditions that limit cancer cells' adaptability, survival, and growth. Fasting could increase the effectiveness of cancer treatments and limit adverse events."[16]

   Also, a 2012 article reported that "Short-term starvation (or fasting) protects normal cells, mice, and potentially humans from the harmful side effects of a variety of chemotherapy drugs."[17] The authors continue: "Cycles of starvation were as effective as chemotherapeutic agents in delaying progression of different tumors."[18]

- **Better brain health.** What's good for your body is often good for your brain as well. Intermittent fasting has been shown to increase levels of a brain hormone called brain-derived neurotrophic factor (which is important for neuron survival and growth).[19]

Do I have your buy-in yet?

If you're still skeptical, let me dangle this carrot in front of you. Black coffee (in addition to tea and water) won't break your fast.[20, 21] This means that when you wake up and are in your fasting window, you're still allowed that cup of Joe!

According to the United States Department of Agriculture (USDA), plain black coffee contains around two calories per cup.[22] This caloric intake isn't likely to initiate any significant metabolic change that would result in a break to your fast. Also, as previously mentioned, moderate coffee consumption has a lot of health benefits[23, 24, 25] (likely resulting from the high antioxidant content of coffee[26]). Be sure to choose organic and pesticide-free coffee—and, although it's more work, consider buying whole beans and grinding them yourself to reduce chemical exposure and toxic mold.

A research study determined that over 90 percent of the beans grown in Brazil were contaminated with mold before they were processed.[27] Dave Asprey, the founder of Bulletproof Coffee, explains in his book *Head Strong* that "Mold toxins form in coffee because the coffee industry saves money by harvesting coffee cherries and then letting them sit in unfiltered water for a couple of days to soften the pulp around the seed. During that time, uncontrolled fermentation creates mold toxins."[28]

However, there's only so much you can control in your life. If freeze-dried, pre-ground instant coffee is your go-to cup, I'd rather you drank that while fasting than not fast at all.

PART III HAS revealed a lot of strategies you could use to improve your health and well-being. To discover *your* optimal, you needn't incorporate all the lifestyle strategies discussed. You must simply begin—begin shifting the needle of your health in a positive way by choosing a few methods capable of altering your thoughts and behaviors. That's where Part IV comes in.

In Part IV you'll work to further clarify your obstacles, the root(s) of those obstacles, and the methods and strategies you'll employ to initiate sustainable change. Before you proceed to Part IV, take a moment to go over the material in Part III.

Summary Points for Part III

- To become better in any dimension of health we must often push beyond our typical limits, then take the necessary recovery time to come back stronger.

- Negative emotions will quickly drain your total energy resources.

- The ability to swiftly move from an emotion that isn't serving you to one that is, is a skill, and like any skill, it can be developed.

- The quality of your life is determined by the state you spend most of your time in.

- Your superpower is that you possess the ability to positively change someone's vibrational state.

- One of the ways people lose time, energy, and special moments is by living a life of disconnect and hurry.

- With practice and dedication, you can improve the speed of your decision-making and the number of decisions you can handle in a day before decision fatigue sets in.

- We are programmed to believe that the accumulation of more will lead to what we all desire, happiness.

- If you tie your perceived happiness to an outcome, then you'll always want to expedite the process.

- Approximately 50 percent of life satisfaction is attributed to genetics. This suggests that the other 50 percent is variable, which means you have a great deal of control over it.

- You must strive for a consistent and sustainable boost to your baseline level of happiness. An authentic shift must be derived from your psychology and your physiology.

- Hedonic happiness is what you feel when something makes you happy.

- Eudaemonic happiness is the feeling you get when you live in accordance with your spirit.

- A more fulfilled life requires you to discover (and implement) more ways that you can boost your eudaemonic happiness. Think of things that align with your spirit, with the deepest sense of who you are or who you want to become.

- Strengthening your vagal tone helps in the conservation of energy—while also enhancing your sense of calm, relaxation, and connectedness within your body.

- Most people battle with their natural rhythms and over time the result is more and more internal fatigue—which results in the body and mind not getting what it needs, when it needs it.

- There are many ways you can support the quantity and quality of sleep you get. Prior to embarking on your sleep journey, consider your nutritional choices, bedroom dynamics, timing and amount of exercise, medications, supplements, and your typical emotional state.

- Starting your day groggy, sluggish, and exhausted is something too many people experience daily and accept as an inevitability.

- One the most important ways you can enhance your immune system is by ensuring your lymphatic system is circulating efficiently.

- Heat as a hormetic stress has been proven to increase cardiovascular health, growth hormone, and heat shock proteins, while also sensitizing the brain to endorphins and improving overall life longevity.

- Cold-water therapy has been proven to produce a large increase in norepinephrine within the brain—this helps with focus, attention, and mood.

- Cold therapy has also been shown to increase mitochondria, adiponectin, the immune system, and your feelings of alertness and energy, as well as healing the blood-brain barrier, activating brown adipose tissue, and decreasing inflammation.

- Intermittent fasting can enhance your physiology and psychology in numerous ways.

PART IV

Developing Your Blueprint

"Our destiny is not written for us, but by us."
—BARACK OBAMA

WELCOME TO WHERE the rubber meets the road and you strategize the implementation of your upgraded health and wellness intentions. Congratulations on getting here! I'm excited for you to take this next step! You've done a great deal of introspection throughout the first three parts of this book and now it's time for us to act on that introspection with intention.

Part IV is largely a workbook. Don't be scared. When it's complete, you'll have defined your purpose and priorities as well as your mission and vision, and will hold in your hands your unique blueprint for health and happiness.

You'll begin with the body, identifying the ways you'll revitalize your physiology and therefore provide a boost to your energy levels and the functioning of your immune system. As stated earlier, a healthy body, one that's robust with vital energy, is the foundation from which growth can be achieved.

Next, you'll evaluate and strategize the improvement in your mental and emotional well-being. This chapter is essential for sustainable health and wellness enhancement—and if you're seeking to better your professional life, it will help with that as well.

Then you'll reflect on your spiritual journey and purpose in life. Change in these areas requires deep thought on the forces that govern your daily decisions, contemplation on the legacy you want to leave behind, and willingness to take actionable steps that you're continually evolving.

BE REALISTIC WITH YOURSELF

I love it when people shoot for the stars and want to change everything–it shows that they're desperate for a lifestyle adjustment. However, this strategy works only on the rarest of occasions.

Before committing (which is what you're doing as you write down your plans), think of all the variables in your life that could interfere with the consistent action required to turn your new behaviors into an ingrained and fixed staple of your life.

Consider your commitments (such as work deadlines and vacations), the resources accessible to you (such as money), and your time-related availability to make certain lifestyle modifications. I'm providing you with this advice and caution because I want sustainable change for you–which is possible only with proper planning. You can achieve *all* of your aspirations if you pursue them using a methodological approach, one that is both ambitious *and* realistic. To do this you must create rituals.

Rituals are highly specific actions that you carry out at precise times and that therefore eventually become automatic or habitual. Incorporating healthy rituals will allow you to grow in a particular area without enduring excessive stress and energy loss before the event has even taken place. For instance, if you go for a run every morning, and have been doing so for a long time, you don't overthink the run and try to talk yourself out of it but just put on your shoes and begin running. In other words, you don't expend any extra mental energy before the act has taken place. Therefore, you have not drained any resources before you needed to.

Conversely, if you want to take up running, and have wanted to for years, but you haven't properly planned how to establish this ritual you likely spend a lot of time thinking and talking about doing it. That time spent thinking about a task that you haven't done yet is draining you of precious energy.

You can achieve *all* of your aspirations
if you pursue them using a methodological
approach, one that is both ambitious
and realistic.

WHEN IT COMES to new habit formation, the approach my wife and I take is to plan our yearly goals on a giant six-foot-wide calendar—this provides a clear visual that helps us to rationalize our decision-making. If there are multiple goals we want to achieve (especially related to our daily life and routines), we add them strategically, one per month. This ensures that each individual objective is dealt with in relative isolation.

If we try to make too many changes at once, we run the risk of burning out and not solidifying them into our routine. With the one-goal-per-month program, we have to focus only on adding to or transforming one element of our lives.

With this strategy, the previous goals we set will have become routinized, as we gave them their own 30 days to become a part of our life. They don't get in the way of the next one we're pursuing because once something becomes routine it requires little conscious thought (or mental energy).

Lauren and I work better with absolutes. As an example, when I was still consuming alcohol more than just a few times per year, I made it a practice to do dry January. Rather than simply reducing the amount I drank—say, by allowing myself a single glass of wine with dinner, which could open the door to a possible second glass—I knew the decision had been made for me at the start of the month. My brain works best with an all-or-nothing mindset. It's easy and quick. I love it.

This approach works for me because it eliminates mental negotiations—my boundaries have been set. This all-or-nothing approach may not be the best one for you, or even advisable for you. That said, are there *certain* changes that would work better for you with an all-or-nothing mindset?

Maybe you don't require this level of binary, black-and-white thinking, but perhaps you could reflect on past attempts to improve your health-related routines and mindset, then determine whether stricter boundaries would have increased adherence.

For me, one month is the time it takes for the sustainable addition of a new behavior—but the time it takes to routinely adopt a habit is highly variable among people. Researchers have found that it takes 66 days before health habits become automatic but that the range for individuals is 18 to 254 days.[1] This finding reinforces my recommendation to add new habits slowly. In time, you'll know how long you require for habits to become part of your lifestyle and can adjust your inclusion schedule accordingly.

You'll notice that some of the topics and questions in Part IV of this book are similar to those raised in Parts I through III. This is intentional. Revisiting the topics through a slightly modified lens may get you thinking about them in a different way and may elicit different responses. Chances are, though, your answers will be the same, and this confirmation of your understanding of yourself will provide you with greater insight into where you are, where you want to be, and how you'll get to where you want to be.

CHAPTER 18

Revitalizing Your Body

"Everything we do speaks to our genes—the food we eat, our relationships, our environment."—DR. MARK HYMAN

DO YOU BELIEVE that your body and the organs residing in it are currently operating in a harmonious flow-state? If your answer is yes, you likely wake up refreshed each morning, don't "require" stimulants to function, and feel fully present and mentally clear as you navigate each day. Albeit rare in today's world, there are people who have a body that functions on this level. This isn't chance, fluke, or good fortune: they have done the work necessary to ensure that their body is receiving, and absorbing, the fuel it needs to thrive—while prohibiting the excessive influx of bodily disruptors (such as toxins) that inundate our society.

I know you want healthy organs, a pain-free body, and abundant physical energy. These wishes become possibilities with the adoption of healthy habits and routines—ones that revitalize and continuously nourish your cells.

Cellular Health and Reducing Your Toxicity

When I ask students where energy comes from, the consensus is that it comes from food. For our purposes, this is incorrect. Think about it . . . When you eat, do you feel energized afterwards? Likely not. Food provides the chemical energy that can eventually be used to aid metabolism, but this delivery of macronutrients (carbohydrates, fats, and proteins) is likely accompanied by ingredients (fillers, pesticides, hormones, etc.) that prevent you from enjoying abundant energy and youthful vitality. So, then, where does energy come from? From your cells! There are nearly

37 trillion cells in your body,[1] and how they function will determine how energetic you feel.

Your cells require oxygen, water, glucose (sugar), minerals, and proper waste removal to survive.[2, 3] An issue in any of these entities will impede your cells' ability to do their job, resulting in a system (your body) that is in disharmony—and since toxins are so prevalent, it can be hard for your detoxification system to keep up with the demands you're putting on it. This toxic accumulation may be the root cause of the unexplained fatigue, persistent inflammation, sleep issues, and so on that many people experience.

It may seem counterintuitive, but cells are created, and cells die; this is a normal part of our physiology. But are cells dying prematurely? Could they survive longer, and in a healthier state, if we lived a cleaner life by optimizing the delivery of water, oxygen, and other nutrients—and drastically reducing the ingestion of toxins while aiding in cellular waste removal? The answer is *yes*.

In fact, in the early 1900s it was believed that chicken cells, and by extension, human cells, could live forever if they were given what they required, and not poisoned by their own environment.[4] Although this was a revolutionary discovery at the time, it isn't completely accurate. Since then, "no one has ever succeeded in serially propagating chick fibroblasts beyond one year."[5] Human cells have a limited capacity to divide and propagate, "after which they become senescent,"[6] which is referred to as the "Hayflick limit."

Regardless, humans don't live in a controlled laboratory, devoid of toxins and other physiological disruptors. Cellular renewal is normal and necessary; however, your priority should be to keep your cells as healthy as possible while they're active within you and to support your immune and detox system so they can be removed and eliminated when it's appropriate.

To start the cleansing of your cellular environment, and the other components of your physiology, you must make toxin reduction a primary consideration (since our physiological function is the foundation on which optimal is possible). Remember, a sick and toxic body will not result in an optimized human—it's not possible.

With simple modifications, you can begin to reduce your toxic load and ease the burden on your detoxification system. See Part II of this book for an in-depth explanation of the toxins in your life. To summarize: from the air you breathe, the water you drink, and the food you eat, to the items you wear, the bed you sleep in, and the beauty products and household cleaners you use, you are inundated with toxic invaders. With this in mind, what can you do to reduce your toxic load?

From the Dirty Dozen foods you eat, to the kitchen cleansers you use, list everything that can be modified or eliminated. An easy way to do this is to move mentally through your home, room by room. Doing this exercise is one surefire way to increase your energy level and the capabilities of your immune system.

Room	Item	Modified or Eliminated	Modification Strategy
EXAMPLE: Bathroom	Deodorant	M	Switch to aluminum-free deodorant

Boosting the Immune System

A weak immune system may be genetically inherited or the result of the environment and your lifestyle. Regardless, there are ways you can improve it. The simple act of reducing the toxic load within your body will immediately lessen the burden on your immune system—this is a great jump-start to rebuilding the capacity and strength of your immune system.

There are many other ways you can support this hard-working set of organs as they do the dirty work of recognizing and eliminating foreign invaders. From the list given in the table, circle the method(s) you are able and willing to employ on a regular basis—each of these has been proven to enhance the functioning of your immune system. Refer to Part III for information on the precise way each of them does so.

After making your selections, indicate on the weekly calendar the day and time you'll use each method, along with your strategy for doing so.

Physical activity and exercise	Rebounding
Dry skin brushing	Massage therapy
Foam rolling	Apple cider vinegar
Eating more water-rich foods	Improved hydration
Supplementation	Increased fiber intake
Sauna use	Wearing loose clothing

Day	Chosen Strategies and Their Timing
Monday	
Tuesday	
Wednesday	
Thursday	
Friday	
Saturday	
Sunday	

By now you're aware of the positive correlation between a healthy gut and your baseline happiness, your immune system capability, and your energy level. It's time to critically evaluate whether your immune system is performing suboptimally and to choose the ways you'll begin supporting it. We'll start with the gut.

Supporting the Gut

Your gastrointestinal system is one of your main contact points with the outside world. What you eat or drink can enter your bloodstream and wreak havoc on your physical and mental health. This is why it's so important to know what you're ingesting.

When you're young your body can stay (mostly) on top of unfamiliar intruders, but the body has a limit, and as people age their detox system is increasingly overworked from years of chronic buildup and neglect.[7]

Gut-related issues may be apparent (such as diarrhea, constipation, or bloating) or somewhat disguised (such as low energy, general fatigue, and unhappiness). Discovering the exact etiology of your unwanted symptoms isn't always necessary; what *is* necessary for optimal well-being is a healthy gut. How you rate the symptoms below, and how you answer the questions that follow, will help to indicate your level of gut dysfunction.

Check all that apply.

Symptom	MILD	MODERATE	SEVERE
Fatigue			
Memory issues			
Brain fog			
Constipation			
Diarrhea			
Low libido			
Bloating and/or excessive flatulence			
Joint pain			
Abdominal pain			
Cramps and/or other menstrual irregularities			
Vaginal burning, itching, or discharge			
Insomnia			
Skin redness (rash)			

These questions *may* further determine whether your symptoms are gut related.

Question	YES	NO
Have you ever taken antibiotics for an extended period?		
Do you have memory or concentration problems (brain fog)?		
Do you have chronic constipation, gas, diarrhea, abdominal pain, or bloating?		
Does your tongue have a thick white coating?		
Are your symptoms worse after you eat certain foods?		
Are your symptoms worse on days that are humid and/or damp?		
Do you crave carbohydrates such as sugar and breads?		
Have you ever had a chronic fungal infection on your skin or nails?		
Are you excessively bothered by tobacco smoke?		
Do you have consistently high stress in your life?		
Are you taking oral contraceptives?		
Do you have uncontrolled diabetes?		
Do you have a weakened immune system?		
Do you have recurring genital or urinary tract infections?		

There's no specific scoring on these questionnaires to determine with precision whether your issues are restricted to your gut. But the more severe the symptoms, the greater the chances that your issues are gut related.

Regardless, you should do what you can to improve your gut's function—your immune system, happiness level, and sense of wellness rely on it.

Choose the strategies you'll commit to. If you need justification for their inclusion, refer to Part II.

Strategy	Immediate Implementaion (YES or NO)
Chew more	
Avoid liquid with meals	
Consume bone broth	
Eat fermented foods (such as yogurt, sauerkraut, kombucha, kefir)	
Reduce red and processed meat	
Consume more polyphenols (such as blueberries, green tea, cocoa, almonds, grapes)	
Increase ginger intake	
Drink apple cider vinegar	
Rebound 10 minutes per day	
Reduce stress	
Drink more water	
Increase fiber intake (via fruits, vegetables, and whole grains)	
Eat prebiotic foods (such as garlic, onions, leeks, asparagus, oats, flaxseeds)	
Eat high probiotic foods (such as yogurt, sauerkraut, kefir, miso, kimchi) or take a probiotic supplement	
Supplement with known gut supporters such as zinc, l-glutamine, and licorice root	
Record the foods that cause gas, bloating, or any other gut-related problems	
Consult a naturopath, dietitian, or some other gut-related specialist	

In addition to the above gut-health suggestions, you should aim to move your body more, either through traditional exercise or by increasing your physical activity each day. Humans were designed to move, not to sit for excessively long periods.

Move!

What if there was a drug that could control your weight, combat health conditions and diseases, improve your mood, boost your energy, improve your sex life, *and* promote better sleep. How much would you pay for it? $50? $100? $1,000? Well, you can have it all . . . for nothing!

It will take a little sweat equity to see the returns, but that's an incredibly small price to pay. Consistent physical activity and exercise is like a magic pill. And no, you don't need to train like a professional athlete to reap the rewards.

According to Jonathan Myers in the article "Exercise and Cardiovascular Health," "the greatest gains in terms of mortality are achieved when an individual goes from being sedentary to becoming moderately active . . . Surprisingly, an individual's fitness level was [found to be] a more important predictor of death than established risk factors such as smoking, high blood pressure, high cholesterol, and diabetes."[8]

A study published in the *New England Journal of Medicine* followed 6,213 men over a six-year period. It looked at the comparative risk of death (after allowing for age adjustments) as it related to level of physical fitness. The researchers discovered that "Healthy adults who are the least fit have a mortality risk that is 4.5 times that of the most fit."[9] Additionally, "For every 1-MET increase in exercise capacity, there was a 12 percent improvement in survival."[10]

To provide some context, 1-MET represents approximately 10 percent of the average person's aerobic fitness level. What this means is that relatively small increases in aerobic capacity can have a major impact on your health and longevity.

So, then, how will you commit to moving more? Here are a few suggestions, but feel free to brainstorm the ways that suit your lifestyle and interests.

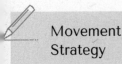

Movement Strategy	Date(s) of Inclusion (Daily or Weekly)	Duration (Min.)
Yoga		
Jogging		
Brisk walking		
Cycling		
Begin a sport		
Stop taking the elevator		
Weight training		
Register for an event		
Hire a qualified trainer		
Other:		
Other:		
Other:		

One of the ways I motivate clients to move more is to have them register for an event. Based on ability, it could be a short fun run, a triathlon, or anything in between. When someone chooses an event, puts down their money, writes it on a calendar, and tells their family and friends, it increases the level of accountability and the chances of retention. And do what you can to recruit other people to join you—this may enhance the fun, excitement, and motivation!

I usually recommend an event that's about three months away—that should provide enough time for positive habit adoption. Bonus: as you train and become fitter, you're less likely to ingest foods or drinks that reduce your training capacity; it may be the domino you're looking for!

Take some time to research events that may be of interest to you. To make it even more appealing, choose one that's in a city you've been wanting to visit—this will provide some added excitement. To get you really thinking about this, I've included a table for you to fill out on the events you are going to do.

Training for an event (if you choose to do one) or simply increasing the amount of time you're physically active will have you reaping rewards. Immediately following your exercise you'll feel a happy influx

Event	Date	Location	People Who May Join In

of endorphins and an improvement in your energy level, something we all want! Also, since your body uses adenosine triphosphate to move, it creates additional adenosine which increases your drive to sleep at night and therefore reduces the time it takes to fall asleep (as well as providing a potential boost in the amount of deep sleep you achieve).[11, 12]

So many benefits!

With your drive to sleep increased due to the additional movement during the day, let's explore how you can double down and further enhance your nightly slumber.

Improving Your Sleep and Waking

Many people are so accustomed to waking up tired from a poor night's sleep that they view it as an inevitability rather than an issue requiring attention. Sleep inertia, which typically lasts 30 to 60 minutes, is a term used to describe "a temporary disorientation and decline in performance and/or mood after awakening from sleep. People can show slower reaction time, poorer short-term memory, and slower speed of thinking, reasoning, remembering, and learning."[13]

Caffeine is a popular method of reducing the time spent in sleep inertia,[14] but, as previously mentioned, some people overconsume caffeine as their body becomes progressively accustomed to it. Your aim should be to find a variety of ways (morning light, cold water exposure, movement, etc.) to reduce the inertia. Additionally, you should focus on minimizing sleep inertia by improving the amount of deep, restful sleep you achieve each night.

To determine your nightly sleep architecture, you must track your sleep stages. This is not a prerequisite for improvements, but it does reduce trial and error by providing insight as to what worked and what didn't.

I religiously track my sleep analytics each night to gain knowledge as to how my diet, lifestyle, and sleep hygiene impact sleep quality. I pay particular attention to the time spent in stages 3 and 4 (deep sleep, which improves restfulness, growth, and functioning of the immune system).

There are numerous steps you can take to improve the quality and duration of your sleep. Refer to the sleep information in Part III (page 197) and indicate what you plan to implement (or eliminate) to enhance your sleep. Once you've identified the changes you'll be making, write down your new sleep hygiene strategy. Indicate the timing of each step and be meticulous about its adoption for at least the next seven days. As the week progresses, notice how your energy levels improve—that should be enough to make you diligently continue.

What I'll implement (or reduce/eliminate):

1.

2.

3.

4.

5.

6.

7.

8.

New sleep routine:

Time	Activity

If you improve your sleep, it stands to reason that you'll be waking up more refreshed. However, if you're used to waking up groggy, and perhaps unhappy that your day is about to begin, then it's time for a change. Life is a gift!

Your objective should be to wake up excited and motivated, because if you take a few moments to reflect you'll notice that you have so much to be grateful for.

On my vision board (which is beside my bed) I have this quote: "Be the kind of man that when your feet hit the floor each morning the devil says, 'Oh shit, he's up!'" This is a reminder to me of the good I intend to project to the world. My life is a blessing and I am grateful for the opportunity to provide support to those who require it.

Now that your sleep will be improving, here are a few suggestions I have for when you wake up, to ensure that you're energized and ready to start the day:

1. Invest in a wake-up light to use as your alarm.

2. Wake up at least 15 minutes before you "need" to. Use the extra time to drink a glass of water (ideally with ½ teaspoon of Himalayan sea salt unless it's medically contraindicated), set your intention for the day, pray or meditate, and revel in all you are grateful for.

3. Move your body through physical activity shortly after waking.

4. Have a cold shower or plunge.

In addition to the strategies mentioned, you should consider other ways to enhance your physiology or reduce the energy loss you typically experience (such as by spending too much time in a sympathetic state).

Alternative Methods for Energy Generation

Eating well, exercising, reducing your toxic load, and participating in flow-inducing activities are just a few of the ways you can generate the energy and capacity your body needs to meet your day and then some—if you want abundant energy, I urge you to consider making these a part of your life.

There are many more methods you can use to preserve energy and build capacity. Remember, you are your greatest experiment. Continue to seek ways to improve your mind, body, and spirit. From the list below, choose the strategies you will begin implementing, then be precise about the strategy you'll employ (for instance, intermittent fasting, 16/8 method).

Energy Preservation and Enhancement Technique	Inclusion (YES or NO)	Specific Strategy
Intermittent fasting		
Hot therapy		
Cold therapy		
Nordic Cycle		
Traditional Chinese Acupuncture (TCA)		
Tapping (EFT)		
Mindfulness meditation		
Immersion in nature		

| Visualization |
| Vagus stimulation (deep breathing) |
| Vagus stimulation (singing/humming) |

Next, you're going to construct your optimal daily blueprint and anticipate roadblocks that may arise. Being anticipatory, rather than reactionary, is essential to keep yourself going on this journey when life and distractions begin to test you—and they will. I guarantee it.

You can use this optimally constructed day as a reference. Perhaps you'll only hit 80 percent of its timelines and objectives, but 80 percent of optimal is much better than 80 percent of average. Aim high!

Living an Ideal Day

If time, money, and responsibilities weren't an issue, I could easily follow a routine that fully optimizes my physical and mental health. But with a family, career, and all the tasks and situations that come our way, we can't always achieve our ideal. That said, most people aren't even scratching the surface of ideal.

I regularly remind myself of the famous Voltaire quote "Don't let the perfect be the enemy of the good." Perhaps some days you can execute 100 percent according to plan but on other days you need to adjust and know that "good" is more than acceptable.

I want to provide you with my (current) optimal schedule along with a brief justification for why I chose these actions and behaviors. It may help to explain why people include certain health habits and offer guidance for your creation of *optimal*. And remember, I'm only human, just like you. I've outlined this optimal schedule for myself but, as previously mentioned, it's something to aim for. I certainly can't live it every day, but having it plotted out helps me to return to it when I do have the time and resources to engage with what I truly want for myself.

In addition to my regular 16-hour food restriction, I aim to have one 24-hour period during the week when I don't consume any

Time	Activity	Justification
5:15 a.m.	Wake-up (with light, rather than just noise) and have 1.5 cups (400 mL) of water with 0.5 teaspoons (2.5 mL) of pink Himalayan sea salt Priming (mindfulness, prayer, gratitude, setting intentions for the day)	Getting up before my kids lets me begin the day in a quiet house, which allows me to set my intentions for how I want the day to unfold. The progressive increase in light (over 20-30 minutes) allows my body to slowly release adrenaline and cortisol into my blood,[15, 16] which results in my waking up more refreshed. The water replaces some of what I lost during sleep. The salt aids in the function of my adrenal glands by providing 84 minerals and trace elements. It also temporarily raises my blood pressure, which is good for people with any level of adrenal fatigue since this is a physiological necessity when we wake up. So now I've enhanced my adrenal glands' ability to raise blood pressure and therefore reduced my burden on them. Priming reminds me that each day is a gift that shouldn't be taken for granted and sets my bodily vibration and energy in a positive way.
5:30-6:30 a.m.	Gentle exercise (light jog or yoga)	Since cortisol (stress hormone) levels are highest in the morning,[17] I don't want an intense workout that exacerbates them further. To reduce sleep inertia, cortisol is beneficial— but once the inertia has subsided, I want to begin decreasing it. This is especially important for people who are chronically tired or stressed. Morning movement is essential to wake the bodily processes and provide a positive hormonal boost. If my day permits, I'll choose gentle exercise for my morning workout so I can reduce my cortisol levels.[18]

Time	Activity	Justification
6:30–6:40 a.m.	Rebound	To aid in the movement of my lymphatic fluid and boost my immune system.
6:40–7:00 a.m.	Cold plunge and shower	To enjoy the wonderful effects of cold hormesis—namely, the distinct rise in the brain's norepinephrine level.
7–8 a.m.	Play with my kids before they go to school	No justification required!
8–9 a.m.	Be outside in nature (yard work, outdoor chores, dog walking, etc.)	The healing power of nature can improve your life in many ways. If you can do this barefoot (or wearing earthing shoes), you'll enhance the benefits by exposing yourself to the earth's negative ions and therefore helping to release some of your accumulated positive ions.
9 a.m.–1 p.m.	Read, write, develop lectures, or problem-solve	Since the brain is most efficient during this time, I use it for creativity, writing, and problem-solving.
(10:55 a.m.)	1 cup (250 mL) of water with half a lemon (just the juice) and 1 tablespoon (5 mL) of apple cider vinegar	Both will aid in the digestion of the food I'm about to eat.
(11 a.m.)	Eating window opens	Bodily digestion levels are rising.

Time	Activity	Justification
1:00–2:30 p.m.	Nap/rest	If I'm tired enough for sleep, I'll aim for a 90-minute nap. Choosing 90 minutes increases the likelihood that I'll go through a complete sleep cycle (otherwise I may have to wake up from a deep sleep, which, as you've likely experienced, can make you feel worse than you did pre-nap).
		It takes between 60 and 110 minutes (with 90 being the average) to complete a sleep cycle.[19]
		If 90 minutes isn't feasible, set an alarm for 20 minutes to get a brief nap that doesn't allow the body to slip into a deep sleep.
		The afternoon "lull" you experience is a normal part of our circadian rhythm.[20] Top companies realize this and provide rest or sleep rooms/pods for their employees.
2:30–3:00 p.m.	Walk and play with my dog (Jasper)	This is beneficial for several reasons: it gets me outside and into nature, I'm fully present and mindful as we play, the dog's goofiness makes me laugh, and he gets the physical exercise he needs.
3–4 p.m.	Intense workout (resistance training, interval training, or playing a sport such as tennis, basketball, or squash)	With certain biological processes (reaction time, cardiovascular efficiency, muscular strength) rising around now, it's the ideal time for a hard workout.
		Note: This ideal exercise time is slightly earlier than the one listed in Part III because I wake up (and go to bed) earlier than the average person. This timing also ensures that I'm available when my kids return from school.

Time	Activity	Justification
4:00–5:15 p.m.	No food (until dinner) Play with my kids	Not eating for a few hours after a workout will maximize human growth hormone (which positively influences bone density and muscle mass, among other bodily processes).[21, 22] Occasionally I'll eat shortly after an afternoon workout, but I forego carbohydrates since they cause an insulin upsurge, which suppresses HGH.[23]
5:15–6:00 p.m.	Dry skin brush Nordic Cycle (hot, cold, relax, repeat)	To exfoliate my skin and provide more lymphatic movement. To enjoy all the wonderful effects of hormetic stresses (discussed at length in Part III). I wait at least an hour after my afternoon workout before doing the Nordic Cycle. I don't want to blunt the positive adaptations that post-exercise inflammation can provide (such as repairing damaged muscle fibers and replenishing the depleted cellular energy).[24, 25]
6–7 p.m.	Family dinner (last meal of the day)	This is the only meal of the day that includes carbohydrates. Because of the hard workout two hours prior, I've upregulated insulin sensitivity[26] and the activity of Glut-4 transporters[27]— this means that a higher percentage of the glucose (sugar) molecules will be stored in my muscle and liver, ready to be used in tomorrow's workouts.
7–9 p.m.	Socialize, watch a movie, have a fire, unwind	With this "free" time after my kids go to bed without a fuss (like I said, this is "ideal"), my wife and I hang out with friends, watch a movie, or do anything that relaxes or connects us.

Time	Activity	Justification
9-10 p.m.	Read Write in our gratitude journal Pray Meditate on the things I see on my vision board	Avoiding screens and intentionally doing things that ramp up my parasympathetic nervous system will ensure that I drift off to sleep more quickly. Focusing on what's good in my life and expressing gratitude to God for my blessings helps my mindset before I embark on my sleep journey.

calories—usually going from dinner one evening to dinner the next evening without eating or drinking calories. I do this to enhance the regenerative capacity of my intestinal stem cells.[28] For me this is beneficial for two reasons:

1. My history of GI issues (which likely stemmed from chronic antibiotic use and too much stress) negatively impacted my gut health.

2. The regeneration of intestinal stem cells slows down as we age[29] (and even though I don't feel it, my chronological age does begin with a four . . .).

I encourage you to create an optimal day based on your current life stage. Use the information in this book to help you choose where to prioritize your focus and commitment. Remember, don't let perfect be the enemy of good. If it seems too overwhelming to incorporate all the strategies you desire, perhaps you could select a few ideals—one for now, one for three months from now, and one for six months from now.

Time	Activity

Time	Activity

You should also develop a strategy for success to ensure that old patterns, thoughts, or behaviors don't sabotage your plan. It might involve buying only healthy groceries, joining a running group, enlisting a family member or friend to keep you accountable, or hiring a coach. Anticipate roadblocks and strategize ways to eliminate or overcome them.

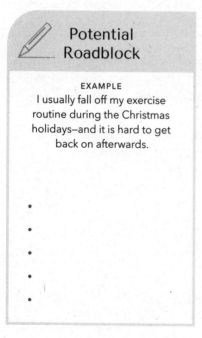

Potential Roadblock	Strategy for Success
EXAMPLE I usually fall off my exercise routine during the Christmas holidays—and it is hard to get back on afterwards.	**EXAMPLE** Plan fun activities that ensure I stay active (such as tobogganing), and schedule workouts with people (for added accountability) for immediately after the holidays.
•	•
•	•
•	•
•	•
•	•

CHAPTER 19

Mental Paradigm and Your Emotional Well-Being

"Talk to yourself like you would to someone you love."—BRENÉ BROWN

THE BEHAVIORAL PATTERNS in your life are often dictated by your mental and emotional state. Your thoughts have the ability to instill confidence and self-assurance—as well as to sow doubt and uncertainty. The inner-self talk you're accustomed to may have existed for decades, which could reduce your confidence in the idea that these patterns can be positively altered. I'm here to tell you that it *is* possible.

To begin, you must draw up a plan (which is what you're doing here). Failure to plan will inevitably result in a return to your typical way of thinking and behaving. It's time to break the cycle!

Let's begin.

Default Pattern and Changing Your Emotional State

What are the emotions that dominate your life? Emotions dictate the satisfaction you experience each day, so you must pay attention when they arise. And yes, you can learn to positively shift your habitual and unwanted emotions—this will, however, require a mental paradigm shift.

When working with clients, I provide scenarios that many people encounter daily. I want to know what they believe—through honest introspection—their emotion(s) would be in those situations (you'll remember that I outlined a couple of these scenarios in Part III). Additionally, for the first week I work with a client, I ask them to write down every time they notice the arrival of an unwanted emotion—what the situation was and how the symptoms manifested in their mind (racing thoughts, reduced clarity, etc.) and body (increased heart rate, upset stomach, etc.).

One of my first priorities with clients is improvement in their daily energy level; this provides the foundation on which we build. Unwanted and negative emotions result in energy leaks that diminish my clients' overall mental and physical capacity. Also, it's very unlikely that you're experiencing an optimal level of personal and professional growth if you're consistently frustrated, fearful, and overwhelmed by self-doubt.

From the list below, identify the unwanted emotions that arrive too often and stay too long. The objective isn't to deny any emotion but to understand when it has overstayed its welcome and contributed to your mental and physical fatigue.

Anger	Disappointment	Fear
Anxiety	Disgust	Guilt
Apathy	Envy	Irritation
Confusion	Exasperation	Sadness
Contempt	Frustration	Worry

Unwanted emotions:

1.

2.

3.

4.

Conversely, what are the emotions (joy, gratitude, etc.) that you wish to cultivate? Don't start with a long list; pick one (maybe two) to begin with.

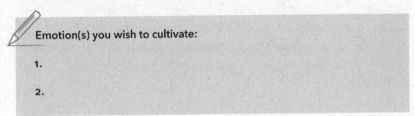

Emotion(s) you wish to cultivate:

1.

2.

Achieving a sustained emotional shift requires diligence. Remember, it takes time to transform something into a sustained habit (one that's initiated with little or no conscious effort).

When you notice an emotion that's unwanted, you must first change your state. The fastest way to change your emotional state is via a physical shift, which could be as gentle as deep, mindful breaths or as intense as cold-water exposure—each situation may require a different strategy.

From the list (or draw up your own), determine which methods you'll implement when unwelcome emotions or thoughts suddenly arise.

Immersing in nature	Meditation	Listening to music
Prayer	Dancing	Sleep
Cold-water exposure	Sauna	Watching a movie
Yoga	Physical activity	Deep breathing
Journaling	Positive incantation	Singing
Talking to a friend		

Choose only a few methods to start. You can add more later, but you don't want decision fatigue when choosing a strategy; you want immediate implementation.

1.

2.

3.

Perhaps there are consistent scenarios in your life that cause a negative emotional state. For instance, maybe you get frustrated and yell when your kids bicker with one another, you get angry when there's excessive traffic, or you experience anxiety during meetings at work.

If there are specific and repeated scenarios, list them, then brainstorm possible solutions to use when you feel the unwanted thoughts or emotions creeping in.

Scenario	Change Strategy

I use all the strategies indicated, some daily and others sporadically, to positively shift my emotions. When I'm short on time and a quick transition is required, I usually opt for deep, mindful breaths or music therapy.

If you populated the music and movie chart in Part III, you'll remember that I included a lot of categories that correlate with the mood you wish to elicit. Rather than have you write them all again, I want you to focus on the "happy" and "goofy" music categories—I find that these tend to help in the quick transition from an unwanted emotional state.

For a more rapid transition, add dancing and singing to your music. Get goofy and unbridled, and don't stop moving until you feel the shift (it will come, I promise!).

Mood I Want to Elicit	Movie(s)	Song(s)
HAPPY (LAUGHING)		
GOOFY		

Affirmations and Incantations (Yes, They *Can* Work!)

Positive self-talk should be a regular part of your day, but you likely spend more time criticizing yourself than building yourself up. This is a mistake, as it will only cement the things you currently dislike about yourself.

Below, write out five affirmations that you can say aloud several times every day. But it's not enough for you to just say the words; for your affirmations to have as much impact as possible, you must become emotionally connected with them and they must be written and spoken in the present tense.

Here are a few examples of positive affirmations that I've used over the years:

- God is guiding my life.
- My spirit is strong.
- My body is healthy.
- My mind is clear.
- My soul is tranquil.
- I am overflowing with joy, happiness, and positivity.
- I am blessed with an incredible family and wonderful friends.
- I have strength in my heart and clarity in my mind.
- I am a warrior for my family.
- I am the architect of my life.
- I am always relaxed and calm.
- I am assertive and powerful.

- I make decisions quickly.
- I find solutions to problems.
- I can conquer any challenge.

Your turn (feel free to use mine if they resonate with you):

Affirmation #1

Affirmation #2

Affirmation #3

Affirmation #4

Affirmation #5

Now that you have a framework, you want to build an incantation—this consists of an impactful description of the person you envision yourself as. It's meant to inspire and drive you toward a new paradigm, one that reflects your optimal life.

You must write, rewrite, and rewrite some more, to create an incantation that you feel inspired to shout each day. It's time to become someone who your future self will be proud of. Your incantation must reflect your highest sense of self—who you want to become.

Here's my current incantation. I project it aloud, two or three times, after each morning workout.

Joseph's incantation:

This is my year of full expression where I expand my audience. I am open, I am joyful, I am balanced.

My decisions reflect my standard of abundant energy and youthful vitality. I push past my comfort zone every day—this gives me a clean body, a happy mind, and a fulfilled soul.

My book, my story, my voice, and my passion elevate people to take action and build momentum in their pursuit of unstoppable energy, overflowing joy, and deep fulfillment. God provides me with abundance so blessings can flow through me.

I am fully present with those who are in front of me; I give them my time and energy. I seek the little moments and memories, and I create connection with those who are important to me.

My purpose in life is to grow and connect with my family and friends—and to elevate the energy and joy of those who seek higher standards.

It took several drafts before I found the wording and structure that resonated with my soul. Take your time as you reflect and write. The words you speak must be intentional and positive—you want to be feeding your subconscious the version of yourself that brings you the most joy, fulfillment, and inspiration!

Draft:

Incantation:

My friend Karissa Kouchis, a world-renowned life strategist, taught me how to connect with my words. She expanded my comfort zone by encouraging me to get out of my head and into my physiology. It wasn't until I had removed any sense of inhibition (that someone might hear or judge me) that I felt the most connected.

Once I experienced that enhanced sense of connection between my mind, body, and spirit, I was hooked! So just as she advised me to do, I encourage you to get excited! Get loud! Get emotionally connected! Incantations are like affirmations on steroids. Don't just read it: get up and move, jump, and project your voice!

To heighten the experience, play a song in the background as you read your incantation aloud. I play the instrumental version of the song "Good Life" by OneRepublic as I emphatically project outwardly. I've read mine so many times that whenever I hear the song my brain immediately begins the incantation.

What song would you like to pair with your incantation?

Song:

Raising the Vibrational State of Others

It's great if you're diligent and work hard on consistently changing your emotional state and therefore the vibration you're projecting to the world. However, those closest to you, whether they are members of your household or the people you interact with regularly, may act as an anchor in this endeavor.

Although it's not your duty to change people—which can be an exhausting and futile task—you want to ensure that their consistent vibrational state isn't adversely affecting you.

Ideally, you're unaffected by the emotional state of others, but that's not typically the case. We're positively and negatively influenced by the people closest to us. You must protect your personal growth by recognizing patterns (in yourself and others) and anticipating them. If you know your partner is usually exhausted and frustrated after a long day at work, you can anticipate this and do things that might spark joy in them—such as the gesture of a romantic dinner, flowers, or a drawn bath.

You can also be diligent about raising their vibrational state. An easy and accessible way of doing so is to give them honest compliments. This will (most likely) raise their vibration and affect how they interact with you. Think about it: if you're having a "bad" day and then receive a genuine compliment from someone, I bet it will positively shift your day.

Are there people in your life who consistently, and negatively, impact your vibration and flow? If so, list them below and brainstorm their positive attributes.

Person	Positive Attributes

Further to this exercise, consider the people you spend the most time with. Their consistent emotional state, work ethic, aspirations, and approach to life will have an impact on you. You must choose them carefully.

"The Power of Five"

"Great minds discuss ideas; average minds discuss events; small minds discuss people."—ELEANOR ROOSEVELT

Did you know that if you grow a pumpkin in a jar it will grow into the shape of the jar? For most, this is a metaphor for the people who surround them. I'm sure by now you've heard someone say that you're the average (in terms of intelligence, earnings, creativity, ambition) of the five people with whom you spend the most time. As I tell my students, if you spend time with a bunch of donkeys, you'll be a donkey; if you spend time with a bunch of thoroughbreds, you'll be a thoroughbred.

Best-selling author James Altucher, in his article "The Power of Five," takes it even farther: "You are the average of the five people around you . . . You are the average of the five things that inspire you the most . . . My thoughts are the average of the five things I think about . . . My body and mind are the average of the five things I 'eat' . . . I am the average of the five things I do to help people each day."[1]

Regarding the people in your life, how much thought have you given to their inclusion?

List the five people with whom you spend the most time. They could be family members, coworkers, or friends. Take some time to think of them, then reflect on their decisions, outlook on life, and ambitions. In this connected world, consider those with whom you interface digitally as well. Don't limit yourself to in-person contacts.

1.

2.

3.

4.

5.

After looking at the above list, ask yourself what it says about your level of positivity, leadership, and confidence. Put yourself right in the middle of this group and that's likely where you'll land. Are you satisfied with the personality traits, ambitions, and values of the people you listed? If not, what character traits do you wish the people around you had more of? List them below.

1.

2.

3.

4.

5.

Do you believe the people you listed have the capability and/or desire to grow with you?

It's okay if they don't, but perhaps you should expand your social circle to include people who align with your current or desired values and traits. This is crucial since it's been proven from the Framington Studies that smoking,[2] obesity,[3] happiness,[4] and even loneliness[5] are, in part, dependent on those within your social circle.

With a little reflection you'll realize there are people who bring you joy, comfort, and support, and there are others who cause undue stress and anxiety in your life.

Before you make any snap decisions on who you want to remain closest to, consider leading from the front by changing yourself and then noticing the reaction of those around you. The people you thought would be the least supportive might surprise you—it may be the inspiration they're looking for to transform their own life.

For myself, I don't need a relationship to be a 50-50 giving and receiving of time, energy, and resources. Truthfully, I'm comfortable providing more of those things. However, if the relationship is skewing 80-20, then I begin to reconsider their presence in my life. This 80-20 rule of mine is even more rigid now that I have a family and am very cognizant of the energy I'm willing to expend on people.

This is not to say I mentally clock every conversation or encounter, but I can certainly feel a distinct imbalance after months (or even years) of encounters with particular individuals. Eventually I begin to question whether they're a true friend who has my best interests at heart, or if I've turned into a commodity for them—simply a place to get their needs met.

One caveat I have is if the family member or friend is going through a difficult time such as a mental health crisis, divorce, or death of a loved one. In these circumstances I feel blessed and grateful that I can provide comfort and a soft landing—80-20 or even 100-0 is okay in these situations.

Removing people from my life with kindness and grace hasn't always been easy. Sometimes it happens organically and sometimes there must be an initiation. For many, fear causes the avoidance of difficult conversations and confrontations. You must be the architect of your life. You must be okay disappointing people; otherwise you'll bend to everyone's expectations of you, which could pull you farther away from your desired life.

Don't let fear and anxiety dictate the path in life that you choose.

Fighting Fear and Anxiety

Fear and anxiety restrict too many people from living the rich (don't think just in terms of money) and fulfilled life they deserve. The negative impact, which is daily for some, must be removed or managed if *optimal* is what you seek.

With honest introspection you may realize that you have a considerable number of fears and anxieties—but don't let this overwhelm you. With habit change, paradoxical intention, and counselling (if needed), you can remove these fears and anxieties and begin to lift the burden of their existence in your life.

To begin, list your fears or phobias; then spend time thinking and, more importantly, feeling the impact they've made. This distinction between *feeling* and *thinking* mustn't be overlooked—the catalyst for change has more to do with emotion than intellect.

Fears or Phobias	Life Impact

"You can't change the people around you, but you can change the people around you."–UNKNOWN

Next, write down all the people, places, things, and/or events that cause undue anxiety within your body and mind. I say "undue" anxiety because a certain level is normal and healthy—your goal isn't to remove it entirely, just to understand the pattern of its arrival and determine whether it's healthy or unhealthy.

Then you must determine whether it should be eliminated (such as removing a toxic person from your life) or reformed. This is an important distinction, one that you must take time to consider. Your first instinct should be to change yourself and the way you view and experience the situation or person. Don't immediately jump to removal as this may leave you with a life that's less than optimal. For instance, if having to address an audience causes you significant anxiety yet you have a passion to be a teacher, you must reform this response so you can realize your dream, expand your comfort zone, and have a self-actualized life where your full potential is reached.

Person/Place/Thing/Event	Eliminated or Reformed

Success in overcoming fears and anxieties is very individual. Some may be able to use their will and a consistent routine to do so, while others might require therapy with a trained professional. Only you know the strategy that's necessary for sustainable change.

Although overcoming fears and anxieties may take more time than you'd like, there are things you can do in the meantime to reduce their negative impact on your physiology. On the next page, consider the strategies you indicated as causing a positive emotional shift within you (listed earlier in this chapter), as well as any other ways of creating calm within your body and mind, then enter them in the strategy column for fear and anxiety reduction. Next to each entry, indicate whether you're going to commit to this technique every day or periodically.

For instance, when I began my teaching career, I had anxiety before each class. My coworkers would tell me, "You look the same age as the students!" This left me feeling that I needed to prove my worth by overworking (at the expense of my mental and physical health). What if the students asked me questions that I couldn't answer? What if they thought I was underqualified? The anxiety I felt fueled me, but also left me exhausted. It fueled me by ensuring that I was very prepared for each class, but the way I voraciously researched and prepared left me drained. As my first semester of teaching progressed, I did a few things that helped dramatically:

1. I took deep, mindful breaths before the class began.
2. I avoided caffeine.
3. If I didn't know the answer to a question, I didn't worry. No one knows everything. I shifted my approach to confidently telling them I'd find the answer and deliver it next class.

Note: As you may remember, I still ended up burning out by the end of my first year of teaching—this was the result of working at two post-secondary institutions while trying to manage a side business. It doesn't matter how diligent you are at anxiety reduction if your overall work-load is beyond a recoverable capacity.

In the table, enter your strategies for minimizing the impact of your fears and anxieties.

Strategy for Fear and Anxiety Reduction	Daily (D) or Periodically (P)

One of the ways I lessened anxiety was by reducing the volume of commitments and tasks I'd grown accustomed to. The time I saved allowed me to slow down and properly prepare for each commitment.

Simplify Your Life

As previously mentioned, the tasks you're doing right now (working, raising kids, household chores, social engagements) aren't likely being done at a faster pace than they would have been generations ago—the problem is that you've likely stacked too many things together. In doing so, your brain is stressed because you always feel a step behind, and your body is stressed because you've built in such a small amount of time for rest, recuperation, and fun.

In years past, multigenerational and communal living was more common, which meant there were often more people to share daily tasks and reduce the mental, and perhaps physical, toll that may be experienced by our present-day living arrangements.

If communal living isn't desirable, or even possible, for you, and you struggle to keep up with your daily demands, then it's time to explore ways to simplify.

Ask yourself what (or who) you can eliminate or modify to simplify your life. Are there things that have unnecessarily robbed you of time or space (social media, TV, poor decision-making, etc.) or have caused life-related complexity (such as out-of-date work practices)? If so, consider altering, reducing, or eliminating them.

This isn't easy, I understand. You may have to create boundaries and have difficult conversations—but if you envision and crave getting more out of life, you need to become comfortable challenging yourself and possibly disappointing people. Your objective is to create space which will provide you with the opportunity for more connection, presence, and levity—you know, the juice in life!

Person or Thing	Reduce or Eliminate	Strategy

The creation of space in your life will naturally increase your daily flow, but you must remain steadfast or modern society will continually find ways of consuming your attention and therefore reducing your flow, and likely your happiness.

In addition to reducing the excessive demands placed on you, you must learn to limit overthinking; this can also rob you of joy and presence.

Harnessing and Enhancing Flow

We live in a connected world, one that demands almost all of our attention. Often, this leaves people stutter-stepping through life, constantly shifting tasks and having their attention diverted this way and that. A part of optimal living is finding times to quiet the distractions in your life that are keeping you from operating in flow. Determining the activities that reduce the constant "inner chatter," and therefore promote flow, is critical to protecting your energy reserves.

For me, a simple way to harness flow is to play sports. In those moments when I'm not thinking about anything other than the activity, I'm completely present. This state is good for both my body and my brain, as both get recharged and strengthened.

What are the activities or situations that induce a flow-like experience in you?

Here are some common examples. Choose your activities and when you can do each one. Can you commit to it daily, or is periodically better (every Saturday, for instance)?

Watching a movie	Playing with kids or pets	Gardening
Playing a sport	Conversing with friends	Knitting
Meditating	Journaling or writing	Art
Exercising	Singing	Dancing
Reading	Driving	Sex

Flow-Inducing Activity	Daily (D) or Periodically (P)
	○
	○
	○
	○
	○

Another way our daily flow gets hijacked is through overindulgence and overconsumption. An unhealthy balance in any area of your life will result in less time spent on the other things. Sometimes we're privy to the unfavorable role those things we overindulge in play in our lives, and sometimes we're oblivious to their negative grasp on us. List the areas in which you overconsume (TV, social media, food, caffeine, etc.), as indicated in Part I.

1.

2.

3.

Now that you've identified your overindulgences, reflect on the steps you'll take to diminish or eliminate them from your life altogether. For instance, can you limit yourself to a specific amount of time (e.g., 30 minutes) and a specific time of day (e.g., after dinner) to engage with them? Or should you take a hard-line approach and close off all your sources of overconsumption to affect a meaningful and lasting change? Only you know what's required—so be honest and use the space provided to write down the actions you'll take.

Source of Overindulgence	Plan to Reduce or Eliminate

Reduce Your Daily Decisions

Decision fatigue is another flow-jacker—and it may be the main contributor to your mental exhaustion at the end of each day. Although you can't rid yourself of decision-making completely, you can ensure that the mundane and ordinary decisions you need to make don't contribute to your fatigue.

Neil Pasricha, author of *The Happiness Equation*,[6] challenges his readers with questions on this topic. Read them and answer with as many responses as you can. Consider involving others in your household as well—the comradery and accountability may help to increase retention.

1: What can you *automate* so you never have to think about it again (or at least only think about it periodically)?

Automate	Solution
EXAMPLE: Clothing	Have a specific outfit for each day of the week

2: What can you *regulate* so you do it during specific times and windows?

✏ Regulate	Solution
EXAMPLE: Email	Check email only at a specific time of day, for a specific length of time

3: What can you *effectuate* as something you simply do?

✏ Effectuate	Solution
EXAMPLE: Waking up	Immediately put my feet on the floor when my alarm goes off—and never hit the snooze button again

Another way to decrease the mental drain of decision fatigue is outsourcing. Think of all the decisions you make from week to week. Are there any you can delegate someone else to take on?

Indicate any decisions (what to watch or to eat, where to go on dates, social plans, etc.) you'd be happy to outsource to a family member, friend, or maybe even an app (I'm sure one exists). It doesn't matter what the decision is—if it routinely causes ambiguity, then consider including it.

Decision	Who (or What) Will Manage It Going Forward

The decisions you listed are likely "light" in nature—as you probably wouldn't outsource any that might have a dramatic effect on the trajectory of your life; those should be reserved for just you. With this in mind, do you have a structure for the approach you take when making bigger decisions? If not, that's okay!

You can strategize this improvement in Chapter 20. These are the decisions that crop up periodically and must be prioritized and approached deliberately. For most, decisions are made based on the happiness they believe will stem from them. But there will always be another "big" decision to make. So stop delaying your happiness—focus on your emotional control and the way you approach each day.

Your typical emotional "home," as well as the amount of flow you experience daily, is your baseline level of happiness. Considering this, would people describe you (or would you describe yourself) as a happy person?

Regardless of whether you answered *yes* or *no* (but definitely if you answered *no*), a happiness boost is something that can benefit you (and the people around you) every day.

Establishing a New Baseline of Happiness

The human brain is constantly on the lookout for what's wrong (as this was necessary for survival for millennia), which is why we gloss over things that bring us joy and happiness while obsessively ruminating over our misfortunes or concerns.

With diligence you can train your brain to "hold onto" happy moments for longer—doing so with regularity may increase your baseline level of happiness. Rick Hanson, author of *Hardwiring Happiness*, suggests the following:[7]

1. When you feel happy, grateful, or appreciated, sit with that feeling (for at least a few slow breaths) rather than letting it quickly pass. Hold onto the positive emotion and soak it in.

2. Try to feel the happiness throughout your entire body.

3. Focus on what's enjoyable about the experience you just had.

Hanson's suggestion is designed to help your brain "hardwire" the positive experiences—which increases the neural connections associated with happy and pleasant thoughts. Stop glossing over compliments, accomplishments, or anything that makes you feel happy, proud, or grateful. Lean into them.

Additionally, you must stop delaying your happiness for a "future" moment when everything aligns. "As soon as" has become a life motto for millions. These aren't necessarily delusional people; they're just the product of a society that celebrates breadth over depth—one that convinces people what it will take to achieve happiness. Please don't forget the story about the Mexican fisherman (see page 166). Joy, contentment, and happiness may be right in front of you, but the societal hedonic treadmill keeps you grinding every day, never reaching "as soon as," and therefore never experiencing the peace of a contented life.

Do you currently have any "as soon as" scenarios?

List them and ponder what your life would look like if you eased up on your "as soon as" timeline, eliminated the thought that this will lead to eternal happiness, and got off the treadmill and opted to walk (metaphorically . . . or perhaps literally) through life. As you strategize how you might remedy your "as soon as" scenarios, consider that it might be a mental shift you need to make, or maybe there's something practical you can do to slow your pace and create space within your life.

Example: As soon as I graduate from college I can get a job, slow down, and be happy.

Solution: If I delay my graduation by one semester, it will allow me to complete my schoolwork at a sustainable pace—and it will create the space I need to visit with friends, exercise, and relax, all of which make me happy.

1. As soon as _____.

    If I let go of this thought, what will happen (e.g., the pressure on me will be reduced, I'll have more free time, etc.)?

    _____.

2. As soon as _____.

    If I let go of this thought, what will happen?

    _____.

3. As soon as _____.

    If I let go of this thought, what will happen?

    _____.

Also, in Western society most of us are taught to associate self-worth with our career title. This puts undue pressure on our youth and subconsciously teaches them to be "realistic" about their dreams and to choose a career that carries a lot of clout. Many also elect to expedite this process as much as possible because of the delusion that their happiness depends on it.

Working hard and having career ambitions is good—but ensure that the path you're on is something you want. Sadly, many young people spend no more than a few minutes determining the job that will make them happy and fulfilled. They're bombarded with questions such as "What do you want to be when you're older?," which can lead them to formulate a response that sounds the most impressive to our mainstream, Western ears.

Challenge yourself to ask kids, and even adults, what they want their life to look like. Do they see themselves traveling, serving the less fortunate, creating beautiful art? Maybe they do dream of climbing the corporate ladder or even running a Fortune 500 company, and that's okay as well. The point is you must determine for yourself what a happy and optimal life looks like.

Since occupation plays such a large role in our lives, give some thought to your ideal position. Rather than chronically searching for advancement and climbing the corporate ladder (without ever questioning whether you really want a promotion), give it some thought and maybe ask people in positions "above" you what it's like.

You may determine that your current position, given the specific time-related duties and responsibilities it entails, aligns very well with your life outside of work. If you were "promoted" you'd likely have to sacrifice aspects of your personal life to accommodate the added responsibilities and time commitments. Is that something you have space for?

Current job:

Ideal job:

Will this position entail more working hours and cause additional stress? If yes, is it worth it?

Laughter 2.0

When was the last time you had a genuine belly laugh? Can you remember the month, or even the year? For your sake, I hope belly laughs occur daily and are easily triggered—but that's not the reality for most. At some point in our adult life the societal wet blanket will most likely increase inhibition and dampen the spirit.

A primary objective for you should be an increase in your day-to-day baseline level of happiness, as well as a surge in the number of belly laughs you experience (which is nearly impossible if your daily emotions are negative). There are many ways you can achieve a shift in your baseline happiness.

From the list below, circle which, if any, you're able and willing to implement regularly. Next, indicate on the weekly calendar the day and time you will accomplish each, along with the strategy for doing so. If my examples don't resonate with you, feel free to make your own list.

Example: Quality sleep is necessary to energize my body and mind, which leads to increased levels of happiness each day. I'm committed to stopping the use of electronics one hour before bed, going to sleep at 10 p.m., and leaving my phone (on airplane mode) outside the room.

Sauna	Nordic Cycle	Morning sunlight
Cold therapy	Physical activity	Practicing gratitude
Daily meditation	Praying	Better sleep hygiene
Improved nutrition		Playing with my kids or pets
Living for a deeper purpose		Increased social connection
More immersion in nature		Being kinder to myself

Day	Time and Strategy
Monday	
Tuesday	
Wednesday	
Thursday	
Friday	
Saturday	
Sunday	

Shifting your happiness baseline is easier than producing belly laughs— those can't be scheduled. However, you can increase the likelihood of belly laughter by creating space and opportunities for them. Below are some ways you can increase the likelihood of more belly laughter in your life. This list is far from exhaustive so please add to it. Think of all the people, situations, or events that could contribute to the influx of the cheek-hurting, sidesplitting discomfort that comes only from intense belly laughter.

- Reduce my chronically overwhelming to-do list.

- Prioritize my health by eating well, improving sleep hygiene, and exercising.

- Call up old friends and reminisce.

- Spend more time playing with kids or animals.

- Watch stand-up comedy.

ACT AS IF

Your thoughts have the ability to cause a physical response in your body. In 1981 a team of researchers led by Harvard psychologist Ellen Langer took two groups of men, all in their seventies and eighties, to a New Hampshire monastery to conduct what they called The Counterclockwise Experiment.[8] The researchers separated the men into two groups. Group one stayed for one week and were asked to act as if they were young men living in the 1950s. Group two also stayed for one week; these men were instructed to remain in the present but to spend time reminiscing about the 1950s. Additionally, both groups were surrounded by mementos that reflected the 1950s. Langer and her colleagues wanted to see if there was a biological impact of "acting as if."

Both groups of men took physical and cognitive tests before and after the experiment. After just one week both groups showed significant changes in all categories, demonstrating improvements in physical strength, manual dexterity, posture, perception, memory, cognition, taste sensitivity, hearing, vision, and intelligence. Amazing!

Although both groups showed positive changes, the men who acted as if they were in the 1950s demonstrated significantly more improvements.

Dr. Langer's results prove that visualization works. She explains that our mindset about our beliefs and perceptions plays a significant role in how old or young we feel. The visualization of a healthy body can transmit healing frequencies all over our body. Conversely, destructive and distorted visualizations can contribute to illness and disease.

What is your view of your body and mind? How often do you think (or say) things such as "I'm too old to do that"?

By "acting as if," you can influence the biological age and ability of your mind and body. Keep this in mind and make sure you don't limit yourself based on age. It's a cliché, but age really is just a number!

Visualization

Our subconscious mind is where sustainable change is derived from, and since it communicates predominantly with pictures, visualization is a key tool you can use to help optimize your life.

We visualize every day—some people are intentional about it while others aren't. You must learn to use this immensely powerful gift since it could help or hinder your performance, perceived self-image, and life satisfaction.

Unfortunately, most people inadvertently use visualization for bad, not good. They might envision themselves doing poorly in an upcoming presentation, striking out at their next at bat, or failing their driving test. This type of visualization is often done repetitively, which further ingrains the negative view that our subconscious has of us and therefore makes our reticular activating system (RAS) focus on what could go wrong.

Let's use visualization and get our RAS and subconscious mind working for us! Before you write out the first few visualizations you want to work on, let's look at some important guidelines to make it as effective as possible.

- **Visualize yourself succeeding with your goal.** Whatever your ambitions are, picture yourself as already having achieved them. Picture yourself in the situation: How do you feel? How are the people around you responding to your achievement? Try to feel your emotions.

- **Establish triggered visuals.** Our minds have the ability to connect experiences we've had. A faint smell, a certain noise, or a song may trigger a powerful memory. You can use your brain's ability to enhance the success of your visualizations by creating your own triggers. For instance, perhaps you can listen to a song while visualizing something positive. In time, that song may automatically conjure up the emotions and images you've curated.

- **Create a vision board.** As we'll see, this can be a very effective way to remind your brain of the goals you have.

- **Create a "happy place."** When you notice anxiety, doubt, or any unhelpful emotion emerge, having a "happy place" where one of your visualizations can take you will help you to move into a more positive state. For instance, perhaps you're a big sports fan and one of your goals is to be more of a leader. You could play a motivating song and picture yourself inspiring the other players to give everything they have—and then you lead them to victory.

- **Convert your desires into beliefs**. Removing words such as "try" and "want" from your vocabulary (or at least using them less) will help to ensure that your goals are reached. "I will" is a much more powerful phrase.

When I've worked with people who have sustained injuries, the ones who recover the most quickly are typically those who always use language that suggests they *will* get better—and in some cases they're stronger than ever after recovery. Typically, athletes fit this description more than the average person; at least that's my observation.

The same can be said of people with chronic diseases. If you believe you'll never get better, your chances of making a full recovery are much less. According to a study conducted at Johns Hopkins University, "researchers suspect that people who are more positive may be better protected against the inflammatory damage of stress . . . hope and positivity help people make better health and life decisions and focus more on long-term goals. Studies also find that negative emotions can weaken immune response."[9]

Furthermore, Johns Hopkins expert Lisa R. Yanek found that "positive people from the general population were 13 percent less likely than their negative counterparts to have a heart attack or other coronary event."[10] Yanek and her colleagues conclude that there's "definitely a strong link between 'positivity' and health"[11] and that having a positive attitude "improves outcomes and life satisfaction across a spectrum of conditions—including traumatic brain injury, stroke and brain tumors."[12]

- **Add sensory experiences to your visualizations**. As discussed, it's not enough to simply have the visualization. To get the most benefit, you must provide your visualization with as many sensory experiences and details as possible: What do you hear or smell during your visualization? Additional details will help your subconscious believe it's true and therefore solidify it as reality.

- **Add positive energy to every instance of visualization.** Doubt will creep in from time to time. Don't get discouraged when this happens. Similar to when you meditate, your focus will inevitably drift back into thought, and that's okay—the key is to bring yourself back to the present moment in a non-judgmental way. When negativity or doubt invades your visualization, simply infuse an extra dose of positivity and picture yourself rising to whatever circumstance or challenge you aim to conquer.

Additionally, you can use the past to the benefit of future performance. We all remember conversations, presentations, or circumstances that went poorly. We often replay these negative scenarios in our head over and over, and many people tend to exaggerate what went wrong, which only serves to cement their belief that it was a failure.

This constant rehearsing and visualization of yourself doing poorly will make the subconscious believe that poor performance is inevitable—and the more you rehearse, the more the poor performance becomes ingrained as a part of who you are. So stop dwelling negatively on the past!

When unhelpful memories come up, visualize how you'd handle them now. For instance, let's say you went on a date with someone you were really interested in but because of nerves and your tendency toward shyness you couldn't relax and let your date get to know who you really are. Bring yourself back to that situation in your mind, but instead of reflecting on how you wished it had gone (which is what most people do), see yourself talking and acting in a way that makes you feel good. Notice how the person's verbal responses and body language toward you are different now that you're relaxed, confident, and able to fully be you.

Don't just do this once—repetition is the key!

It's going to take a full commitment to undo all the years of internal negative self-talk, regret, and worry, and to feed your subconscious the narrative that will make you happiest. Just as one salad won't make you miraculously healthy, one bout of visualization won't instantly change the way your subconscious has you responding in various situations.

Your subconscious will believe what it's told, so be diligent in feeding it the positive qualities you want to have and the goals you intend to achieve. How you see yourself will be reflected in how others see you. If you're overly critical and negative about who you are, this will be reflected in the way you project yourself to the world.

If you see yourself as weak, the world will *not* view you as strong.

If you see yourself as a follower, the world will *not* view you as a leader.

If you see yourself as negative, the world will *not* see you as positive.

How and what you think can be seen in the way you carry yourself. Someone who's proud, happy, and joyful isn't likely to be walking around with slouched shoulders and with their head down. Someone who's angry isn't going to walk around with a smile on their face (unless it's a frightening smile . . .).

At this point you know which character traits you'd like to reduce and which ones you'd like to bolster. List the character traits you desire most, as well as the visualization you could use to conjure and create an environment and situation where you're using that trait.

What you write down doesn't have to be your final version. You'll notice that your brain will build on the scenario—it will continually evolve. As long as it's positive, let it do so. What you write in the table will serve as the base to begin with.

Character Trait	Visualization
EXAMPLE: Decisive leadership	Picture yourself in a meeting with coworkers and your boss. Everyone is looking to you for advice and the best course of action. You answer confidently every time. You feel the trust they have in your leadership and the fact that they're captivated by your words. Your body language is open (shoulders back, standing tall) and your eye contact is engaging.

"A strong, positive self-image is the best possible preparation for success."

—JOYCE BROTHERS

To initiate the spark to visualize what you desire, I strongly suggest you create a vision board. It may seem juvenile for you to have one in your house, but this couldn't be farther from the truth! You want to stack the odds of success in your favor—this is one of the ways to do that. Don't let the concept make sense just in your mind. Take action and do something about it!

Create Your Vision Board

The more you can filter images that reflect happiness, positivity, and success into your brain, the greater your chances of achieving your goals. Follow the steps below and *dream big!*

Once the vision board is completed, you should consciously and unconsciously look at it multiple times per day. Have it in a place where you'll regularly notice it, such as in your bedroom, on your fridge, or in your office. Placing it in your line of sight will allow your subconscious to consistently notice it. You should also view it intentionally—remember, your subconscious is a goal-seeking organism that doesn't distinguish between real and imagined. Look at the images and words and see yourself as having already reached those goals.

By acting as if you already possess what's on your board (certain personality traits, a particular job, a healthy lifestyle, etc.), you will enable your subconscious, along with your RAS, to work to bring it to fruition by attracting (helping you notice) the things and the people necessary for this.

Step 1: Ask Questions
Write down everything you desire (character traits, how you want to look, where you want to work, what you want out of life, etc.). Make your goals S.M.A.R.T. (Specific, Measurable, Attainable, Relevant, Time-Bound).

If you're struggling with specificity, think about these questions before you begin:

What do you see as constituting an optimal life?

Think of yourself as a very old person. Now reflect on your life—what accomplishments do you wish you'd realized?

What brings you fulfillment in life?

These are very "big" questions. It may be useful for you to break them down further:

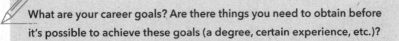

What are your career goals? Are there things you need to obtain before it's possible to achieve these goals (a degree, certain experience, etc.)?

Are there any skills you want to learn (play the guitar, speak a foreign language, etc.)?

How do you want others to remember you? Do you want to be remembered as kind, generous, funny, thoughtful, a leader, et cetera?

What are your relationship goals? Be specific: What do you want those with whom you have relationships to look like? What would you like their personality traits to be? How do you want to spend quality time together?

Now that you have a bit more framework, write out your goals and the things you'd like to include on the board:

-
-
-
-
-
-
-
-

Note: If you like, you can make two vision boards, one personal and one professional.

Step 2: Decide on Your Format and Location

A vision board can be on posterboard, corkboard, or any other material that can be hung on your wall. Alternatively, you might choose to do it electronically. If it's a physical board (which I usually recommend), decide on the place in your home where you want to display it.

Material:

Location:

Step 3: Collect Images

Find positive images that reflect your goals. While the subconscious mind will hear words, it operates in pictures—that's why we dream in pictures and not words. It's okay to have some positive words and affirmations as well, but remember, it's easier to get emotionally connected to an image and to subsequently see yourself in that situation. But having both is beneficial.

You can find images online and in magazines. There are even books made specifically for creating a dream board. In addition to these images, you can print some of your personal pictures. Perhaps you want to regain the physique you once had, or you want to move to a destination that you once visited.

Step 4: Put It Together and Hang It

Before you paste anything on your board, play around with the composition of the images and words. Find an arrangement that makes you feel the most connected. Once it's completed, hang it in the location you've chosen.

Step 5: View It Intentionally

You want to make it part of your routine to regularly look at your board. Find a time in your day that you can stick to. My wife and I spend five minutes before bed looking at our boards. We envision ourselves already possessing what we see—and we get as emotionally connected as we can. It works!

Lauren and I have achieved so many beautiful things that were once on our vision boards. Often, the images have ended up matching our eventual reality almost identically. ☺

CHAPTER 20

Defining Your Purpose and Engaging Your Spirit

"There is no greater gift you can give or receive than to honor your calling.
It's why you were born. And how you become most truly alive."

—OPRAH WINFREY

WHAT MOTIVATES YOUR decisions, actions, and path in life? Do you live an intentional life, or do you haphazardly approach each day, going through the motions until it's time to sit on the couch once again?

Too many people lack guidance in their decision-making, choose hedonic happiness, and have no defined purpose. There are certain very important life-related questions that many people neglect to answer—I'm going to prompt you with those questions. I hope you've already given them considerable thought. But if you haven't, that's okay. That's why you're here!

To become self-actualized, you must ensure that you're living in alignment with the version of yourself that makes you happiest. It's time to make it happen. It's time to discover just who that person is. Failure to do so may cause a level of disintegration that will lead to decades of unfulfillment.

Purpose and Passion

You might know your purpose and you might not. Most people associate their purpose with their occupation, and that does make some sense. However, I'd like to challenge you to think beyond that. Your career will most likely encompass a portion of your passion, perhaps a large portion, but I don't believe it should be the entire thing.

To determine whether there's a correlation between your current profession and your passions (or life's purpose), answer the following questions.

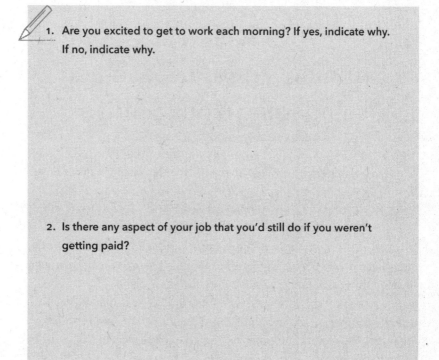

1. Are you excited to get to work each morning? If yes, indicate why. If no, indicate why.

2. Is there any aspect of your job that you'd still do if you weren't getting paid?

I hope there's at least an aspect of your job that ignites and inspires you. But even if there isn't (yet), you can begin incorporating passion and purpose into your life outside of work. It's time to think beyond your career—to determine your life's mission and the values you want to live by.

Neil Pasricha uses the question "What do you do on a Saturday morning when you have nothing to do?" to help people discover their "authentic passion." He asks his readers, "Do you go to the gym? Do you record yourself playing guitar? Take whatever answer you have and then wildly brainstorm ways you can pursue opportunities that naturally spew from that passion."[1] Pasricha believes that this one question, "What do you do on a Saturday morning when you have nothing to do?," will lead you to come up with hundreds of ideas. You can begin to filter these and eventually reach a higher level of personal and professional passion.

What do you do on a Saturday morning when you have nothing to do?

I invite you to write down all the things you typically do on a Saturday morning when you have nothing that you *have* to do. As for my friends with young children, I'm guessing you don't have that Saturday morning freedom at the moment (but don't worry . . . eventually you will). So, instead, think about what you did *before* you had kids.

1.

2.

3.

4.

5.

When you look at your list, is there any correlation between what you do for a living and what you wrote down? This is important because it's very unlikely that you're fulfilled, energized, and living optimally if you spend 40 or more hours per week in a job that you have very little passion for.

Identifying your passions is a shortcut to discovering your purpose. For me, an ideal Saturday morning (if I had no responsibilities) would involve hanging out with my wife and kids, playing a sport, and soaking up some sun while chatting with a friend about health, supplements, energy, biohacks, et cetera. These passions relate to my purpose—which, I've discovered, is to move my body, play, connect, learn, and grow. I've forged my life in such a way that I have a job that lets me live my purpose and pursue my passions. For that I'm very grateful.

From the passions you've outlined above, can you distill your purpose? Write down what comes to mind.

If your job fits within your purpose and passions, congratulations! You're one step closer to living optimally. If it doesn't, fear not! You don't necessarily need to quit your job and start over (something very few people have the luxury of doing). You may be able to shift your current position (or your mindset about the job) so that it brings you a tad more joy and fulfillment.

Even if quitting your job isn't a possibility, take some time to fantasize about the career you'd choose if you could do anything you wanted. There are so many more options today than there were just a few decades ago. With the explosion in online and virtual careers, people can create their own jobs, schedule, and work-related duties. Perhaps your desired profession is as traditional as high-school biology teacher, or you may long for something that's unique and individualized. The purpose here is to ignore your conservative and rational brain and fantasize about a career that most aligns with your passions.

What career would you choose if you could do anything you wanted?

Perhaps you don't even want to associate yourself with the word "career," because you feel it is too tied to the traditional—but for simplicity I'll continue to use it. So close your eyes and dream for a minute.

> ✏️ **Write down your optimal career and/or describe what you'd like your day-to-day responsibilities to be:**

Even if you have no intention of leaving your current position, the process of determining your ideal day-to-day responsibilities, coupled with their inclusion on your vision board, will give your subconscious the goal of moving you into closer alignment with that reality.

Turn off your skeptical brain and do the work—your life is too important to blindly trudge from one day to the next with little thought to how it can be improved. Great ideas don't just appear; they're manifested. You need to be open and receptive to possibilities. A skeptical brain will close the door to these possibilities.

Let's now build on the creation of a purposeful career by revamping the purpose that drives you each day (assuming it's not your job). To do so, we can learn from the residents of Okinawa, Japan.

In Okinawa the average life expectancy is eight years longer for women than it is in America.[2] Okinawans also have a longer disability-free life expectancy than any other culture on Earth.[3] What are they doing differently, and can we incorporate it into our lives?

Researchers were able to determine that residents of blue zones, where there's a disproportionate number of centenarians, live longer for a multitude of reasons; researchers refer to the reasons as the "Power 9."[4] Here's a summary of the Power 9:

1. **Move naturally.** Instead of going to gyms, participating in marathons, and lifting weights, many blue zone residents engage in a lot of manual work such as gardening, chores, and yard work.

2. **Purpose.** Okinawans call it *ikigai* and Nicoyans call it *plan de vida*—they both translate to "why I wake up in the morning."

3. **Downshift.** These cultures still experience stress, but they actively reduce it by (depending on the culture) praying, napping, and having a happy hour.

4. **80% rule.** The Okinawans stop eating when they're 80 percent full, and they often eat their smallest meal in the early evening and then don't eat for the rest of the day.

5. **Plant slant.** The diet of these cultures favors plant-based, with limited meat intake.

6. **Wine @ 5.** Most blue zone cultures drink alcohol (typically wine) regularly, but moderately (one to two glasses per day) with friends and/or with food.

7. **Belong.** The vast majority of centenarians belong to a faith-based community.

8. **Loved ones first.** These communities are more likely to live with or near aging parents—and they commit to a life partner.

9. **Positive association.** Residents of these communities choose social circles that encourage healthy behaviors.

Let's learn some more from the people of Okinawa. While people in the West believe that a life of hard work will be rewarded with retirement, Okinawans don't even have a word for retirement. Okinawans purpose in life is not reserved for their working years—their purpose permeates every facet of their lives. This isn't to say that their purpose won't change over time, but the spirit of having a specific daily intention remains.

Ikigai (pronounced "icky guy") essentially means "the reason you wake up in the morning." Let's dissect the word: iki = life and gai = worth, so together they mean "life worth living." Put another way, it's the thing that motivates you the most.

Okinawans are encouraged to determine their ikigai and then use it to drive their decision-making. The ikigai of a 100-year-old fisherman is to feed his family, and the ikigai of a 102-year-old woman is to hold her great-great-great granddaughter.

You may be asking, How does having an ikigai lead to a longer life? Researchers from Tohoku University Graduate School of Medicine sought to find the answer. They spent seven years studying the longevity of 43,391 Japanese adults and determined that the "subjects who did not find a sense of ikigai were associated with an increased risk of all-cause mortality. The increase in mortality risk was attributable to cardiovascular disease and external causes, but not cancer."[5] At the end of the seven years, 95 percent of the people with an ikigai were still living, versus 83 percent of the other participants. It was also found that the participants who had an ikigai were more likely to be married, educated, and employed; they also had higher levels of self-rated health and lower levels of stress.

So, then, what's your reason for waking up each day? What's your ikigai?

Take some time to think about your answer—this is a process that shouldn't be rushed. I recommend finding a quiet time in your day, getting in to a relaxed, parasympathetic state through meditation, and asking this question with no sense of urgency. Perhaps the answer will come quickly and with clarity, or maybe it will take several intentional attempts before the answer is clear. Enjoy the process as you ponder the question. This should be exciting!

Use the space below to brainstorm your thoughts before you decide on the driving force that inspires you to begin each day.

My ikigai is:

With your ikigai clearly defined, write it on a piece of paper and put the paper beside your bed. In time you won't need a daily reminder, but when you first start looking at your life through this lens (getting out of bed with purpose) it can be helpful to have your purpose as the first thing you see in the morning.

Before we go on, I invite you to take a break, reflect, and thank yourself for the deep, introspective work you're engaging in. Don't gloss over the gift you're giving yourself. You're doing the hard and meaningful work to improve your life—I applaud that and so should you. You are worth it!

When you're ready, proceed to the next step on your journey: your spirituality. Everyone has a spiritual self, one that must be nurtured for you to achieve optimal life alignment.

Discovering Your Spiritual Self

"No man or woman is an island. To exist just for yourself is meaning-less. You can achieve the most satisfaction when you feel related to some greater purpose in life, something greater than yourself."—DENIS WAITLEY

When some people hear the word "spiritual" they automatically associate it with God or religion. It could reflect a relationship to God, or it may simply represent a deep set of values and principles they choose to live by. When you feel connected to a distinct purpose in life, the actions you take will be in close alignment with who you truly are.

Think about your typical decision-making. Is it based, at least in part, on a set of principles by which you choose to live your life? Even if you're a self-described atheist, it's still important to have a creed that helps to govern your decisions. It could simply be that you follow your values and treat others as you wish to be treated.

If you're unfulfilled in life, one of the reasons could be that your decision-making is haphazard and lacking guidance from the values or life principles you align with. Are there any decisions (big or small) you've made in the past year that, upon reflection, went against your values and beliefs?

Think of circumstances in the near future when you know you'll be challenged to make a decision that may not align with your faith or values. Write down what comes to mind.

Note: If you lack clarity on the values that govern your life, don't worry—there's an activity coming up that's designed to help. You can return to this exercise if need be.

In times of doubt and uncertainty, some people move away from spiritual alignment, which pulls them farther from their goal of happiness and fulfillment. Growth in this area typically requires you to tie yourself to a purpose that goes beyond just serving yourself. The sooner you reconnect and realign with your values and morals, the sooner you can begin to heal and grow your spiritual health.

If growing your spirituality hasn't been a priority up to this point, it's time to ask yourself some difficult questions. The answers to these questions will help form the backbone of your aligned life. Consider them carefully, answering with as much detail as possible.

1. Beyond your family, what gives your life meaning?

2. Is your purpose driven by external motivators (money, power, fame, recognition, etc.) or internal motivators (giving, advancing God's kingdom, connection, etc.)?

3. Is there anyone you know who lives a very purposeful life? Think about those who have a clearly defined mission (which could be charity work, improving their community, enhancing their health, investing in the next generation, or anything that constantly motivates them). What are their character traits?

The questions you answered are designed to prompt conscious thought on the road map you use to navigate life. If they were difficult to answer, or, upon reflection, you're unhappy with the truth in the answers, that's okay! The activities you're about to do will guide you in discovering your optimal spiritual blueprint.

We'll begin with the values you use to govern your thoughts, behaviors, and decisions. Ideally, they align with your purpose and your life's mission.

Identifying Your Values

Your values are strongly held beliefs about what you consider to be important. They help you to navigate life with clarity. For instance, if honesty is one of your core values, then no matter how hard it is to tell the truth on occasion, you'll spend little time worrying about what you should do when confronted with an opportunity to be dishonest, because you know what you must do: tell the truth.

According to *The Power of Full Engagement* by Jim Loehr and Tony Schwartz,[6] your values are your "road map for action"; therefore, you must think about which values are the most motivating to you, because they'll influence the daily choices and actions you take. Loehr and Schwartz reflect on the reality that too often people's behavior is expedient rather than value-driven—that people tend to do what makes them feel good in the moment instead of letting their intrinsic values guide them.

To help define your values, think of the ones that you'd like to pass on to your children or that you hope the next generation will possess or embody. Do you want your children to value hard work and perseverance above all else? Or is dedication and loyalty what you'll preach most?

Another way to approach this question is by envisioning someone you look up to. What are this person's values and character traits? Take a moment to think of a person you admire (it can even be someone you've never met), then write down their character traits. If it's too hard to narrow it down to just one person, combine the traits of a few people.

Name(s):

Character traits:

To help you to define your values, I've provided you with a list. From these, pick 8–10 that you identify with or wish to cultivate. This isn't supposed to be easy, so take your time, reflect, and choose with purpose.

Perseverance	Logic	Consistency	Conviction
Discretion	Accomplishment	Acceptance	Accountability
Freedom	Reputation	Cleanliness	Confidence
Determination	Diversity	Resilience	Enthusiasm
Simplicity	Generosity	Intuition	Power
Faith	Optimism	Action	Authenticity
Modesty	Balance	Mastery	Dreaming
Daring	Aggressiveness	Imagination	Calm
Playfulness	Intelligence	Dynamism	Adventure
Approachability	Wealth	Originality	Poise
Growth	Patience	Obedience	Bravery
Peace	Serenity	Service to others	Respect for others

Responsibility   Fitness   Silence   Tradition

Collaboration   Organization   Frugality   Self-awareness

Professionalism   Experience   Wisdom   Politeness

Fairness   Education   Sincerity   Punctuality

Justice   Rest   Conservation   Longevity

Community   Dependability   Consideration   Compassion

Open-mindedness   Concern for others   Commitment   Loyalty

Courage   Creativity   Empathy   Excellence

Family   Friendship   Freedom   Knowledge

Generosity   Genuineness   Happiness   Harmony

Health   Honesty   Humour   Integrity

Kindness

My values:

1.

2.

3.

4.

5.

6.

7.

8.

9.

10.

Another way to distill your values and define your purpose is to think of yourself at the end of your life. Reflect on what you've already accomplished and what you want to accomplish from this point forward. Think in terms of character traits you wish to possess, things you want to achieve, and how you want to be remembered. Reflect on these issues and then write your future obituary.

It may feel a bit morbid, but don't let this exercise frighten you. We're all going to die someday (hopefully many, many years down the road). This exercise is designed to help you unveil the legacy you wish to leave—how you made people feel, what you achieved, and what you left behind.

It likely goes without saying, but when you compose your obituary, write all your future accomplishments and character traits as having taken place or having existed.

Name:

Born: **Died:**   (make yourself live to 100)

Clarifying Your Mission Statement

Now that you've isolated your purpose and passion, narrowed down the values you wish to govern your life, and pondered the legacy you wish to leave, it's time to construct a mission statement for your life (if you prefer, you can divide it into two: personal and professional).

Your statement doesn't have to include the exact words you have chosen as your values, but it should encompass the spirit of their meaning. This activity will help to shape the blueprint of your life and how you plan to invest your energy. Below you will see my mission statement as well as those from a few well-known people and companies that I respect.

Joseph Gibbons

To honor my mind with positivity, joy, and information, my body with healthy food and exercise, and my spirit by serving the Lord's purpose.

Maya Angelou

My mission in life is not merely to survive, but to thrive; and to do so with some passion, some compassion, some humor, and some style.

Tony Robbins

To humbly serve our Lord by being a loving, playful, powerful, and passionate example of the absolute joy that is available to us the moment that we rejoice in God's gifts and sincerely love and enjoy all his creations.

Richard Branson

To have fun in my journey through life and learn from my mistakes.

Mahatma Gandhi

I shall not fear anyone on Earth. I shall fear only God. I shall not bear ill will toward anyone. I shall not submit to injustice from anyone. I shall conquer untruth by truth. And in resisting untruth, I shall put up with all suffering.

TED

Spread ideas.

Nike

Bring inspiration and innovation to every athlete in the world. If you have a body, you are an athlete.

NOW IT'S TIME to write your mission statement. This isn't about getting the wording just perfect, and it doesn't have to be the final draft. This is a reflective exercise meant to give meaning to the decisions that shape your life.

Begin by writing some key words or phrases that have arisen from your purpose, values, ikigai, or anything else you have brainstormed or penned prior to this. I've left space for a few drafts of your mission. You want its wording and flow to inspire and influence how you approach each day. Take your time, revisit when necessary, and create something beautiful.

Key words or phrases:

Draft 1:

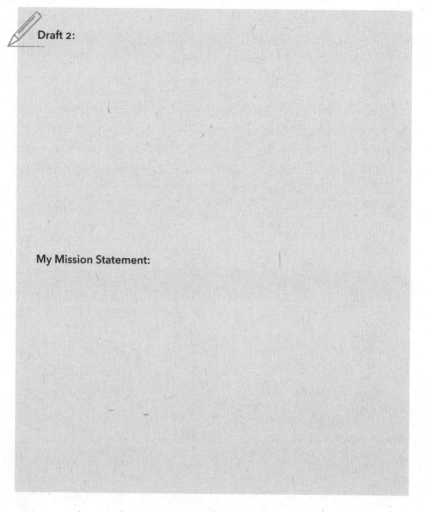

Draft 2:

My Mission Statement:

Take it a step farther. Spread your newfound sense of direction and guidance by gathering together the members of your household and creating a family mission statement. With equal say, the prioritization of family values, and an honest discussion of how you (as a family) will journey together, build a mission statement that motivates and inspires each one of you equally. When it's complete, frame it and display it proudly. You're taking real, meaningful action, and that should be celebrated!

CHAPTER 21

The Motivation to Keep Going

"For me, becoming isn't about arriving somewhere or achieving a certain aim. I see it instead as forward motion, a means of evolving, a way to reach continuously toward a better self. The journey doesn't end."

—MICHELLE OBAMA

WHAT A JOURNEY! Are you pumped up? I hope so. I'm excited about what lies ahead for you. I started this book by telling you that discovering your optimal self wasn't going to be easy—and I'm sure you'll attest to that: for all the good that Part IV of this book has brought, it's been incredibly challenging.

The questions asked of you, and about you, are the most difficult questions you'll likely ever encounter. They called for deep introspection and compassionate, considered thought. If you're like me, you found it scary. It likely was a difficult, emotional, but ultimately rewarding experience. And I'll bet you were exhausted afterward.

Be proud of yourself. I'm proud of you. Don't shrug it off. You've done the hard work of getting to the core of who you are—your purpose, passions, values, and mission in life. Whoa! That's impressive.

I encourage you to sit with whatever it is you're feeling right now. Really feel it. You've earned it. I also encourage you to come back to Part IV and review it from time to time. This will remind you of your goals, hopes, and dreams, and will keep you pointed at _your_ North Star. It will also enable you to see if, over time, some things have changed. Just as the world keeps on turning, life changes, and you will too. Remember the people of Okinawa? Their ikigai changes throughout life. Be open to change.

Unbroken

I hope my journey has given you hope that no matter where you are, you can design a life that enables you to thrive. I began researching out of desperation. I was clinging to any thread of hope I could as my health deteriorated. I spent years oscillating between extremes, feverishly hunting for the path, the cure, and the answer to my unexplained ailments. I knew there had to be a better way, but at times the mental cloud and physical exhaustion seemed too severe to overcome. But I persisted. You should too.

Optimal is never guaranteed. You must be open, willing to evolve and adapt, or the current of society will wash you back to where you once were. My hope is that this book has taught you to become a better swimmer, more impervious to the clutches of temptation and external dependence.

The outcome of my third breakdown, which was the initiation of a depersonalization disorder, is a persistent reminder of the life I used to lead. When symptoms arise, I immediately reflect on that period in 2017 when I thought my brain was shutting down. I remember how scared I was.

My journey since then, although very rocky at times, has been transformational. The biggest hurdle for me to conquer was my tendency to overwork as a means to suppress my emotions. This tendency was so deeply rooted in my subconscious that it still requires continuous diligence on my part not to fall back into my bad habits. I don't consider myself healed; I consider myself aware. I'm aware of my habitual tendencies and I use that to fuel my decision-making.

I'll never burn out again.

I'll share my fears, emotions, and vulnerabilities with those I trust.

These are the promises I've made to myself. Self-awareness, the ability to take constructive criticism, and the willingness to adapt have ensured that I keep these promises. As you progress and grow, be kind to yourself. You're going to have days that lack flow, and that's okay. I have difficult and frustrating days, but the knowledge that I've accrued, along with my values and mission in life, ensure that they're farther and farther apart. I'm aware. I'm responsive. I'm diligent.

I believe in you.

CONCLUSION

Full Transparency

THIS IS IT, the end of my book. Am I afraid to write the conclusion? Yes. I've been struggling for weeks trying to summarize my message, to ignite a fire and passion in you to take control of your life and to get you moving toward optimal. But that's not why I took so long to write this section. In fact, I have a tinge of guilt about that. My hesitation came from fear. I'm sad to admit it, but it's true.

As I sit here reflecting on my health journey, I'm reminded about what this book has meant to me. It's been a source of comfort when my mental, physical, and spiritual health struggled. It's something I could control when the outside forces seemed overwhelming.

The knowledge I acquired in researching and writing has brought me from burnout and despair to abundant energy and vitality with a newfound enthusiasm for life. My hesitancy in writing this conclusion comes from mourning the culmination and completion of the book—because it has meant so much to me over the years.

However, by choosing to focus on my mission, I've stopped operating from a place of unconscious fear. Writing the conclusion has filled me with gratitude for what this journey has taught me. I feel truly blessed for that. I'm grateful for all the ups and downs, the challenges and the triumphs. They blend together to form my life's experience, and each day that experience expands. To quote Michelangelo, "I am still learning."

This book isn't about teaching you to become so rigid in your routines and habits that you systematize your entire life in the pursuit of perfection—it's about determining your priorities and therefore opening you up to discovering your optimal self. What works for me may not work for you. What works in this season of life may not work a few months or years down the road. Any time you decide that you need to rethink, recharge, revitalize, rediscover, or re-anything in your life, this book can always be returned to.

You have everything you need to elevate your mindset, adopt healthier routines, and reach your potential. Never settle for mediocrity—you deserve better than that.

JOSEPH GIBBONS

Acknowledgments

THE REALIZATION OF this book would not have been possible without the contributions of so many—without their guidance, patience, expertise, and loving grace, I never would have seen this dream come to fruition. Thank you to all who have had a hand in making this book.

To my beautiful wife, Lauren, I owe you the most gratitude. When my physical and mental health were declining, you never ceased to believe in me. You have connected with my soul on a level that no one ever has, and your presence in my life is my most cherished gift. Every day, I am in awe of your ability to live with tenacity, grace, compassion, and warmth. You are a blessing in this world—a bright light and a soft landing for those who need it. Thank you, God, for bringing this woman into my life.

To my miracles, Jakoby and Elijah, you are my source of motivation. You motivate me to pursue balance, seek levity, and remain playful.

Jakey, you epitomize joy. You are spontaneous, lively, and a beautiful reminder to live in the moment and fully enjoy the presence of those around you.

Elijah, you astonish me. You are the most curious, engaging, and empathetic person I know. You impress and amaze me every day.

I have also been blessed with the support of so many others on my journey with this book and the discovering of my optimal life. Humber College, you have provided me with the tools and resources to mature as a professional. Tony Robbins and Karissa Kouchis, you have influenced and inspired me to embrace everything that life offers, viewing it as a blessing and learning to grow, transform, and evolve from it. Tony Evans, you have been my spiritual guide; your teachings have deepened my faith and taught me how to expand my relationship with God. And to all the unspecified people who have made up my life's experience, I thank you.

References

INTRODUCTION

1. B.B. Fredholm, K. Bättig, J. Holmén, A. Nehlig, and E.E. Zvartau, "Actions of caffeine in the brain with special reference to factors that contribute to its widespread use," *Pharmacological Reviews* 51, no. 1 (1999): 83–133.

2. A. Capritto, "Need more coffee to stay awake? Here's why," CNET, April 7, 2021. https://www.cnet.com/health/nutrition/caffeine-tolerance-why-you-need-more-and-more-coffee-to-get-a-boost/

3. C. Drake, T. Roehrs, J. Shambroom, and T. Roth, "Caffeine effects on sleep taken 0, 3, or 6 hours before going to bed," *Journal of Clinical Sleep Medicine* 9, no. 11 (2013): 1195–1200. doi: 10.5664/jcsm.3170

4. K.Y. Ryu and J. Roh, "The effects of high peripubertal caffeine exposure on the adrenal gland in immature male and female rats," *Nutrients* 11, no. 5 (2019): 951. doi: 10.3390/nu11050951

5. U.S. Food and Drug Administration, *Spilling the beans: How much caffeine is too much?* (FDA, December 12, 2018). https://www.fda.gov/consumers/consumer-updates/spilling-beans-how-much-caffeine-too-much#:~:text=For%20healthy%20adults%2C%20the%20 FDA,associated%20with%20dangerous%2C%20negative%20effects

6. M. Górecki and E. Hallmann, "The antioxidant content of coffee and its in vitro activity as an effect of its production method and roasting and brewing time," *Antioxidants* 9/10, no. 4 (2020): 308. doi: 10.3390/antiox9040308

7. J.H. O'Keefe, J.J. DiNicolantonio, and C.J. Lavie, "Coffee for cardioprotection and longevity," *Progress in Cardiovascular Diseases* 61, no. 1 (2018): 38–42. doi: 10.1016/j.pcad.2018.02.002

8. A. Iriondo-DeHond, J.A. Uranga, M.D. Del Castillo, and R. Abalo, "Effects of coffee and its components on the gastrointestinal tract and the brain–gut axis," *Nutrients* 13, no. 1 (2020): 88. doi: 10.3390/nu13010088

9. *Decaf coffee*, Caffeine Informer (n.d.). https://www.caffeineinformer.com/caffeine-content/coffee-decaf-brewed

10. *The complete guide to Starbucks caffeine*, Caffeine Informer (n.d.). https://www.caffeineinformer.com/the-complete-guide-to-starbucks-caffeine

CHAPTER 1: THE PAINFUL WAY I CAME TO FIND MY PATH

1. Brené Brown, *Brené on ffts*, April 22, 2022. https://brenebrown.com/podcast/brene-on-ffts/

2. P. Nelson, *There's a hole in my sidewalk: The romance of self-discovery* (New York: Atria, 2018).

CHAPTER 2: HARD TRUTHS

1. Napoleon Hill, *Think and grow rich* (New York: Tarcher, 2007).

2. Y.B. Zhang, X.F. Pan, J. Chen, A. Cao, L. Xia, Y. Zhang, J. Wang, H. Li, G. Liu, and A. Pan. "Combined lifestyle factors, all-cause mortality and cardiovascular disease: A systematic review

and meta-analysis of prospective cohort studies," *Journal of Epidemiology and Community Health* 75, no. 1: 92–99. doi: 10.1136/jech-2020-214050

3. M.E. Lean and L. Te Morenga, "Sugar and type 2 diabetes," *British Medical Bulletin* 120, no. 1 (2016): 43–53. doi: 10.1093/bmb/ldw037

4. J. Rehm, B. Taylor, S. Mohapatra, H. Irving, B. Baliunas, J. Patra, and M. Roerecke, "Alcohol as a risk factor for liver cirrhosis: A systematic review and meta-analysis," *Drug and Alcohol Review* 29, no. 4 (2010): 437–45. doi: 10.1111/j.1465-3362.2009.00153.x

5. L.A. Loeb, V.L. Ernster, K.E. Warner, J. Abbotts, and J. Laszlo, "Smoking and lung cancer: An overview," *Cancer Research* 44, no. 12 (1984): 5940–58. Erratum in *Cancer Research* 46, no. 10 (1986): 5453.

6. J.L. Heileson, "Dietary saturated fat and heart disease: A narrative review," *Nutrition Review* 78, no. 6 (2020): 474–85. doi: 10.1093/nutrit/nuz091

7. H. Avey, K.B. Matheny, A. Robbins, and T.A. Jacobson, "Health care providers' training, perceptions, and practices regarding stress and health outcomes," *Journal of the National Medical Association* 95, no. 9 (2003): 833, 836–45.

8. A. Nerurkar, A. Bitton, R.B. Davis, R.S. Phillips, and G. Yeh, "When physicians counsel about stress: Results of a national study," *Journal of the American Medical Association, Internal Medicine* 173, no. 1 (2013): 76–77. doi: 10.1001/2013.jamainternmed.480

9. Christopher Krueger, "Muffin madness: Health conscious snackers stir up new yen for old favorite," *Los Angeles Times,* July 31, 1988.

10. See note 9.

11. C.L. Birmingham, J. Su, J.A. Hlynsky, E.M. Goldner, and M. Gao, "The mortality rate from anorexia nervosa," *International Journal of Eating Disorders* 38, no. 2 (2005): 143–46. doi: 10.1002/eat.20164

12. Brené Brown, *Brené on ffts,* April 22, 2022. https://brenebrown.com/podcast/brene-on-ffts/

CHAPTER 3: BURNOUT

1. R. Prem, B. Kubicek, S. Diestel, and C. Korunka, "Regulatory job stressors and their within-person relationships with ego depletion: The roles of state anxiety, self-control effort, and job autonomy," *Journal of Vocational Behavior* 92 (2016): 22–32. https://doi.org/10.1016/j.jvb.2015.11.004

2. Mayo Foundation for Medical Education and Research, *Know the signs of job burnout* (Mayo Clinic, 2021). https://www.mayoclinic.org/healthy-lifestyle/adult-health/in-depth/burnout/art-20046642

3. O. Sovijärvi, T. Arina, and J. Halmetoja, *Biohacker's handbook: Upgrade yourself and unleash your inner potential* (Tallinn: Biohacker Center, 2018).

4. N. Pasricha, *The happiness equation: Want nothing + do anything = have everything* (London: Vermilion, 2017).

5. Terry Edward MacDougall, "Yoshida Shigeru and the Japanese transition to liberal democracy," *International Political Science Review* 9, no. 1 (1988): 55–69. doi:10.1177/019251218800900105

6. K. Iwasaki, M. Takahashi, and A. Nakata, "Health problems due to long working hours in Japan: Working hours, workers' compensation (Karoshi), and preventive measures," *Industrial Health* 44, no. 4 (2006): 537–40. doi: 10.2486/indhealth.44.537

7. M. Ishikawa, "Relationships between overwork, burnout and suicidal ideation among resident physicians in hospitals in Japan with medical residency programmes: A nationwide questionnaire-based survey," *British Medical Journal* 10/12, no. 3 (2022): e056283. doi: 10.1136/bmjopen-2021-056283

8. K. Nishiyama and J.V. Johnson, "*Karoshi*—death from overwork: Occupational health consequences of Japanese production management," *International Journal of Health Services* 27, no. 4 (1997): 625–41. https://doi.org/10.2190/1jpc-679v-dynt-hj6g

9. K. Wada, H. Eguchi, and D. Prieto-Merino, "Differences in stroke and ischemic heart disease mortality by occupation and industry among Japanese working-aged men," *SSM Population Health* 15, no. 2 (2016): 745–49. doi: 10.1016/j.ssmph.2016.10.004

10. See note 4.

11. James E. Loehr and Tony Schwartz, *The power of full engagement: Managing energy, not time, is the key to high performance and personal renewal* (New York: Free Press, 2005).

CHAPTER 4: FEAR, WORRY, ANXIETY, AND STRESS

1. S.A. Vreeburg, F.G. Zitman, J. van Pelt, R.H. Derijk, J.C. Verhagen, R. van Dyck, W.J. Hoogendijk, J.H. Smit, and B.W. Penninx, "Salivary cortisol levels in persons with and without different anxiety disorders," *Psychosomatic Medicine* 72, no. 4 (2010): 340–47. doi: 10.1097/PSY.0b013e3181d2f0c8

2. K. Golonka, J. Mojsa-Kaja, M. Blukacz, M. Gawłowska, and T. Marek, "Occupational burnout and its overlapping effect with depression and anxiety," *International Journal of Occupational Medicine and Environmental Health* 32, no. 2 (2019): 229–44. doi: 10.13075/ijomeh.1896.01323

3. M. Lourel and N. Gueguen, "Une méta-analyse de la mesure du burnout à l'aide de l'instrument MBI [A meta-analysis of job burnout using the MBI scale]," *Encephale* 33, no. 6 (2007): 947–53. doi: 10.1016/j.encep.2006.10.001

4. V.E. Frankl, H.S. Kushner, and W.J. Winslade, *Man's search for meaning* (Boston: Beacon, 2007).

5. L.M. Shin and I. Liberzon, "The neurocircuitry of fear, stress, and anxiety disorders," *Neuropsychopharmacology* 35, no. 1 (2020): 169–91. doi: 10.1038/npp.2009.83

6. E.T. Higgins, "Beyond pleasure and pain," *American Psychologist* 52, no. 12 (1997): 1280–300. doi: 10.1037//0003-066X.52.12.1280

7. W.W. Tryon, "Possible mechanisms for why desensitization and exposure therapy work," *Clinical Psychology Review* 25, no. 1 (2005): 67–95. doi: 10.1016/j.cpr.2004.08.005

8. T. Robbins, *How to make progress in life by learning how to feel good* (tonyrobbins.com, April 29, 2019). https://www.tonyrobbins.com/leadership-impact/feel-good-now/

9. C. Doughty, *Death positive movement: The order of the good death* (Death Positive Movement | The Order of the Good Death, n.d.). Retrieved December 2, 2022, from https://www.orderofthegooddeath.com/death-positive-movement/

10. M.C. Reddan, T.D. Wager, and D. Schiller, "Attenuating neural threat expression with imagination," *Neuron* 4 (2018): 994–1005. doi: 10.1016/j.neuron.2018.10.047

11. Tony Evans, *Overcoming the consequences of worry and anxiety* (Tony Evans Sermon [Video], January 25, 2018). https://www.youtube.com/watch?v=0aOLVAQFYEC

12. *King James Bible* (Oxford: Oxford University Press, 2008/1769).

13. S. Regan, *12 universal laws and how to use them to unlock a more spiritual life* (mindbodygreen, November 8, 2022). https://www.mindbodygreen.com/articles/the-12-universal-laws-and-how-to-practice-them

14. H. Yaribeygi, Y. Panahi, H. Sahraei, T.P. Johnston, and A. Sahebkar, "The impact of stress on body function: A review," *EXCLI Journal* 21, no. 16 (2017): 1057–72. doi: 10.17179/excli2017-480

15. O. Sovijärvi, T. Arina, and J. Halmetoja, *Biohacker's handbook: Upgrade yourself and unleash your inner potential* (Tallinn: Biohacker Center, 2018).

16. L. Thau, J. Gandhi, and S. Sharma, "Physiology, cortisol" [updated August 29, 2022], *StatPearls* (Treasure Island, FL: StatPearls Publishing, 2022). https://www.ncbi.nlm.nih.gov/books/NBK538239/

17. E.S. Epel, B. McEwen, T. Seeman, K. Matthews, G. Castellazzo, K.D. Brownell, J. Bell, and J.R. Ickovics, "Stress and body shape: Stress-induced cortisol secretion is consistently greater among women with central fat," *Psychosomatic Medicine* 62, no. 5 (2000): 623–32. doi: 10.1097/00006842-200009000-00005

18. U.S. Department of Health and Human Services, NIH *study shows how insulin stimulates fat cells to take in glucose* (National Institutes of Health, October 2, 2015). https://www.nih.gov/news-events/news-releases/nih-study-shows-how-insulin-stimulates-fat-cells-take-glucose

CHAPTER 5: THE SUBCONSCIOUS MIND

1. M. Szegedy-Maszak, *Mysteries of the mind* (Mysteries of the Mind, n.d.). http://webhome.auburn.edu/~mitrege/ENGL2210/USNWR-mind.html
2. A. Urmston, *Parts of the mind and their primary functions* (Urmston Hypnotherapy and Psychotherapy, n.d.). https://www.urmstonhypnotherapy.com/parts-of-the-mind-and-their-primary-functions/
3. B.S. McEwen, "Early life influences on life-long patterns of behavior and health," *Mental Retardation and Developmental Disabilities Review* 9, no. 3 (2003): 149–54. doi: 10.1002/mrdd.10074
4. J. Murphy, *The power of your subconscious mind* (Brooklyn, NY: Brownstone, 2022).
5. M. Karefilakis, *The conscious and subconscious mind* (Kare Psychology, 2019). https://karepsychology.com.au/the-conscious-and-subconscious-mind/#:~:text=The%20conscious%20mind%20is%20your,day%20in%20the%20conscious%20mind
6. B. Tracy, *The power of your subconscious mind* (2022). https://www.briantracy.com/blog/personal-success/understanding-your-subconscious-mind/
7. G. Marra, *9 interesting facts about your subconscious mind* (Gail Marra Hypnotherapy, May 26, 2022). https://www.gailmarrahypnotherapy.com/9-interesting-facts-about-your-subconscious-mind/
8. A. Morin, *How kids develop cognitive skills* (Understood, December 9, 2020). https://www.understood.org/en/articles/how-kids-develop-thinking-and-learning-skills
9. S.B. Johnson, R.W. Blum, and J.N. Giedd, "Adolescent maturity and the brain: The promise and pitfalls of neuroscience research in adolescent health policy," *Journal of Adolescent Health* 45, no. 3 (2009): 216–21. doi: 10.1016/j.jadohealth.2009.05.016
10. J. Kucera, "I guess your subconscious mind just can't take a joke: Why self-deprecating humor may bring you more harm than laughs," *Watkins MIND BODY SPIRIT Magazine*, January 13 (2020). https://www.watkinsmagazine.com/self-deprecating-humor
11. MediLexicon International, "Placebos: The power of the placebo effect," *Medical News Today*, n.d. https://www.medicalnewstoday.com/articles/306437
12. S. Kemsley, "The effects of bitter placebos on cognitive tests," *Psychology and Behavioral Sciences* 5, no. 4 (2016): 98. https://www.sciencepublishinggroup.com/journal/paperinfo?journalid=201&doi=10.11648%2Fj.pbs.20160504.14
13. See note 11.
14. See note 11.
15. See note 11.
16. A.J. de Craen, P.J. Roos, A.L. de Vries, and J. Kleijnen, "Effect of colour of drugs: Systematic review of perceived effect of drugs and of their effectiveness," *British Medical Journal* 313, no. 7072 (1996): 1624–26. doi: 10.1136/bmj.313.7072.1624
17. B. Jones, *Chickens laying eggs: CIT Freshers Week with comedy hypnotist Barry Jones September 24th, 2015*. YouTube, October 9, 2015. https://www.youtube.com/watch?v=sDaUUpEeuW4&list=PLzlGCJ02FlkQwL3_BIbsgkEQRreKq3450
18. K. von Sponneck, *Eating an onion thinking it's an apple under hypnosis | stage hypnotist Kris Von Sponneck*. YouTube, August 2, 2022. https://www.youtube.com/watch?v=0tYtROwOKlU
19. G.H. Montgomery, D. David, G. Winkel, J.H. Silverstein, and D.H. Bovbjerg, "The effectiveness of adjunctive hypnosis with surgical patients: A meta-analysis," *Anesthesia and Analgesia* 94, no. 6 (2002): 1639–45. doi: 10.1097/00000539-200206000-00052
20. American Psychological Association, *About division 30* (2014). https://www.apadivisions.org/division-30/about

21. Y. Li, "Modern epigenetics methods in biological research," *Methods* 187 (2021): 104–13. doi: 10.1016/j.ymeth.2020.06.022

22. See note 21.

23. *What is epigenetics? The answer to the nature vs. nurture debate.* Center on the Developing Child at Harvard University (October 30, 2020). https://developingchild. harvard.edu/resources/what-is-epigenetics-and-how-does-it-relate-to-child-development/#:~:text=During%20development%2C%20the%20DNA%20that,have%20rearrange%20those%20chemical%20marks

24. See note 23.

25. B. Greenfield, *Boundless: Upgrade your brain, optimize your body and defy aging* (Victory Belt Publishing, 2020).

26. See note 25.

27. L.D. Kubzansky and R.C. Thurston, "Emotional vitality and incident coronary heart disease: Benefits of healthy psychological functioning," *Archives of General Psychiatry*, 64, no. 12 (2007): 1393–1401. doi: 10.1001/archpsyc.64.12.1393

28. B.L. Fredrickson, "The broaden-and-build theory of positive emotions," *Philosophical Transactions of the Royal Society* 29, no. 359 (2004): 1367–78. doi: 10.1098/rstb.2004.1512

29. P.O. Sun, E.T. Walbeehm, R.W. Selles, H.P. Slijper, D.J.O. Ulrich, and J.T. Porsius, "Patient mindset and the success of carpal tunnel release," *Plastic Reconstructive Surgery* 147, no. 1 (2021): 66e–75e. doi: 10.1097/PRS.0000000000007441

30. N.A. Huebschmann and E.S. Sheets, "The right mindset: Stress mindset moderates the association between perceived stress and depressive symptoms," *Anxiety, Stress and Coping* 33, no. 3 (2020): 248–55. doi: 10.1080/10615806.2020.1736900

31. P. Kaliman, M.J. Alvarez-López, M. Cosín-Tomás, M.A. Rosenkranz, A. Lutz, and R.J. Davidson, "Rapid changes in histone deacetylases and inflammatory gene expression in expert meditators," *Psychoneuroendocrinology* 40 (2014): 96–107. doi: 10.1016/j.psyneuen.2013.11.004

32. See note 31.

33. B.H. Lipton, *The biology of belief: Unleashing the power of consciousness, matter and miracles* (Hay House, 2016).

34. B. Lipton, *Researchers show how meditation can change your genes* (Guided Mindfulness Meditation Course & Lessons Online, n.d.). https://www.thewayofmeditation.com.au/meditation-can-change-your-genes

35. See note 34.

36. N. Choi, *Visualization: What the science says* (November 30, 2020). https://toat.com/blogs/wellness/visualization-what-science-says

37. A. Filgueiras, E.F. Quintas Conde, and C.R. Hall, "The neural basis of kinesthetic and visual imagery in sports: An ALE meta-analysis," *Brain Imaging Behavior* 12, no. 5 (2018): 1513–23. doi: 10.1007/s11682-017-9813-9

38. See note 37.

39. B. Yates, "Watch: 'The will to do it,'" *Huffington Post*, October 20, 2013. https://www.huffpost.com/entry/eft-tapping_b_3839655

40. B. Proctor, *Are you the star in your own movie?* (YouTube, June 4, 2020). https://www.youtube.com/watch?v=OPkD5hW_3GY

41. L. Brown, *The graveyard is the richest place on Earth - Les Brown - this speech will give you goosebumps!* (YouTube, July 14, 2020). https://www.youtube.com/watch?v=YgjNfn8nlj8

CHAPTER 7: TOXIC OVERLOAD, IMMUNITY, AND YOUR DETOXIFICATION SYSTEM

1. K. Nowak, W. Ratajczak-Wrona, M. Górska, and E. Jabłońska, "Parabens and their effects on the endocrine system," *Molecular Cell Endocrinology* 474 (2018): 238–51. doi: 10.1016/j.mce.2018.03.014

2. P.D. Darbre, "Aluminium, antiperspirants and breast cancer," *Journal of Inorganic Biochemistry* 99, no. 9 (2005): 1912–19. doi: 10.1016/j.jinorgbio.2005.06.001

3. S. Frothingham, *Deodorants vs. antiperspirants: Health benefits and risks* (Healthline, October 4, 2019). https://www.healthline.com/health/deodorant-vs-antiperspirant#deodorants

4. Environmental Protection Agency, *The inside story: A guide to indoor air quality* (EPA, n.d.). https://www.epa.gov/indoor-air-quality-iaq/inside-story-guide-indoor-air-quality

5. M. Schade, *Volatile vinyl - the new shower curtain's chemical smell* (Academia.edu, October 15, 2016). https://www.academia.edu/29180491/Volatile_Vinyl_the_New_Shower_Curtains_Chemical_Smell

6. CBC/Radio Canada, "Plastic shower curtain smell may be toxic: Study" (*CBC News*, June 12, 2008). https://www.cbc.ca/news/science/plastic-shower-curtain-smell-may-be-toxic-study-1.703815#:~:text=Polyvinyl%20chloride%20(PVC)%20shower%20curtains,the%20study%20by%20the%20U.S.%2D

7. Roundtable on Environmental Health Sciences, Research, and Medicine; Board on Population Health and Public Health Practice; Institute of Medicine, *Identifying and reducing environmental health risks of chemicals in our society: Workshop summary.* Washington: National Academies Press, October 2, 2014.

8. S. Buchanan, J. Rizzo, A. Rolfes, and C. Hafer, *Toxic chemicals found in minority cord blood* (Environmental Working Group, November 29, 2022). https://www.ewg.org/news-insights/news-release/toxic-chemicals-found-minority-cord-blood

9. R.A. Bernhoft, "Mercury toxicity and treatment: A review of the literature," *Journal of Environmental Public Health* (2012): 460508. doi: 10.1155/2012/460508

10. L. Patrick, "Lead toxicity, a review of the literature. Part 1: Exposure, evaluation, and treatment," *Alternative Medicine Review* 11, no. 1 (2006): 2–22.

11. Cancer Council, *Testicular cancer: Causes, symptoms and treatments* (Cancer Council, 2020). https://www.cancer.org.au/cancer-information/types-of-cancer/testicular-cancer

12. Johns Hopkins Medicine, *Testicular cancer statistics* (Johns Hopkins Medicine, November 19, 2019). https://www.hopkinsmedicine.org/health/conditions-and-diseases/testicular-cancer/testicular-cancer-statistics#:~:text=Testis%20cancer%20is%20most%20common,20%20to%2040%20years%20old

13. H. Gao, B.J. Yang, N. Li, L.M. Feng, X.Y. Shi, W.H. Zhao, and S.J. Liu, "Bisphenol A and hormone-associated cancers: Current progress and perspectives," *Medicine* 94, no. 1 (2015): e211. doi: 10.1097/MD.0000000000000211

14. A. Gore, *Chemicals in our daily lives are hurting us - here's how* (Save the Corals, February 26, 2020). https://savethecorals.club/the-oxybenzone-magazine/chemicals-in-our-daily-lives-hurting-us-abc-science

15. *Estrogen: Hormone, function, levels and imbalances* (Cleveland Clinic, August 2, 2022). https://my.clevelandclinic.org/health/body/22353-estrogen

16. See note 13.

17. D.Y. Kim, S.H. Chun, Y. Jung, D.F.M.S. Mohamed, H.S. Kim, D.Y. Kang, J.W. An, S.Y. Park, H.W. Kwon, and J.H. Kwon, "Phthalate plasticizers in children's products and estimation of exposure: Importance of migration rate," *International Journal of Environmental Research and Public Health* 17, no. 22 (2020): 8582. doi: 10.3390/ijerph17228582

18. Joe Schwarcz, *Turning up the heat on thermal paper receipts* (Montreal: Office for Science and Society, McGill University, February 25, 2020). https://www.mcgill.ca/oss/article/health/turning-heat-thermal-paper-receipts

19. S. Ndaw, A. Remy, D. Jargot, and A. Robert, "Occupational exposure of cashiers to bisphenol A via thermal paper: Urinary biomonitoring study," *International Archives on Occupational and Environmental Health* 89, no. 6 (2016): 935–46. doi: 10.1007/s00420-016-1132-8

20. M.A. Mehlman, "Dangerous and cancer-causing properties of products and chemicals in the oil refining and petrochemical industry: Part I. Carcinogenicity of motor fuels: Gasoline," *Toxicology and Industrial Health* 7, no. 5–6 (1991): 143–52. doi: 10.1177/074823379100700516

21. R. Snyder, "Leukemia and benzene," *International Journal of Environmental Research and Public Health* 9, no. 8 (2012): 2875-93. doi: 10.3390/ijerph9082875

22. V.A. Benignus, "Health effects of toluene: A review," *Neurotoxicology* 2, no. 3 (1981): 567-68.

23. *The Hazards of* DEET (EHANS, Spring 2003). https://www.environmentalhealth.ca/spring03hazards.html

24. See note 23.

25. HauteCoton, *Detox your sleep: 7 toxic chemicals in your bedding and safer alternatives* (HauteCoton, September 11, 2019). https://hautecoton.com/blogs/news/detox-your-sleep-7-toxic-chemicals-in-your-bedding-safer-alternatives

26. W.A. Chiu, J. Jinot, C.S. Scott, S.L. Makris, G.S. Cooper, R.C. Dzubow, A.S. Bale, M.V. Evans, K.Z. Guyton, N. Keshava, J.C. Lipscomb, S. Barone Jr, J.F. Fox, M.R. Gwinn, J. Schaum, and J.C. Caldwell, "Human health effects of trichloroethylene: Key findings and scientific issues," *Environmental Health Perspectives* 121, no. 3 (2013): 303-11. doi: 10.1289/ehp.1205879

27. G.W. Hoyle and E.R. Svendsen, "Persistent effects of chlorine inhalation on respiratory health," *Annals of the New York Academy of Science* 1378, no. 1 (2016): 33-40. doi: 10.1111/nyas.13139

28. *Petroleum distillates: Substance* (Washington: Environmental Working Group, n.d.). https://www.ewg.org/guides/substances/4384-PETROLEUMDISTILLATES/

29. See note 26.

30. Centers for Disease Control and Prevention, *Hydrogen chloride* (Centers for Disease Control and Prevention, October 21, 2014). https://wwwn.cdc.gov/TSP/MMG/MMGDetails.aspx?mmgid=758&toxid=147#:~:text=Ingestion%20of%20concentrated%20hydrochloric%20acid%20can%20also%20cause%20severe%20corrosive,stricture%20formation%20as%20potential%20sequelae.&text=Liver%20damage%20and%20ischemia%20may%20be%20observed.&text=Renal%20failure%20and%20nephritis%20may%20occur

31. *Carcinogens in cosmetics* (Safe Cosmetics, April 26, 2022). https://www.safecosmetics.org/chemicals/known-carcinogens/

32. See note 31.

33. CBC/Radio Canada, FAQs | *Canada's rules for organic food* (CBC News, December 8, 2011). https://www.cbc.ca/news/canada/faqs-canada-s-rules-for-organic-food-1.985587

34. E. Jackson, R. Shoemaker, N. Larian, and L. Cassis, "Adipose tissue as a site of toxin accumulation," *Comparative Physiology* 4, no. 4 (2017): 1085-35. doi: 10.1002/cphy.c160038. Erratum in *Comparative Physiology* 18, no. 3 (2018): 1251.

35. S.C. Segerstrom, "Stress, energy, and immunity: An ecological view," *Current Directions in Psychological Science* 16, no. 6 (2007): 326-30. doi: 10.1111/j.1467-8721.2007.00522.x

36. See note 35.

37. M.J. Marmura, "Triggers, protectors, and predictors in episodic migraine," *Current Pain and Headache Reports* 22, no. 12 (2018): 81. doi: 10.1007/s11916-018-0734-0

38. A.K. Choudhary and Y.Y. Lee, "Neurophysiological symptoms and aspartame: What is the connection?" *Nutritional Neuroscience* 21, no. 5 (2018): 306-16. doi: 10.1080/1028415X.2017.1288340

39. G.H. Sands, L. Newman, and R. Lipton, "Cough, exertional, and other miscellaneous headaches," *Medical Clinics of North America* 75, no. 3 (1991): 733-47. doi: 10.1016/s0025-7125(16)30446-1

40. R. Rettner, *12 worst hormone-disrupting chemicals and their health effects* (LiveScience, January 27, 2022). https://www.livescience.com/40733-hormone-disrupting-chemicals-health.html

41. D.V. Parke and A.L. Parke, "Chemical-induced inflammation and inflammatory diseases," *International Journal of Occupational Medicine and Environmental Health* 9, no. 3 (1996): 211-17.

42. N. Hasan, *6 signs you have a weakened immune system* (Pennmedicine.org, February 15, 2022). https://www.pennmedicine.org/updates/blogs/health-and-wellness/2020/march/weakened-immune-system#:~:text=It%27s%20perfectly%20normal%20for%20adults,Hasan

43. See note 42.
44. A.D. Sperber et al., "Worldwide prevalence and burden of functional gastrointestinal disorders: Results of Rome Foundation Global Study," *Gastroenterology* 160, no. 1 (2021): 99–114. doi: 10.1053/j.gastro.2020.04.014
45. *The gut-brain connection* (Harvard Health, April 19, 2021). https://www.health.harvard.edu/diseases-and-conditions/the-gut-brain-connection#:~:text=A%20troubled%20intestine%20can%20send,GI)%20system%20are%20intimately%20connected
46. Healthline Media, *Improve gut health: Recognize the signs of an unhealthy gut* (Healthline, June 1, 2022). https://www.healthline.com/health/gut-health
47. G. Vighi, F. Marcucci, L. Sensi, G. Di Cara, and F. Frati, "Allergy and the gastrointestinal system," *Clinical and Experimental Immunology* 153, Suppl 1 (2008): 3–6. doi: 10.1111/j.1365-2249.2008.03713.x
48. See note 47.
49. A.N.R. and N.B. Rafiq, *Candidiasis* (Treasure Island, FL: StatPearls Publishing, August 7, 2022).
50. M. Scanlan, *Is your sugar addiction feeding your intestinal candida? A path to natural health* (Naturopathic Doctors, n.d.). https://www.apathtonaturalhealth.com/blog/is-your-sugar-addiction-feeding-your-intestinal-candida#:~:text=When%20you%20have%20an%20organism,crave%20more%20and%20more%20sugar
51. A. Erdogan and S.S. Rao, "Small intestinal fungal overgrowth," *Currents in Gastroenterology Reports* 17, no. 4 (2015): 16. doi: 10.1007/s11894-015-0436-2
52. J.P. Richardson and D.L. Moyes, "Adaptive immune responses to Candida albicans infection," *Virulence* 6, no. 4 (2015): 327–37. doi: 10.1080/21505594.2015.1004977
53. C. Dean, *Dr. Carolyn Dean on yeast and magnesium* (Hotze Health & Wellness Center, January 27, 2022). https://www.hotzehwc.com/blog/dr-carolyn-dean-on-yeast-and-magnesium/
54. N. Terry and K.G. Margolis, "Serotonergic mechanisms regulating the GI tract: Experimental evidence and therapeutic relevance," *Handbook of Experimental Pharmacology* 239 (2017): 319–42. doi: 10.1007/164_2016_103
55. A.L. Roy and R.S. Conroy, "Toward mapping the human body at a cellular resolution," *Molecular Biology of the Cell* 29, no. 15 (2018): 1779–85. doi:10.1091/mbc.e18-04-0260
56. R. Sender, S. Fuchs, and R. Milo, "Revised estimates for the number of human and bacteria cells in the body," *PLOS Biology* 14, no. 8 (2016): e1002533. doi: 10.1371/journal.pbio.1002533
57. J. Cafasso, *How many cells are in the human body? Fast facts* (Healthline, July 18, 2018). https://www.healthline.com/health/number-of-cells-in-body#daily-cell-death
58. D. Bethesda, *Blood groups and red cell antigens* (National Center for Biotechnology Information, 2005). https://www.ncbi.nlm.nih.gov/books

CHAPTER 8: MODERN FOOD AND WATER

1. F. Spritzler, 6 *"toxins" in food that are actually concerning* (Healthline, May 23, 2016). https://www.healthline.com/nutrition/food-toxins-that-are-concerning#TOC_TITLE_HDR_3
2. *EWG's 2022 shopper's guide to pesticides in produce™:* Summary (April 7, 2022). https://www.ewg.org/foodnews/summary.php
3. See note 2.
4. *SmartGreen Post,* "Pesticides, the list of the most contaminated fruits and vegetables," *SmartGreen Post,* March 20, 2021. https://www.smartgreenpost.com/2021/03/20/pesticides-the-list-of-the-most-contaminated-fruits-and-vegetables/
5. See note 4.
6. See note 2.
7. *Scientific American,* "Dirt poor: Have fruits and vegetables become less nutritious?" *Scientific American,* April 27, 2011. https://www.scientificamerican.com/article/soil-depletion-and-nutrition-loss/

8. C. Cuneo, "Is an orange of the 1950's equivalent to 21 of today's oranges?" *soscuisine*, February 16, 2015. https://www.soscuisine.com/blog/orange-1950s-equivalent-21-todays-oranges/#:~:text=An%20orange%20from%20the%201950%27s,The%20iron%20content%20in%20meat%3F

9. D.R. Davis, M.D. Epp, and H.D. Riordan, "Changes in USDA food composition data for 43 garden crops, 1950 to 1999," *Journal of the American College of Nutritionists* 23, no. 6 (2004): 669–82. doi: 10.1080/07315724.2004.10719409

10. See note 9.

11. See note 9.

12. L. Fulkerson, *Forks Over Knives* [documentary] (Forks Over Knives, May 20, 2011). https://www.forksoverknives.com/the-film/

13. R. Patrob, *Diet – where your ancestral heritage is important* (Michael Rose's 55, June 16, 2011). https://55theses.org/2011/06/16/diet-where-your-racial-heritage-is-important/

14. H. Kim, L.E. Caulfield, V. Garcia-Larsen, L.M. Steffen, J. Coresh, and C.M. Rebholz, "Plant-based diets are associated with a lower risk of incident cardiovascular disease, cardiovascular disease mortality, and all-cause mortality in a general population of middle-aged adults," *Journal of the American Heart Association* 8, no. 16 (2019): e012865. doi: 10.1161/JAHA.119.012865

15. Y. Zheng, Y. Li, A. Satija, A. Pan, M. Sotos-Prieto, E. Rimm, W.C. Willett, and F.B. Hu, "Association of changes in red meat consumption with total and cause specific mortality among US women and men: Two prospective cohort studies," *British Medical Journal* 12, no. 365 (2019): 2110. doi: 10.1136/bmj.l2110

16. *5 surprising polyrhachis ant benefits* (Healthy Huemans, September 17, 2021). https://healthyhuemans.com/polyrhachis-ant-benefits/

17. J. Kou, Y. Ni, N. Li, J. Wang, L. Liu, and Z.H. Jiang, "Analgesic and anti-inflammatory activities of total extract and individual fractions of Chinese medicinal ants Polyrhachis lamellidens," *Biological and Pharmaceutical Bulletin* 28, no. 1 (2005): 176–80. doi: 10.1248/bpb.28.176. PMID: 15635188

18. See note 16.

19. T. Duan, N. Bi, and M. Huang, "The treatment of intrauterine growth retardation with ant polyrhachis vicina roge," *Zhonghua Fu Chan Ke Za Zhi* 34, no. 5 (1999): 290–92.

20. K. Doheny, *Drugs in our drinking water?* (WebMD, March 10, 2008). https://www.webmd.com/a-to-z-guides/features/drugs-in-our-drinking-water#:~:text=According%20to%20the%20investigation%2C%20the,out%20in%20urine%20or%20feces

21. G.C. White, *The handbook of chlorination* (Van Nostrand Reinhold, 1986).

22. C.M. Villanueva, F. Fernánde, N. Malats, J.O. Grimalt, and M. Kogevinas, "Meta-analysis of studies on individual consumption of chlorinated drinking water and bladder cancer," *Journal of Epidemiology and Community Health* 57, no. 3 (2003): 166–73. doi: 10.1136/jech.57.3.166. Erratum in *Journal of Epidemiology and Community Health* 59, no. 1 (2005): 87.

23. Centers for Disease Control and Prevention, *Water fluoridation basics* (Centers for Disease Control and Prevention, October 1, 2021). https://www.cdc.gov/fluoridation/basics/index.htm#:~:text=For%20adults%2C%20drinking%20water%20with,Less%20severe%20cavities

24. R. Ullah, M.S. Zafar, and N. Shahani, "Potential fluoride toxicity from oral medicaments: A review," *Iranian Journal of Basic Medical Sciences* 20, no. 8 (2017): 841–48. doi: 10.22038/IJBMS.2017.9104

25. P. Grandjean, "Developmental fluoride neurotoxicity: An updated review," *Environmental Health* 18, no. 1 (2019): 110. doi: 10.1186/s12940-019-0551-x

26. M. Bhatia, "Is RO (reverse osmosis) drinking water really harmful?" *Times of India* blog, June 29, 2021. https://timesofindia.indiatimes.com/readersblog/manufocus/is-ro-reverse-osmosis-drinking-water-really-harmful-34395/

27. Doctors Beyond Medicine, *World Health Organization issues reverse osmosis water warning* (n.d.). https://www.doctorsbeyondmedicine.com/listing/world-health-organization-issues-reverse-osmosis-water-warning

28. Doctors Beyond Medicine, *What water should I drink* (n.d.). https://www.doctorsbeyondmedicine.com/listing/what-water-should-i-drink

29. CBC/Radio Canada, "Plastic bottles leach chemicals into water: Study," CBC *News*, December 21, 2006. https://www.cbc.ca/news/plastic-bottles-leach-chemicals-into-water-study-1.605134#:~:text=The%20longer%20water%20is%20stored,chemical%2C%20a%20new%20study%20suggests

30. WestchesterGov.com, *Bisphenol-A (BPA): BPA and phthalates* (White Plains, NY: Westchester County, n.d.). https://health.westchestergov.com/bisphenol-a-and-phthalates#:~:text=Bisphenol%2DA%20(commonly%20known%20as,sippy%20cups%2C%20pacifiers%20and%20teethers

31. See note 30.

32. B.A. Bauer, *What is BPA, and what are the concerns about BPA?* Mayo Clinic, March 8, 2022. https://www.mayoclinic.org/healthy-lifestyle/nutrition-and-healthy-eating/expert-answers/bpa/faq-20058331#:~:text=Exposure%20to%20BPA%20is%20a,2%20diabetes%20and%20cardiovascular%20disease

33. See note 30.

34. S. Eladak, T. Grisin, D. Moison, M.J. Guerquin, T. N'Tumba-Byn, S. Pozzi-Gaudin, A. Benachi, G. Livera, V. Rouiller-Fabre, and R. Habert, "A new chapter in the bisphenol A story: Bisphenol S and bisphenol F are not safe alternatives to this compound," *Fertility and Sterility* 103, no. 1 (2015): 11–21. doi: 10.1016/j.fertnstert.2014.11.005

35. See note 32.

CHAPTER 9: LEARNING THE LANGUAGE OF THE GI SYSTEM

1. P. Enck et al., "Irritable bowel syndrome," *Nature Reviews Disease Primers* 24, no. 2 (2016): 16014. doi: 10.1038/nrdp.2016.14

2. Y. Endo, T. Shoji, and S. Fukudo, "Epidemiology of irritable bowel syndrome," *Annals of Gastroenterology* 28 no. 2 (2015): 158–59.

3. American Optometric Association, *Do no harm: A case study on overprescribing* (November 5, 2020). https://www.aoa.org/news/clinical-eye-care/public-health/case-study-on-overprescribing?sso=y#:~:text=The%20case%20study%20defines%20overprescribing,with%20limited%20potential%20to%20benefit.%E2%80%9D

4. I.B. Moura, A. Grada, W. Spittal, E. Clark, D. Ewin, J. Altringham, E. Fumero, M.H. Wilcox, and A.M. Buckley, *Profiling the effects of systemic antibiotics for acne, including the narrow-spectrum antibiotic sarecycline, on the human gut microbiota.* Frontiers, May 9, 2022. https://www.frontiersin.org/articles/10.3389/fmicb.2022.901911/full

5. J. Maret-Ouda, S.R. Markar, and J. Lagergren, "Gastroesophageal reflux disease," *Journal of the American Medical Association* 324, no. 24 (2020): 2565. doi:10.1001/jama.2020.21573

6. National Institute of Diabetes and Digestive and Kidney Diseases, *Definition and facts for gallstones* (U.S. Department of Health and Human Services, November 2017). https://www.niddk.nih.gov/health-information/digestive-diseases/gallstones/definition-facts

7. Celiac Disease Foundation, *What is celiac disease?* (n.d.). https://celiac.org/about-celiac-disease/what-is-celiac-disease/

8. Beyond Celiac: Together for a Cure, *Celiac disease: Fast facts* (November 14, 2022). https://www.beyondceliac.org/celiac-disease/facts-and-figures/#:~:text=An%20estimated%201%20in%20133,celiac%20disease%20to%20be%201.6%25

9. See note 8.

10. Crohn's & Colitis Foundation, *Causes of Crohn's disease* (n.d.). https://www.crohnscolitisfoundation.org/what-is-crohns-disease/causes

11. Crohn's and Colitis Foundation of America, *The facts about inflammatory bowel diseases* (New York: Crohn's and Colitis Foundation of America, 2014).

12. See note 11.

13. National Institute of Diabetes and Digestive and Kidney Diseases, *Treatment for irritable bowel syndrome* (U.S. Department of Health and Human Services, November 2017). https://www.niddk.nih.gov/health-information/digestive-diseases/irritable-bowel-syndrome/treatment#:~:text=Doctors%20may%20treat%20irritable%20bowel,find%20the%20right%20treatment%20plan

14. H.Y. Qin, C.W. Cheng, X.D. Tang, and Z.X. Bian, "Impact of psychological stress on irritable bowel syndrome," *World Journal of Gastroenterology* 20, no. 39 (2014): 14126–31. doi: 10.3748/wjg.v20.i39.14126

15. H.G. Veloso, *FODMAP diet: What you need to know* (Johns Hopkins Medicine, December 29, 2021). https://www.hopkinsmedicine.org/health/wellness-and-prevention/fodmap-diet-what-you-need-to-know#:~:text=When%20people%20say%20%E2%80%9CFODMAP%20diet,and%20which%20foods%20reduce%20symptoms

16. C. Canavan, J. West, and T. Card, "The epidemiology of irritable bowel syndrome," *Clinical Epidemiology* 4, no. 6 (2014): 71–80. doi: 10.2147/CLEP.S40245

17. A. Fox, P.H. Tietze, and K. Ramakrishnan, "Anorectal conditions: Hemorrhoids," FP *Essentials* 419 (2014): 11–19.

18. A.T. Hawkins et al., "Diverticulitis: An update from the age old paradigm," *Current Problems in Surgery* 57, no. 10 (2020): 100862. doi: 10.1016/j.cpsurg.2020.100862

19. See note 18.

20. T.H. Lee et al., "Aging, obesity, and the incidence of diverticulitis: A population-based study," *Mayo Clinic Proceedings* 93, no. 9 (2018): 1256–65. doi: 10.1016/j.mayocp.2018.03.005

21. See note 18.

22. UCSF Health. (2022, June 24). *Anal fissures*. ucsfhealth.org. https://www.ucsfhealth.org/education/anal-fissures

23. National Institute of Diabetes and Digestive and Kidney Diseases, *Your digestive system and how it works* (U.S. Department of Health and Human Services, December 2017). https://www.niddk.nih.gov/health-information/digestive-diseases/digestive-system-how-it-works#:~:text=The%20digestive%20process%20starts%20in,down%20starches%20in%20your%20food

24. T. Bhatia, *Using collagen to heal and seal a leaky gut* (Dr. Taz, MD, Integrative Medicine, June 1, 2021). https://doctortaz.com/heal-leaky-gut-with-collagen/

25. D.J. Axe, *Bone broth benefits for joints, gut, skin* (Dr. Axe, December 16, 2022). https://draxe.com/nutrition/bone-broth-benefits/

26. N. Larsen, C. Bussolo de Souza, L. Krych, T. Barbosa Cahú, M. Wiese, W. Kot, K.M. Hansen, A. Blennow, K. Venema, and L. Jespersen, "Potential of pectins to beneficially modulate the gut microbiota depends on their structural properties," *Frontiers in Microbiology* 10 (2019): 223. doi: 10.3389/fmicb.2019.00223

27. N. Alammar, L. Wang, B. Saberi, J. Nanavati, G. Holtmann, R.T. Shinohara, and G.E. Mullin, "The impact of peppermint oil on the irritable bowel syndrome: A meta-analysis of the pooled clinical data," BMC *Complementary and Alternative Medicine* 19, no. 1 (2019): 21. doi: 10.1186/s12906-018-2409-0

28. L. Zong, Y. Qu, D.X. Luo, Z.Y. Zhu, S. Zhang, Z. Su, J.C. Shan, X.P. Gao, and L.G. Lu, "Preliminary experimental research on the mechanism of liver bile secretion stimulated by peppermint oil," *Journal of Digestive Disorders* 12, no. 4 (2011): 295–301. doi: 10.1111/j.1751-2980.2011.00513.x

29. I. Lete and J. Allué, "The effectiveness of ginger in the prevention of nausea and vomiting during pregnancy and chemotherapy," *Integrative Medical Insights* 31, no. 11 (2016): 11–17. doi: 10.4137/IMI.S36273

30. J. Leech, *11 scientifically proven health benefits of ginger* (Healthline, March 18, 2021). https://www.healthline.com/nutrition/11-proven-benefits-of-ginger#6.-Can-help-treat-chronic-indigestion

31. E. Cronkleton, *Ginger for arthritis: Does it work?* (Healthline, April 4, 2017). https://www.healthline.com/health/ginger-for-arthritis#:~:text=Ginger%20has%20 anti%2Dinflammatory%2C%20antioxidant,way%20as%20COX%2D2%20inhibitors

32. D. Yagnik, V. Serafin, and A. Shah, "Antimicrobial activity of apple cider vinegar against Escherichia coli, Staphylococcus aureus and Candida albicans: Downregulating cytokine and microbial protein expression," *Scientific Reports* 8, no. 1 (2018): 1732. doi: 10.1038/s41598-017-18618-x

33. S. Moore, *Rebounding – Superfood Sarah* (Sarah Moore Health, December 28, 2015). http://www.sarahmoorehealth.com/blog/tag/rebounding

34. Integrated Health Blog, *Rebounding for detoxification* (Washington: National Integrated Health Associates, May 29, 2012). https://info.nihadc.com/integrative-health-blog/bid/56530/Rebounding-for-Detoxification

35. Cellercise, *How many minutes per day should you rebound?* (October 31, 2021). https://cellercise.com/blog/how-many-minutes-per-day-should-you-rebound/#:~:text=Ten%20 minutes%20of%20rebounding%20offers,effectiveness%20of%20your%20other%20 workouts

36. Cleveland Clinic, *Gut-brain Connection: What it is, behavioral treatments* (March 12, 2020). https://my.clevelandclinic.org/health/treatments/16358-gut-brain-connection#:~:text=This%20%E2%80%9Ccrosstalk%E2%80%9D%20in%20 communication%20between,regulate%20the%20body%27s%20immune%20response

37. Harvard Health, *The gut-brain connection* (April 19, 2021). https://www.health.harvard.edu/diseases-and-conditions/the-gut-brain-connection#:~:text=Therefore%2C%20a%20 person%27s%20stomach%20or,GI)%20system%20are%20intimately%20connected

38. Colleen De Bellefonds, *Everything you need to know about how stress can impact your gut health* (Well + Good, November 9, 2022). https://www.wellandgood.com/stress-gut-health/

39. K. Gunnars, *FODMAP 101* (Healthline, December 15, 2021). https://www.healthline.com/nutrition/fodmaps-101

40. A. Shil and H. Chichger, "Artificial sweeteners negatively regulate pathogenic characteristics of two model gut bacteria, *E. coli* and *E. faecalis*," *International Journal of Molecular Science* 22, no. 10 (2021): 5228. doi: 10.3390/ijms22105228

41. Alexa Lardieri, *Study: Artificial sweeteners toxic to digestive gut bacteria* (CNBC, October 4, 2018). https://www.cnbc.com/2018/10/03/artificial-sweeteners-are-toxic-to-digestive-gut-bacteria-study.html

42. See note 41.

43. Y.M. Chang, M. El-Zaatari, and J.Y. Kao, "Does stress induce bowel dysfunction?" *Expert Review of Gastroenterology and Hepatology* 8, no. 6 (2014): 583–85. doi: 10.1586/17474124.2014.911659

44. J. Gonenne, T. Esfandyari, M. Camilleri, D.D. Burton, D.A. Stephens, K.L. Baxter, A.R. Zinsmeister, and A.E. Bharucha, "Effect of female sex hormone supplementation and withdrawal on gastrointestinal and colonic transit in postmenopausal women," *Neurogastroenterology and Motility* 18, no. 10 (2006): 911–18. doi: 10.1111/j.1365-2982.2006.00808.x

45. M.M. Heitkemper and L. Chang, "Do fluctuations in ovarian hormones affect gastrointestinal symptoms in women with irritable bowel syndrome?" *Gender Medicine* 6 (Suppl 2) (2009): 152–67. doi: 10.1016/j.genm.2009.03.004

46. D. Vandeputte, G. Falony, S. Vieira-Silva, R.Y. Tito, M. Joossens, and J. Raes, "Stool consistency is strongly associated with gut microbiota richness and composition, enterotypes and bacterial growth rates," *Gut* 65, no. 1 (2016): 57–62. doi: 10.1136/gutjnl-2015-309618

47. B. Jani and E. Marsicano, "Constipation: Evaluation and management," *Missouri Medicine* 115, no. 3 (2018): 236–40.

48. Y. Li, J. Cui, Y. Liu, K. Chen, L. Huang, and Y. Liu, "Oral, tongue-coating microbiota, and metabolic disorders: A novel area of interactive research," *Frontiers of Cardiovascular Medicine* 20, no. 8 (2021): 730203. doi: 10.3389/fcvm.2021.730203

49. Rosie Fitzmaurice, "How your tongue can show signs of gut problems and why you should scrape it every day," *Evening Standard*, August 23, 2019. https://www.standard.co.uk/lifestyle/tongue-scraping-diagnosis-wellbeing-a4083956.html

50. The Wellness Principle, *How to diagnose a tongue in traditional Chinese medicine* (The Wellness Principle, August 22, 2022). https://www.tcmwellnessprinciple.com/blog/traditional-chinese-medicine-tongue-diagnosis#:~:text=The%20ideal%20tongue%20should%20be,a%20clue%20to%20an%20imbalance

51. H.J. Miller, "Dehydration in the older adult," *Journal of Gerontological Nursing* 41, no. 9 (2015): 8–13. doi: 10.3928/00989134-20150814-02

52. Calm Clinic, *Anxiety issues and bowel problems* (March 1, 2021). https://www.calmclinic.com/anxiety/symptoms/bowel-problems

53. R. Gao, Y. Tao, C. Zhou, J. Li, X. Wang, L. Chen, F. Li, and L. Guo, "Exercise therapy in patients with constipation: A systematic review and meta-analysis of randomized controlled trials," *Scandinavian Journal of Gastroenterology* 54, no. 2 (2019): 169–77. doi:10.1080/00365521.2019.1568544

54. E.P. de Oliveira and R.C. Burini, "The impact of physical exercise on the gastrointestinal tract," *Current Opinion in Clinical Nutrition and Metabolic Care* 12, no. 5 (2009): 533–38. doi: 10.1097/MCO.0b013e32832e6776

55. S. Bunyavanich and M.C. Berin, "Food allergy and the microbiome: Current understandings and future directions," *Journal of Allergy and Clinical Immunology* 144, no. 6 (2019): 1468–77. doi:10.1016/j.jaci.2019.10.019

56. S.J. Lewis and K.W. Heaton, "Stool Form Scale as a useful guide to intestinal transit time," *Scandinavian Journal of Gastroenterology* 32, no. 9 (1997): 920–24. doi: 10.3109/00365529709011203

57. M.R. Blake, J.M. Rake, and K. Whelan, "Validity and reliability of the Bristol Stool Form Scale in healthy adults and patients with diarrhoea-predominant irritable bowel syndrome," *Alimentary Pharmacology and Therapeutics* 44, no. 7 (2016): 693–703. doi: 10.1111/apt.13746

PART III: SELF-OPTIMIZATION

1. World Health Organization, *Constitution of the World Health Organization* (Geneva: WHO, 1947). https://www.who.int/about/governance/constitution#:~:text=Health%20is%20a%20state%20of,belief%2C%20economic%20or%20social%20condition

CHAPTER 10: ENERGY MANAGEMENT

1. Centers for Disease Control and Prevention, *Rhabdomyolysis* (U.S. Department of Health and Human Services, April 22, 2019). https://www.cdc.gov/niosh/topics/rhabdo/

2. Alan S. Cowen and Dacher Keltner, *Self-report captures 27 distinct categories of emotion bridged by continuous gradients* (U.S. National Library of Medicine, September 5, 2017). https://pubmed.ncbi.nlm.nih.gov/28874542/

3. Soryu Forall, *The Center for Mindful Learning*, 2021. https://www.centerformindfullearning.org/

4. Harriet Cabelly, *Rebuild life now*, October 15, 2018. https://rebuildlifenow.com/

5. Tara L. Kraft and Sarah D. Pressman, "Grin and bear it," *Psychological Science* 23, no. 11 (2012): 1372–78. doi:10.1177/0956797612445312

CHAPTER 11: ENERGY FIELDS AND VIBRATIONAL FREQUENCY

1. H. Treugut, M. Köppen, B. Nickolay, R. Füß, and P. Schmid, "Kirlian-Fotografie: Zufälliges Oder Personenspezifisches Entladungsmuster?" *Complementary Medicine Research* 7, no. 1 (2000): 12–16. doi:10.1159/000057163
2. Rachael Towne, "What is Kirlian photography? Aura photography revealed," *Light Stalking*, March 26, 2020. https://www.lightstalking.com/what-is-kirlian-photography-the-science-and-the-myth-revealed/
3. B. Proctor, *Leave everyone with the impression of increase* (Scottsdale, AZ: Proctor Gallagher Institute, March 23, 2020). https://www.proctorgallagherinstitute.com/video/leave-everyone-with-the-impression-of-increase-bob-proctor
4. "Luke 6:38." Essay. In *King James Bible*, NIV (Nashville, TN: Thomas Nelson, 1991).
5. Roger Nelson, *The Global Consciousness Project* (Princeton, NJ: Trustees of Princeton University, 1998). https://noosphere.princeton.edu/
6. Roger Nelson, *The Global Consciousness Project: Introduction* (Princeton, NJ: Trustees of Princeton University, 1998). https://noosphere.princeton.edu/introduction.html#:~:text=The%20probability%20that%20the%20effect,weak%20to%20be%20reliably%20interpreted
7. Mihaly Csikszentmihalyi, *Flow: The psychology of optimal experience* (New York: Harper and Row, 2009).
8. Napoleon Hill, *Think and grow rich* (Vrindavan, India: Classy Publishing, 2021).
9. Arne Dietrich, "Neurocognitive mechanisms underlying the experience of flow," *Consciousness and Cognition* 13, no. 4 (2004): 746–61. doi:10.1016/j.concog.2004.07.002
10. Tom Peters, "Tom Peters quotes," *BrainyQuote* (Xplore, 2023). https://www.brainyquote.com/quotes/tom_peters_130731
11. Roy F. Baumeister and John Tierney, *Willpower: Rediscovering the greatest human strength* (New York: Penguin, 2012).
12. N. Naqvi, B. Shiv, and A. Bechara, "The role of emotion in decision making: A cognitive neuroscience perspective," *Current Directions in Psychological Science* 15, no. 5 (2006): 260–64. https://doi.org/10.1111/j.1467-8721.2006.00448.x
13. Vanity Fair, "Barack Obama to Michael Lewis on a presidential loss of freedom: 'You don't get used to it—at least, I don't'" (*Vanity Fair*, September 5, 2012). https://www.vanityfair.com/news/2012/09/barack-obama-michael-lewis

CHAPTER 12: HAPPINESS

1. Maharishi University, *Jim Carrey at MIU: Commencement address at the 2014 graduation.* YouTube, 2014. https://www.youtube.com/watch?v=v80-gPkpH6M
2. "Hedonic Treadmill," *Psychology Today*, 2023. https://www.psychologytoday.com/us/basics/hedonic-treadmill#:~:text=The%20hedonic%20treadmill%20is%20the,was%20prior%20to%20these%20experiences
3. Rick Hanson, *Hardwiring happiness* (New York: Random House, 2015).
4. See note 3.
5. Bronnie Ware, "Top five regrets of the dying," *Guardian*, February 1, 2012. https://www.theguardian.com/lifeandstyle/2012/feb/01/top-five-regrets-of-the-dying
6. See note 5.
7. David Lykken and Auke Tellegen, "Happiness is a stochastic phenomenon," *Psychological Science* 7, no. 3 (1996): 186–89. doi:10.1111/j.1467-9280.1996.tb00355.x
8. Martin Seligman, *Flourish: A visionary new understanding of happiness and well-being* (New York: Atria, 2013).
9. Seph Fontane Pennock, "Positive Psychology 1504: Harvard's groundbreaking course," *PositivePsychology.com*, November 26, 2022. https://positivepsychology.com/harvards-1504-positive-psychology-course/

10. Alaa Elassar, "Two years into the pandemic, Yale's 'Happiness' course is more popular than ever," *CNN*, January 23, 2022. https://www.cnn.com/2022/01/23/us/yale-happiness-course-pandemic-wellness/index.html

11. "Happiness," definition and meaning, *Merriam-Webster*, 2023. https://www.merriam-webster.com/dictionary/happiness

12. "Joy," definition and meaning, *Merriam-Webster*, 2023. https://www.merriam-webster.com/dictionary/joy

13. Dan Harris, *10% happier* (New York: It Books, 2014).

14. See note 3.

15. L.S. Berk, D.L. Felten, S.A. Tan, B.B. Bittman, and J. Westengard, "Modulation of neuroimmune parameters during the eustress of humor-associated mirthful laughter," *Alternative Therapies in Health and Medicine* 7, no. 2 (2001): 62–72, 74–76.

16. Ingela Ratledge Amundson, "Smiling through trying times," *Time* magazine special edition: The power of joy, 2021.

17. See note 16.

18. See note 16.

19. See note 16.

20. B.K. Hölzel, S.W. Lazar, T. Gard, Z. Schuman-Olivier, D.R. Vago, and U. Ott, "How does mindfulness meditation work? Proposing mechanisms of action from a conceptual and neural perspective," *Perspectives on Psychological Science* 6, no. 6 (2011): 537–59. doi: 10.1177/1745691611419671

21. M.T. Treadway and S.W. Lazar, "The neurobiology of mindfulness," in *Clinical handbook of mindfulness* (New York: Springer, 2009), 45–57.

22. J. Linder, "5 ways mindfulness practice positively changes your brain," *Psychology Today*, May 9, 2019. https://www.psychologytoday.com/ca/blog/mindfulness-insights/201905/5-ways-mindfulness-practice-positively-changes-your-brain

23. A. Crego, J.R. Yela, M.A. Gómez-Martínez, P. Riesco-Matías, and C. Petisco-Rodríguez, "Relationships between mindfulness, purpose in life, happiness, anxiety, and depression: Testing a mediation model in a sample of women," *International Journal of Environmental Research and Public Health* 18, no. 3 (2021): 925. doi: 10.3390/ijerph18030925

24. C. Crowley, L.R. Kapitula, and D. Munk, "Mindfulness, happiness, and anxiety in a sample of college students before and after taking a meditation course," *Journal of the American College of Health* 70, no. 2 (2022): 493–500. doi: 10.1080/07448481.2020.1754839

25. N. Zarifsanaiey, K. Jamalian, L. Bazrafcan, F. Keshavarzy, and H.R. Shahraki, "The effects of mindfulness training on the level of happiness and blood sugar in diabetes patients," *Journal of Diabetes and Metabolic Disorders* 19, no. 1 (2020): 311–17. doi: 10.1007/s40200-020-00510-7

26. "Practicing daily gratitude to enhance health," *Moravian Manor Communities*, May 31, 2021. https://www.moravianmanorcommunities.org/practicing-daily-gratitude-to-enhance-health/#:~:text=Gratitude%20vibrates%20at%20540%20MHz,the%20healthier%20your%20body%20becomes

27. Paul Olivier and Maria Erving, "Gratitude and appreciation are two of the most powerful emotions you can have," *Maria Erving — Transformational teacher*, September 21, 2019. https://mariaerving.com/gratitude-highest-vibration/

28. Jill Leigh, *What is your vibration?* Energy Healing Institute, May 5, 2021. https://energyhealinginstitute.org/what-is-your-vibration/#:~:text=Guilt%2C%20Joy%20and%20other%20Emotions&text=When%20you%20hold%20yourself%20in,in%20a%20lethargic%20emotional%20quagmire

29. Gilles Varette, "Release the endorphins!" *LinkedIn*, December 23, 2020. https://linkedin.com/pulse/release-endorphins-gilles-varette-mbs-emcc-eia/

30. Dana R. Carney, Amy J.C. Cuddy, and Andy J. Yap, "Power posing," *Psychological Science* 21, no. 10 (2010): 1363–68. doi:10.1177/0956797610383437

31. Daniel Gilbert, *Stumbling on happiness* (London: Harper, 2007).

32. John Maltby, Christopher Alan Lewis, and Liza Day, "Religious orientation and psychological well-being: The role of the frequency of personal prayer," *British Journal of Health Psychology* 4, no. 4 (1999): 363–78. doi:10.1348/135910799168704

33. Andrew B. Newberg, "The neuroscientific study of spiritual practices," *Frontiers in Psychology* 5 (2014). doi:10.3389/fpsyg.2014.00215

34. Joan Domènech-Abella, Elvira Lara, Maria Rubio-Valera, Beatriz Olaya, Maria Victoria Moneta, Laura Alejandra Rico-Uribe, Jose Luis Ayuso-Mateos, Jordi Mundó, and Josep Maria Haro, "Loneliness and depression in the elderly: The role of social network," *Social Psychiatry and Psychiatric Epidemiology* 52, no. 4 (2017): 381–90. doi:10.1007/s00127-017-1339-3

35. Evren Erzen and Özkan Çikrikci, "The effect of loneliness on depression: A meta-analysis," *International Journal of Social Psychiatry* 64, no. 5 (2018): 427–35. doi:10.1177/0020764018776349

36. "About Loneliness," *Mind*, 2023. https://www.mind.org.uk/information-support/tips-for-everyday-living/loneliness/about-loneliness/#:~:text=Feeling%20lonely%20can%20also%20have,sleep%20problems%20and%20increased%20stress

37. Debra Umberson and Jennifer Karas Montez, "Social relationships and health: A flashpoint for health policy," *Journal of Health and Social Behavior* 51 (Suppl 1) (2010). doi:10.1177/0022146510383501

38. Oscar Ybarra, Eugene Burnstein, Piotr Winkielman, Matthew C. Keller, Melvin Manis, Emily Chan, and Joel Rodriguez, "Mental exercising through simple socializing: Social interaction promotes general cognitive functioning," *Personality and Social Psychology Bulletin* 34, no. 2 (2007): 248–59. doi:10.1177/0146167207310454

39. Aislinn Kotifani, "Moai—this tradition is why Okinawan people live longer, better," *Blue Zones*, September 26, 2022. https://www.bluezones.com/2018/08/moai-this-tradition-is-why-okinawan-people-live-longer-better/

40. See note 39.

41. See note 3.

CHAPTER 13: BRIDGING MIND AND BODY

1. Chrissy Sexton, "Electrical ear stimulation may help prevent age-related health issues," *Earth.com*, July 29, 2019. https://www.earth.com/news/electrical-ear-stimulation-health-issues/

2. See note 1.

3. Wei He, Xiaoyu Wang, Hong Shi, Hongyan Shang, Liang Li, Xianghong Jing, and Bing Zhu, "Auricular acupuncture and vagal regulation," *Evidence-Based Complementary and Alternative Medicine* (2012): 1–6. doi:10.1155/2012/786839

4. See note 3.

5. See note 3.

6. Morgan Clond, "Emotional freedom techniques for anxiety," *Journal of Nervous and Mental Disease* 204, no. 5 (2016): 388–95. doi:10.1097/nmd.0000000000000483

7. Brenda Sebastian and Jerrod Nelms, "The effectiveness of emotional freedom techniques in the treatment of posttraumatic stress disorder: A meta-analysis," *EXPLORE* 13, no. 1 (2017): 16–25. doi:10.1016/j.explore.2016.10.001

8. Peta Stapleton, Gabrielle Crighton, Debbie Sabot, and Hayley Maree O'Neill, "Reexamining the effect of emotional freedom techniques on stress biochemistry: A randomized controlled trial," *Psychological Trauma: Theory, Research, Practice, and Policy* 12, no. 8 (2020): 869–77. doi:10.1037/tra0000563

9. See note 6.

10. M. Goyal et al., "Meditation programs for psychological stress and well-being: A systematic review and meta-analysis," *Deutsche Zeitschrift Für Akupunktur* 57, no. 3 (2014): 26–27. doi:10.1016/j.dza.2014.07.007

11. Richard J. Davidson and Jon Kabat-Zinn, "Alterations in brain and immune function produced by mindfulness meditation: Three caveats: Response," *Psychosomatic Medicine* 66, no. 1 (2004): 149–52. doi:10.1097/00006842-200401000-00023

12. Peter Malinowski, Adam W. Moore, Bethan R. Mead, and Thomas Gruber, "Mindful aging: The effects of regular brief mindfulness practice on electrophysiological markers of cognitive and affective processing in older adults," *Mindfulness* 8, no. 1 (2015): 78–94. doi:10.1007/s12671-015-0482-8

13. So-An Lao, David Kissane, and Graham Meadows, "Cognitive effects of MBSR/MBCT: A systematic review of neuropsychological outcomes," *Consciousness and Cognition* 45 (2016): 109–23. doi:10.1016/j.concog.2016.08.017

14. Marta Alda, Marta Puebla-Guedea, Baltasar Rodero, Marcelo Demarzo, Jesus Montero-Marin, Miquel Roca, and Javier Garcia-Campayo, "Zen meditation, length of telomeres, and the role of experiential avoidance and compassion," *Mindfulness* 7, no. 3 (2016): 651–59. doi:10.1007/s12671-016-0500-5

15. Jason C. Ong, Rachel Manber, Zindel Segal, Yinglin Xia, Shauna Shapiro, and James K. Wyatt, "A randomized controlled trial of mindfulness meditation for chronic insomnia," *Sleep* 37, no. 9 (2014): 1553–63. doi:10.5665/sleep.4010

16. Napoleon Hill, *Think and grow rich* (Vrindavan, India: Classy Publishing, 2021).

17. Tiina M. Mäkinen, Matti Mäntysaari, Tiina Pääkkönen, Jari Jokelainen, Lawrence A. Palinkas, Juhani Hassi, Juhani Leppäluoto, Kari Tahvanainen, and Hannu Rintamäki, "Autonomic nervous function during whole-body cold exposure before and after cold acclimation," *Aviation, Space, and Environmental Medicine* 79, no. 9 (2008): 875–82. doi:10.3357/asem.2235.2008

18. See note 17.

19. Sigrid Breit, Aleksandra Kupferberg, Gerhard Rogler, and Gregor Hasler, "Vagus nerve as modulator of the brain–gut axis in psychiatric and inflammatory disorders," *Frontiers in Psychiatry* 9 (2018). doi:10.3389/fpsyt.2018.00044

20. Andrew Weil, "Breathwork," *Katie DiChiara — Wellness Facilitator*, 2023. https://ktdwellness.com/breathwork#:~:text=%E2%80%9CIf%20I%20had%20to%20limit,and%20well%20being%20than%20breathwork.%E2%80%9D

21. Jason Por Tan, Jessica Elise Beilharz, Uté Vollmer-Conna, and Erin Cvejic, "Heart rate variability as a marker of healthy ageing," *International Journal of Cardiology* 275 (2019): 101–3. doi:10.1016/j.ijcard.2018.08.005

22. Preeti Chandra et al., "Predictors of heart rate variability and its prognostic significance in chronic kidney disease," *Nephrology Dialysis Transplantation* 27, no. 2 (2011): 700–709. doi:10.1093/ndt/gfr340

23. Hye-Geum Kim, Eun-Jin Cheon, Dai-Seg Bai, Young Hwan Lee, and Bon-Hoon Koo, "Stress and heart rate variability: A meta-analysis and review of the literature," *Psychiatry Investigation* 15, no. 3 (2018): 235–45. doi:10.30773/pi.2017.08.17

24. M. Buchheit, C. Simon, F. Piquard, J. Ehrhart, and G. Brandenberger, "Effects of increased training load on vagal-related indexes of heart rate variability: A novel sleep approach," *American Journal of Physiology-Heart and Circulatory Physiology* 287, no. 6 (2004). doi:10.1152/ajpheart.00490.2004

25. Suh-Yeon Dong, Miran Lee, Heesu Park, and Inchan Youn, *Stress resilience measurement with heart-rate variability during mental and physical stress*, 40th Annual International Conference of the IEEE Engineering in Medicine and Biology Society (EMBC), 2018. doi:10.1109/embc.2018.8513531

26. Nikki Van der Velden, "The ideal breathing rate to maximize HRV? Research shows it's 5 to 7 breaths per minute," *Moonbird*, October 18, 2021. https://www.moonbird.life/magazine/ideal-breathing-rate/

27. "Self-care: The ingredients for health and happiness," *Health*, January 8, 2021.

28. Mathew P. White, Ian Alcock, James Grellier, Benedict W. Wheeler, Terry Hartig, Sara L. Warber, Angie Bone, Michael H. Depledge, and Lora E. Fleming, "Spending at least 120 minutes a week in nature is associated with good health and wellbeing," *Scientific Reports* 9, no. 1 (2019). doi:10.1038/s41598-019-44097-3

29. Rollin McCraty, Mike Atkinson, Viktor Stolc, Abdullah Alabdulgader, Alfonsas Vainoras, and Minvydas Ragulskis, "Synchronization of human autonomic nervous system rhythms with geomagnetic activity in human subjects," *International Journal of Environmental Research and Public Health* 14, no. 7 (2017): 770. doi:10.3390/ijerph14070770

30. Gaétan Chevalier, Stephen T. Sinatra, James L. Oschman, Karol Sokal, and Pawel Sokal, "Earthing: Health implications of reconnecting the human body to the earth's surface electrons," *Journal of Environmental and Public Health* (2012): 1–8. doi:10.1155/2012/291541

31. Mark Coleman and Karen Bouris, *Awake in the wild: Mindfulness in nature as a path of self-discovery* (Makawao, HI: Inner Ocean, 2017).

CHAPTER 14: SLEEP

1. *Better sleep for a better you*, Sleep Foundation, March 3, 2023. https://www.sleepfoundation.org/

2. Lawrence J. Epstein and Steven Mardon, *The Harvard Medical School guide to a good night's sleep* (New York: McGraw-Hill, 2007).

3. "How sleep influenced 5 major disasters," *Somnology MD*, September 22, 2021. https://www.somnologymd.com/2019/11/disasters-caused-by-lack-of-sleep/#:~:text=Exxon%20valdez%20spill&text=How%20sleep%20was%20Involved%3A%20The%20tanker's%20crew%20had%20been%20working,legally%20when%20the%20accident%20occurred

4. See note 3.

5. Charlie Walker, *Nuclear accidents and sleep deprivation*, May 24, 2017. http://large.stanford.edu/courses/2017/ph241/walker2/

6. Osamu Itani, Maki Jike, Norio Watanabe, and Yoshitaka Kaneita, "Short sleep duration and health outcomes: A systematic review, meta-analysis, and meta-regression," *Sleep Medicine* 32 (2017): 246–56. doi:10.1016/j.sleep.2016.08.006

7. See note 2.

8. See note 2.

9. Linda Searing, "18 percent of U.S. adults use medication to help them sleep," *Washington Post*, February 4, 2023. https://www.washingtonpost.com/wellness/2023/02/07/more-women-use-sleep-medication/

10. Stephanie Watson and Kristeen Cherney, "The effects of sleep deprivation on your body," *Healthline*, December 15, 2021. https://www.healthline.com/health/sleep-deprivation/effects-on-body

11. Hans J. Schmitt, *History of electroencephalography*, 2008 IEEE History of Telecommunications Conference. doi:10.1109/histelcon.2008.4668719

12. *REM sleep behavior disorder*, Mayo Foundation for Medical Education and Research, January 18, 2018. https://www.mayoclinic.org/diseases-conditions/rem-sleep-behavior-disorder/symptoms-causes/syc-20352920

13. See note 2.

14. Gabriele Andreatta and Kristin Tessmar-Raible, "The still dark side of the moon: Molecular mechanisms of lunar-controlled rhythms and clocks," *Journal of Molecular Biology* 432, no. 12 (2020): 3525–46. doi:10.1016/j.jmb.2020.03.009

15. David K. Welsh, Joseph S. Takahashi, and Steve A. Kay, "Suprachiasmatic nucleus: Cell autonomy and network properties," *Annual Review of Physiology* 72, no. 1 (2010): 551–77. doi:10.1146/annurev-physiol-021909-135919

16. "Home," *Chronobiology.com*, September 17, 2021. https://www.chronobiology.com/

17. Michael Breus, "Your personal guide to a better night's sleep," *The Sleep Doctor*, January 30, 2023. https://thesleepdoctor.com/

18. Simon N. Archer, Donna L. Robilliard, Debra J. Skene, Marcel Smits, Adrian Williams, Josephine Arendt, and Malcolm von Schantz, "A length polymorphism in the circadian clock gene PER3 is linked to delayed sleep phase syndrome and extreme diurnal preference," *Sleep* 26, no. 4 (2003): 413–15. doi:10.1093/sleep/26.4.413

19. Michael Breus, *Chronotype quiz*, The Sleep Doctor, December 13, 2022. https://thesleepdoctor. com/sleep-quizzes/chronotype-quiz/

20. Brett A. Dolezal, Eric V. Neufeld, David M. Boland, Jennifer L. Martin, and Christopher B. Cooper, "Interrelationship between sleep and exercise: A systematic seview," *Advances in Preventive Medicine* (2017): 1–14. doi:10.1155/2017/1364387

21. Masahiro Banno, Yudai Harada, Masashi Taniguchi, Ryo Tobita, Hiraku Tsujimoto, Yasushi Tsujimoto, Yuki Kataoka, and Akiko Noda, "Exercise can improve sleep quality: A systematic review and meta-analysis," *PeerJ* 6 (2018): e5172. doi:10.7717/peerj.5172

22. Pei-Yu Yang, Ka-Hou Ho, Hsi-Chung Chen, and Meng-Yueh Chien, "Exercise training improves sleep quality in middle-aged and older adults with sleep problems: A systematic review," *Journal of Physiotherapy* 58, no. 3 (2012): 157–63. doi:10.1016/s1836-9553(12)70106-6

23. Christopher E. Kline, "The bidirectional relationship between exercise and sleep," *American Journal of Lifestyle Medicine* 8, no. 6 (2014): 375–79. doi:10.1177/1559827614544437

24. Teodora Surdea-Blaga, Dana E. Negrutiu, Mariana Palage, and Dan L. Dumitrascu, "Food and gastroesophageal reflux disease," *Current Medicinal Chemistry* 26, no. 19 (2019): 3497–511. doi:10.2174/0929867324666170515123807

25. Soon-Yeob Park, Mi-Kyeong Oh, Bum-Soon Lee, Haa-Gyoung Kim, Won-Joon Lee, Ji-Ho Lee, Jun-Tae Lim, and Jin-Young Kim, "The effects of alcohol on quality of sleep," *Korean Journal of Family Medicine* 36, no. 6 (2015): 294. doi:10.4082/kjfm.2015.36.6.294

26. Ian Clark and Hans Peter Landolt, "Coffee, caffeine, and sleep: A systematic review of epidemiological studies and randomized controlled trials," *Sleep Medicine Reviews* 31 (2017): 70–78. doi:10.1016/j.smrv.2016.01.006

27. Katie Simpson, "Sleep and digestion — how to improve your gut health," *Sleep Advisor*, February 14, 2023. https://www.sleepadvisor.org/sleep-and-digestion/

28. Danielle Pacheco, *How drinking water before bed impacts sleep*, Sleep Foundation, February 2, 2023. https://www.sleepfoundation.org/nutrition/drinking-water-before-bed

29. Alicia Nunez et al., "Smoke at night and sleep worse? The associations between cigarette smoking with insomnia severity and sleep duration," *Sleep Health* 7, no. 2 (2021): 177–82. doi:10.1016/j.sleh.2020.10.006

30. Pamela Foral, Jon Knezevich, Naresh Dewan, and Mark Malesker, "Medication-induced sleep disturbances," *Consultant Pharmacist* 26, no. 6 (2011): 414–25. doi:10.4140/tcp.n.2011.414

31. Patricia J. Murphy, Pietro Badia, Bryan L. Myers, Michelle R. Boecker, and Kenneth P. Wright, "Nonsteroidal anti-inflammatory drugs affect normal sleep patterns in humans," *Physiology and Behavior* 55, no. 6 (1994): 1063–66. doi:10.1016/0031-9384(94)90388-3

32. Greg Potter, "Biohacker Summit 2019 video recordings," *Campwire*, 2019. https://www.campwire.com/sections/20484/modules/95399

33. See note 32.

34. Michael Lazarus, Yo Oishi, Theresa E. Bjorness, and Robert W. Greene, "Gating and the need for sleep: Dissociable effects of adenosine A1 and A2A receptors," *Frontiers in Neuroscience* 13 (2019). doi:10.3389/fnins.2019.00740

35. Joaquim A. Ribeiro and Ana M. Sebastião, "Caffeine and adenosine," *Journal of Alzheimer's Disease* 20 (s1) (2010). doi:10.3233/jad-2010-1379

36. Eric Ralls, "Going to bed angry is bad for your health, study finds," *Earth.com*, September 26, 2017. https://www.earth.com/news/bed-angry-bad-health/

37. *Raise your vibration with appreciation and compassion*, HeartMath Institute, February 21, 2019. https://www.heartmath.org/articles-of-the-heart/ raise-your-vibration-with-appreciation-and-compassion/

38. Alex M. Wood, Stephen Joseph, Joanna Lloyd, and Samuel Atkins, "Gratitude influences sleep through the mechanism of pre-sleep cognitions," *Journal of Psychosomatic Research* 66, no. 1 (2009): 43–48. doi:10.1016/j.jpsychores.2008.09.002

39. Mariangela Rondanelli, Annalisa Opizzi, Francesca Monteferrario, Neldo Antoniello, Raffaele Manni, and Catherine Klersy, "The effect of melatonin, magnesium, and zinc on primary insomnia in long-term care facility residents in Italy: A double-blind, placebo-controlled clinical trial," *Journal of the American Geriatrics Society* 59, no. 1 (2011): 82-90. doi:10.1111/j.1532-5415.2010.03232.x

40. James J. DiNicolantonio, James H. O'Keefe, and William Wilson, "Subclinical magnesium deficiency: A principal driver of cardiovascular disease and a public health crisis," *Open Heart* 5, no. 1 (2018). doi:10.1136/openhrt-2017-000668

41. See note 39.

42. *9 natural sleep aids to help you get more zzz's*, Healthline (n.d.). https://www.healthline.com/nutrition/sleep-aids

43. Siobhan Mendicino, *The 5 best adaptogens for sleep*, Botanical Institute, November 29, 2022. https://botanicalinstitute.org/adaptogens-for-sleep/#:~:text=Adaptogens%20work%20to%20lower%20cortisol,to%20fall%20asleep%20at%20night

44. Martha Hotz Vitaterna, Joseph S. Takahashi, and Fred W. Turek, *Overview of circadian rhythms* (National Institute on Alcohol Abuse and Alcoholism, U.S. Department of Health and Human Services, 2023). https://pubs.niaaa.nih.gov/publications/arh25-2/85-93.htm#:~:text=Light%20represents%20the%20most%20important,For%20comparison%2C%20see%20circadian%20time

45. Shawn K. Elmore, Patricia A. Betrus, and Robert Burr, "Light, social zeitgebers, and the sleep-wake cycle in the entrainment of human circadian rhythms," *Research in Nursing and Health* 17, no. 6 (1994): 471-78. doi:10.1002/nur.4770170610

46. Siegfried Wahl, Moritz Engelhardt, Patrick Schaupp, Christian Lappe, and Iliya V. Ivanov, "The inner clock—blue light sets the human rhythm," *Journal of Biophotonics* 12, no. 12 (2019). doi:10.1002/jbio.201900102

47. Leila Chaieb, Elke Caroline Wilpert, Thomas P. Reber, and Juergen Fell, "Auditory beat stimulation and its effects on cognition and mood states," *Frontiers in Psychiatry* 6 (2015). doi:10.3389/fpsyt.2015.00070

48. See note 2.

49. See note 2.

50. Elizabeth Capezuti, Kevin Pain, Evelyn Alamag, XinQing Chen, Valicia Philibert, and Ana C. Krieger, "Systematic review: Auditory stimulation and sleep," *Journal of Clinical Sleep Medicine* 18, no. 6 (2022): 1697-709. doi:10.5664/jcsm.9860

51. Susie Suh, Elliot H. Choi, and Natasha Atanaskova Mesinkovska, "The expression of opsins in the human skin and its implications for photobiomodulation: A systematic review," *Photodermatology, Photoimmunology and Photomedicine* 36, no. 5 (2020): 329-38. doi:10.1111/phpp.12578

52. *The best temperature for sleep: Advice & tips*, Sleep Foundation, February 13, 2023. https://www.sleepfoundation.org/bedroom-environment/best-temperature-for-sleep#:~:text=The%20best%20bedroom%20temperature%20for,for%20the%20most%20comfortable%20sleep

53. Samantha Prattey and Lisa Walden, "26 best air purifying plants for the home," *Country Living*, October 4, 2022. https://www.countryliving.com/uk/wellbeing/a668/houseplants-to-purify-house-air/

54. *3 ways air quality affects your sleep and how to improve it*, Alaska Sleep Clinic, October 17, 2022. https://www.alaskasleep.com/~alaskasl/3-ways-air-quality-affects-your-sleep-and-how-to-improve-it/

55. Jay Summer, "Which direction is best to sleep in?" *Sleep Foundation*. February 16, 2023. https://www.sleepfoundation.org/sleeping-positions/best-direction-to-sleep#:~:text=According%20to%20ancient%20traditions%20like,your%20feet%20are%20pointed%20north.

56. See note 55.

57. See note 55.

58. J. Leppäluoto, T. Westerlund, P. Huttunen, J. Oksa, J. Smolander, B. Dugué, and M.

Mikkelsson, "Effects of long-term whole-body cold exposures on plasma concentrations of ACTH, beta-endorphin, cortisol, catecholamines and cytokines in healthy females," *Scandinavian Journal of Clinical and Laboratory Investigation* 68, no. 2 (2008): 145–53. doi:10.1080/00365510701516350

59. Nikolai A. Shevchuk, "Adapted cold shower as a potential treatment for depression," *Medical Hypotheses* 70, no. 5 (2008): 995–1001. doi:10.1016/j.mehy.2007.04.052

60. Carolyn J. Heckman, Katherine Liang, and Mary Riley, "Awareness, understanding, use, and impact of the UV index: A systematic review of over two decades of international research," *Preventive Medicine* 123 (2019): 71–83. doi:10.1016/j.ypmed.2019.03.004

61. Mohammed S. Razzaque, "Sunlight exposure: Do health benefits outweigh harm?" *Journal of Steroid Biochemistry and Molecular Biology* 175 (2018): 44–48. doi:10.1016/j.jsbmb.2016.09.004

62. S. Knippenberg, J. Damoiseaux, Y. Bol, R. Hupperts, B.V. Taylor, A.-L. Ponsonby, T. Dwyer, S. Simpson, and I.A. van der Mei, "Higher levels of reported sun exposure, and not vitamin D status, are associated with less depressive symptoms and fatigue in multiple sclerosis," *Acta Neurologica Scandinavica* 129, no. 2 (2013): 123–31. doi:10.1111/ane.12155

63. G.W. Lambert, C. Reid, D.M. Kaye, G.L. Jennings, and M.D. Esler, "Effect of sunlight and season on serotonin turnover in the brain," *Lancet* 360, no. 9348 (2002): 1840–42. doi:10.1016/s0140-6736(02)11737-5

64. Christine Blume, Corrado Garbazza, and Manuel Spitschan, "Effects of light on human circadian rhythms, sleep and mood," *Somnologie* 23, no. 3 (2019): 147–56. doi:10.1007/s11818-019-00215-x

65. M. Kanariou, E. Petridou, E. Vrachnou, and D. Trichopoulos, "Lymphocyte alterations after prolonged sunlight exposure," *Journal of Epidemiology and Biostatistics* 6, no. 6 (2001): 463–65. doi:10.1080/135952201317225499

66. Matthias Wacker and Michael F. Holick, "Sunlight and vitamin D," *Dermato-Endocrinology* 5, no. 1 (2013): 51–108. doi:10.4161/derm.24494

67. Michael F. Holick, "Sunlight and vitamin D for bone health and prevention of autoimmune diseases, cancers, and cardiovascular disease," *American Journal of Clinical Nutrition* 80, no. 6 (2004). doi:10.1093/ajcn/80.6.1678s

CHAPTER 15: IMMUNITY

1. Rachael A. Clark, "Skin-resident T cells: The ups and downs of on site immunity," *Journal of Investigative Dermatology* 130, no. 2 (2010): 362–70. doi:10.1038/jid.2009.247

2. G. Vighi, F. Marcucci, L. Sensi, G. Di Cara, and F. Frati, "Allergy and the gastrointestinal system," *Clinical and Experimental Immunology* 153 (Suppl 1) (2008): 3–6. doi:10.1111/j.1365-2249.2008.03713.x

3. Geoffrey E. Hespe et al., "Exercise training improves obesity-related lymphatic dysfunction," *Journal of Physiology* 594, no. 15 (2016): 4267–82. doi:10.1113/jp271757

4. Andrea Leonard, *The benefits of rebounding in the prevention and management of lymphedema and improving your immune response* (Cancer Exercise Training Institute, March 20, 2020). https://www.thecancerspecialist.com/2019/08/01/the-benefits-of-rebounding-in-the-prevention-and-management-of-lymphedema/#:~:text=The%20movement%20that%20is%20performed,lymphatic%20system%20lacks%20a%20pump

5. Lucia Cugusi, Andrea Manca, Roberto Serpe, Giovanni Romita, Marco Bergamin, Christian Cadeddu, Paolo Solla, and Giuseppe Mercuro, "Effects of a mini-trampoline rebounding exercise program on functional parameters, body composition and quality of life in overweight women," *Journal of Sports Medicine and Physical Fitness* 58, no. 3 (2018). doi:10.23736/s0022-4707.16.06588-9

6. *Exercise on the rebound,* CBS News, January 31, 2002. https://www.cbsnews.com/news/exercise-on-the-rebound/

7. See note 4.

8. Katie Rodan, Kathy Fields, George Majewski, and Timothy Falla, "Skincare bootcamp," *Plastic and Reconstructive Surgery - Global Open* 4 (2016). doi:10.1097/gox.0000000000001152

9. "Dry brushing: Benefits, myths, and how to dry brush," *Medical News Today* (MediLexicon International, February 9, 2022). https://www.medicalnewstoday.com/articles/dry-brushing#benefits

10. Abdullah M.N. Al-Bedah, Ibrahim S. Elsubai, Naseem Akhtar Qureshi, Tamer Shaban Aboushanab, Gazzaffi I.M. Ali, Ahmed Tawfik El-Olemy, Asim A.H. Khalil, Mohamed K.M. Khalil, and Meshari Saleh Alqaed, "The medical perspective of cupping therapy: Effects and mechanisms of action," *Journal of Traditional and Complementary Medicine* 9, no. 2 (2019): 90–97. doi:10.1016/j.jtcme.2018.03.003

11. Tomoo Kondo, Mikiya Kishi, Takashi Fushimi, Shinobu Ugajin, and Takayuki Kaga, "Vinegar intake reduces body weight, body fat mass, and serum triglyceride levels in obese Japanese subjects," *Bioscience, Biotechnology, and Biochemistry* 73, no. 8 (2009): 1837–43. doi:10.1271/bbb.90231

12. Ying Zhao and Yan-Bo Yu, "Intestinal microbiota and chronic constipation," *SpringerPlus* 5, no. 1 (2016). doi:10.1186/s40064-016-2821-1

13. See note 12.

14. Lin Xu, Wenkui Yu, Xiaobo Feng, and Ning Li, "Efficacy of pectin in the treatment of diarrhea predominant irritable bowel syndrome," *Chinese Journal of Gastrointestinal Surgery* 18, no. 3 (2015): 267–71.

15. See note 14.

16. Shaun K. Riebl and Brenda M. Davy, "The hydration equation," *ACSM's Health and Fitness Journal* 17, no. 6 (2013): 21–28. doi:10.1249/fit.0b013e3182a9570f

17. Kelly A. Dougherty, Lindsay B. Baker, Mosuk Chow, and W. Larry Kenney, "Two percent dehydration impairs and six percent carbohydrate drink improves boys' basketball skills," *Medicine and Science in Sports and Exercise* 38, no. 9 (2006): 1650–58. doi:10.1249/01.mss.0000227640.60736.8e

18. Michael N. Sawka, Samuel N. Cheuvront, and Robert Carter, "Human water needs," *Nutrition Reviews* 63 (2005). doi:10.1111/j.1753-4887.2005.tb00152.x

19. Adrian F. Gombart, Adeline Pierre, and Silvia Maggini, "A review of micronutrients and the immune system—working in harmony to reduce the risk of infection," *Nutrients* 12, no. 1 (2020): 236. doi:10.3390/nu12010236

20. Inga Wessels, Martina Maywald, and Lothar Rink, "Zinc as a gatekeeper of immune function," *Nutrients* 9, no. 12 (2017): 1286. doi:10.3390/nu9121286

21. Ángel Julio Romero Cabrera, "Zinc, aging, and immunosenescence: An overview," *Pathobiology of Aging and Age-Related Diseases* 5, no. 1 (2015): 25592. doi:10.3402/pba.v5.25592

22. Bernadeta Szewczyk, "Zinc homeostasis and neurodegenerative disorders," *Frontiers in Aging Neuroscience* 5 (2013). doi:10.3389/fnagi.2013.00033

23. Laura M. Plum, Lothar Rink, and Hajo Haase, "The essential toxin: Impact of zinc on human health," *International Journal of Environmental Research and Public Health* 7, no. 4 (2010): 1342–65. doi:10.3390/ijerph7041342

24. George J. Brewer, Steve H. Kanzer, Earl A. Zimmerman, Eric S. Molho, Dzintra F. Celmins, Susan M. Heckman, and Robert Dick, "Subclinical zinc deficiency in Alzheimer's disease and Parkinson's disease," *American Journal of Alzheimer's Disease and Other Dementias* 25, no. 7 (2010): 572–75. doi:10.1177/1533317510382283

25. Shang-Ru Tsai and Michael R. Hamblin, "Biological effects and medical applications of infrared radiation," *Journal of Photochemistry and Photobiology B: Biology* 170 (2017): 197–207. doi:10.1016/j.jphotobiol.2017.04.014

26. Chun-Chih Lin, Cheng-Lung Lee, and Chia-Chi Lung, "Antioxidative effect of far-infrared radiation in humans," *Public Health Frontiers* 2, no. 2 (2013): 97–102. doi:10.5963/phf0202006

CHAPTER 16: TEMPERATURE THERAPIES AND YOU

1. Rhonda Patrick, Dir., *Hormetic stressors – health benefits of sauna and cold exposure,* YouTube, 2020. https://www.youtube.com/watch?v=-ty6VTNPjqw

2. Christoph Schwarzer, "30 years of dynorphins—new insights on their functions in neuropsychiatric diseases," *Pharmacology and Therapeutics* 123, no. 3 (2009): 353–70. doi:10.1016/j.pharmthera.2009.05.006

3. "How to increase dynorphin release in the sauna?" *Northern Saunas,* January 27, 2020. https://northernsaunas.com/blogs/news/how-to-increase-dynorphin-release-in-the-sauna#:~:text=The%20reason%20why%20you%20should,as%20%22the%20runners%20high%22

4. Lauréline Roger, Fanny Tomas, and Véronique Gire, "Mechanisms and regulation of cellular senescence," *International Journal of Molecular Sciences* 22, no. 23 (2021): 13173. doi:10.3390/ijms222313173

5. See note 1.

6. See note 1.

7. Rhonda P. Patrick and Teresa L. Johnson, "Sauna use as a lifestyle practice to extend healthspan," *Experimental Gerontology* 154 (2021): 111509. doi:10.1016/j.exger.2021.111509

8. Karol Dokladny, Orrin B. Myers, and Pope L. Moseley, "Heat shock response and autophagy—cooperation and control," *Autophagy* 11, no. 2 (2015): 200–13. doi:10.1080/15548627.2015.1009776

9. Olli Sovijärvi, *Heat alteration: Health benefits of traditional sauna & infrared heat room,* Biohacker Center Store, February 21, 2023. https://biohackercenter.com/blogs/biohacking-guides/heat-alteration-health-benefits-traditional-sauna-infrared-room?_pos=1&_sid=698736609&_ss=r

10 J. Leppäluoto, T. Westerlund, P. Huttunen, J. Oksa, J. Smolander, B. Dugué, and M. Mikkelsson, "Effects of long-term whole-body cold exposures on plasma concentrations of ACTH, beta-endorphin, cortisol, catecholamines and cytokines in healthy females," *Scandinavian Journal of Clinical and Laboratory Investigation* 68, no. 2 (2008): 145–53. doi:10.1080/00365510701516350

11. Rhonda Patrick, "Wim Hof on the connection between mental health and embracing the cold," *FoundMyFitness,* 2023. https://www.foundmyfitness.com/episodes/cold-breath-inflammation-mental-health

12. See note 10.

13. Nana Chung, Jonghoon Park, and Kiwon Lim, "The effects of exercise and cold exposure on mitochondrial biogenesis in skeletal muscle and white adipose tissue," *Journal of Exercise, Nutrition and Biochemistry* 21, no. 2 (2017): 39–47. doi:10.20463/jenb.2017.0020

14. Wim Hof, *Cold water immersion (CWI),* Wim Hof Method, 2023. https://www.wimhofmethod.com/cold-water-immersion#:~:text=Scientifically%2C%20it%20has%20been%20proven,tissue%2C%20and%20reduces%20further%20swelling.&text=Cold%20water%20immersion%20can%20be,it%20comes%20to%20weight%20loss

15. M.J. Tipton, N. Collier, H. Massey, J. Corbett, and M. Harper, "Cold water immersion: Kill or cure?" *Experimental Physiology* 102, no. 11 (2017): 1335–55. doi:10.1113/ep086283

16. Kayvan Khoramipour, Karim Chamari, Amirhosein Ahmadi Hekmatikar, Amirhosein Ziyaiyan, Shima Taherkhani, Nihal M. Elguindy, and Nicola Luigi Bragazzi, "Adiponectin: Structure, physiological functions, role in diseases, and effects of nutrition," *Nutrients* 13, no. 4 (2021): 1180. doi:10.3390/nu13041180

17. Anouk A.J.J. van der Lans et al., "Cold acclimation recruits human brown fat and increases nonshivering thermogenesis," *Journal of Clinical Investigation* 123, no. 8 (2013): 3395–403. doi:10.1172/jci68993

18. R.J. Brychta and K.Y. Chen, "Cold-induced thermogenesis in humans," *European Journal of Clinical Nutrition* 71, no. 3 (2016): 345–52. doi:10.1038/ejcn.2016.223

19. Louisa Nicola, "Cold thermogenesis and the brain," *LinkedIn.* July 15, 2020. https://www.linkedin.com/pulse/cold-thermogenesis-brain-louisa-nicola/

20. Geert A. Buijze, Inger N. Sierevelt, Bas C. van der Heijden, Marcel G. Dijkgraaf, and Monique H. Frings-Dresen, "The effect of cold showering on health and work: A randomized controlled trial," *PLOS One* 11, no. 9 (2016). doi:10.1371/journal.pone.0161749

21. P. Srámek, M. Simecková, L. Janský, J. Savlíková, and S. Vybíral, "Human physiological responses to immersion into water of different temperatures," *European Journal of Applied Physiology* 81, no. 5 (2000): 436-42. doi:10.1007/s004210050065

22. Rhonda Patrick, "Cold exposure," *FoundMyFitness*, 2023. https://www.foundmyfitness.com/topics/cold-exposure-therapy#bibid-19d52909634c06d96a9c2cd9482bfdc5

23. John Richter, *The ultimate chest freezer cold plunge DIY guide* (e-Book), Chest Freezer Cold Plunge, October 30, 2019. https://chestfreezercoldplunge.com/product/the-ultimate-chest-freezer-cold-plunge-diy-guide/

24. O. Sovijärvi, T. Arina, and J. Halmetoja, *Biohacker's handbook: Upgrade yourself and unleash your inner potential* (Tallinn: Biohacker Center, 2018).

25. W. Michael Panneton and Qi Gan, "The mammalian diving response: Inroads to its neural control," *Frontiers in Neuroscience* 14 (2020). doi:10.3389/fnins.2020.00524

26. "How we are made to hold our breath and why we will never be seals," *Freedive Wire*, December 28, 2018. https://www.freedivewire.com/mammalian-dive-response/

27. James N. Baraniuk and Samantha J. Merck, "Neuroregulation of human nasal mucosa," *Annals of the New York Academy of Sciences* 1170, no. 1 (2009): 604-9. doi:10.1111/j.1749-6632.2009.04481.x

28. "How the dive reflex protects the brain and heart," *Divers Alert Network*, February 25, 2021. https://dan.org/alert-diver/article/how-the-dive-reflex-protects-the-brain-and-heart/#:~:text=The%20vagus%20nerve%20slows%20down,extremities%20back%20toward%20our%20heart

29. Jason M. Keeler, Hayden W. Hess, Erica Tourula, Tyler B. Baker, Payton M. Kerr, Joel T. Greenshields, Robert F. Chapman, Blair D. Johnson, and Zachary J. Schlader, "Increased spleen volume provoked by temperate head-out-of-water immersion," *American Journal of Physiology-Regulatory, Integrative and Comparative Physiology* 323, no. 5 (2022). doi:10.1152/ajpregu.00111.2022

30. Darija Bakovic, Davor Eterovic, Zana Saratlija-Novakovic, Ivan Palada, Zoran Valic, Nada Bilopavlovic, and Zeljko Dujic, "Effect of human splenic contraction on variation in circulating blood cell counts," *Clinical and Experimental Pharmacology and Physiology* 32, no. 11 (2005): 944-51. doi:10.1111/j.1440-1681.2005.04289.x

31. Aryane Flauzino Machado, Paulo Henrique Ferreira, Jéssica Kirsch Micheletti, Aline Castilho de Almeida, Ítalo Ribeiro Lemes, Franciele Marques Vanderlei, Jayme Netto Junior, and Carlos Marcelo Pastre, "Can water temperature and immersion time influence the effect of cold water immersion on muscle soreness? A systematic review and meta-analysis," *Sports Medicine* 46, no. 4 (2015): 503-14. doi:10.1007/s40279-015-0431-7

32. M. Yamane, N. Ohnishi, and T. Matsumoto, "Does regular post-exercise cold application attenuate trained muscle adaptation?" *International Journal of Sports Medicine* 36, no. 8 (2015): 647-53. doi:10.1055/s-0034-1398652

33. Motoi Yamane, Hiroyasu Teruya, Masataka Nakano, Ryuji Ogai, Norikazu Ohnishi, and Mitsuo Kosaka, "Post-exercise leg and forearm flexor muscle cooling in humans attenuates endurance and resistance training effects on muscle performance and on circulatory adaptation," *European Journal of Applied Physiology* 96, no. 5 (2005): 572-80. doi:10.1007/s00421-005-0095-3

34. See note 22.

35. Antti Mero, Jaakko Tornberg, Mari Mäntykoski, and Risto Puurtinen, "Effects of far-infrared sauna bathing on recovery from strength and endurance training sessions in men," *SpringerPlus* 4, no. 1 (2015). doi:10.1186/s40064-015-1093-5

36. Daniel A. Judelson, Carl M. Maresh, Linda M. Yamamoto, Mark J. Farrell, Lawrence E. Armstrong, William J. Kraemer, Jeff S. Volek, Barry A. Spiering, Douglas J. Casa, and Jeffrey M. Anderson, "Effect of hydration state on resistance exercise-induced endocrine markers of

anabolism, catabolism, and metabolism," *Journal of Applied Physiology* 105, no. 3 (2008): 816–24. doi:10.1152/japplphysiol.01010.2007

37. C. Maresh, M. Whittlesey, L. Armstrong, L. Yamamoto, D. Judelson, K. Fish, D. Casa, S. Kavouras, and V. Castracane, "Effect of hydration state on testosterone and cortisol responses to training-intensity exercise in collegiate runners," *International Journal of Sports Medicine* 27, no. 10 (2006): 765–70. doi:10.1055/s-2005-872932

38. Bill Bachand, "The Nordic Cycle therapy," *Renu Therapy*, March 21, 2022. https://www.renutherapy.com/blogs/blog/the-nordic-cycle-therapy

CHAPTER 17: INTERMITTENT FASTING

1. M.L. Hartman, J.D. Veldhuis, M.L. Johnson, M.M. Lee, K.G. Alberti, E. Samojlik, and M.O. Thorner, "Augmented growth hormone (GH) secretory burst frequency and amplitude mediate enhanced GH secretion during a two-day fast in normal men," *Journal of Clinical Endocrinology and Metabolism* 74, no. 4 (1992): 757–65. https://doi.org/10.1210/jcem.74.4.1548337

2. Tatiana Moro, Grant Tinsley, Antonino Bianco, Giuseppe Marcolin, Quirico Francesco Pacelli, Giuseppe Battaglia, Antonio Palma, Paulo Gentil, Marco Neri, and Antonio Paoli, "Effects of eight weeks of time-restricted feeding (16/8) on basal metabolism, maximal strength, body composition, inflammation, and cardiovascular risk factors in resistance-trained males," *Journal of Translational Medicine* 14, no. 1 (2016). doi:10.1186/s12967-016-1044-0

3. See note 2.

4. Maria M. Mihaylova et al., "Fasting activates fatty acid oxidation to enhance intestinal stem cell function during homeostasis and aging," *Cell Stem Cell* 22, no. 5 (2018). doi:10.1016/j.stem.2018.04.001

5. Abu Shufian Ahmed, Matilda H.C. Sheng, Samiksha Wasnik, David J. Baylink, and Kin-Hing William Lau, "Effect of aging on stem cells," *World Journal of Experimental Medicine* 7, no. 1 (2017): 1. doi:10.5493/wjem.v7.i1.1

6. Mehrdad Alirezaei, Christopher C. Kemball, Claudia T. Flynn, Malcolm R. Wood, J. Lindsay Whitton, and William B. Kiosses, "Short-term fasting induces profound neuronal autophagy," *Autophagy* 6, no. 6 (2010): 702–10. doi:10.4161/auto.6.6.12376

7. Olivier Descamps, Jacqueline Riondel, Véronique Ducros, and Anne-Marie Roussel, "Mitochondrial production of reactive oxygen species and incidence of age-associated lymphoma in OF1 mice: Effect of alternate-day fasting," *Mechanisms of Ageing and Development* 126, no. 11 (2005): 1185–91. doi:10.1016/j.mad.2005.06.007

8. M. Mattson and R. Wan, "Beneficial effects of intermittent fasting and caloric restriction on the cardiovascular and cerebrovascular systems," *Journal of Nutritional Biochemistry* 16, no. 3 (2005): 129–37. doi:10.1016/j.jnutbio.2004.12.007

9. Christian Zauner, Bruno Schneeweiss, Alexander Kranz, Christian Madl, Klaus Ratheiser, Ludwig Kramer, Erich Roth, Barbara Schneider, and Kurt Lenz, "Resting energy expenditure in short-term starvation is increased as a result of an increase in serum norepinephrine," *American Journal of Clinical Nutrition* 71, no. 6 (2000): 1511–15. doi:10.1093/ajcn/71.6.1511

10. Fehime B. Aksungar, Aynur E. Topkaya, and Mahmut Akyildiz, "Interleukin-6, C-reactive protein and biochemical parameters during prolonged intermittent fasting," *Annals of Nutrition and Metabolism* 51, no. 1 (2007): 88–95. doi:10.1159/000100954

11. *The top 10 causes of death* (Geneva: World Health Organization, December 9, 2020). https://www.who.int/news-room/fact-sheets/detail/the-top-10-causes-of-death

12. Krista A. Varady, Surabhi Bhutani, Emily C. Church, and Monica C. Klempel, "Short-term modified alternate-day fasting: A novel dietary strategy for weight loss and cardioprotection in obese adults," *American Journal of Clinical Nutrition* 90, no. 5 (2009): 1138–43. doi:10.3945/ajcn.2009.28380

13. Eleah Stringer, Julian J. Lum, and Nicol Macpherson, "Intermittent fasting in cancer: A role in survivorship?" *Current Nutrition Reports* 11, no. 3 (2022): 500–507. doi:10.1007/s13668-022-00425-0

14. Kelsey Gabel, Kate Cares, Krista Varady, Vijayakrishna Gadi, and Lisa Tussing-Humphreys, "Current evidence and directions for intermittent fasting during cancer chemotherapy," *Advances in Nutrition* 13, no. 2 (2022): 667–80. doi:10.1093/advances/nmab132

15. Alessio Nencioni, Irene Caffa, Salvatore Cortellino, and Valter D. Longo, "Fasting and cancer: Molecular mechanisms and clinical application," *Nature Reviews Cancer* 18, no. 11 (2018): 707–19. doi:10.1038/s41568-018-0061-0

16. Sagun Tiwari, Namrata Sapkota, and Zhenxiang Han, "Effect of fasting on cancer: A narrative review of scientific evidence," *Cancer Science* 113, no. 10 (2022): 3291–302. doi:10.1111/cas.15492

17. Changhan Lee et al., "Fasting cycles retard growth of tumors and sensitize a range of cancer cell types to chemotherapy," *Science Translational Medicine* 4, no. 124 (2012). doi:10.1126/scitranslmed.3003293

18. See note 17.

19. Mark P. Mattson, "Energy intake, meal frequency, and health: A neurobiological perspective," *Annual Review of Nutrition* 25, no. 1 (2005): 237–60. doi:10.1146/annurev.nutr.25.050304.092526

20. Christina M. Sciarrillo, Bryant H. Keirns, Destinee C. Elliott, and Sam R. Emerson, "The effect of black coffee on fasting metabolic markers and an abbreviated fat tolerance test," *Clinical Nutrition ESPEN* 41 (2021): 439–42. doi:10.1016/j.clnesp.2020.11.020

21. Bryant Keirns, Destinee Elliott, Christina Sciarrillo, Nicholas Koemel, Kara Poindexter, and Sam Emerson, "Effect of black coffee on fasting metabolic markers and an abbreviated fat tolerance test," *Current Developments in Nutrition* 4 (2020): 4140639. doi:10.1093/cdn/nzaa049_032

22. "Beverages, coffee, brewed, prepared with tap water," *FoodData Central* (U.S. Department of Agriculture, April 2018). https://fdc.nal.usda.gov/fdc-app.html#/food-details/171890/nutrients

23. James H. O'Keefe, James J. DiNicolantonio, and Carl J. Lavie, "Coffee for cardioprotection and longevity," *Progress in Cardiovascular Diseases* 61, no. 1 (2018): 38–42. doi:10.1016/j.pcad.2018.02.002

24. Karen Nieber, "The impact of coffee on health," *Planta Medica* 83, no. 16 (2017): 1256–63. doi:10.1055/s-0043-115007

25. Kazuo Yamagata, "Do coffee polyphenols have a preventive action on metabolic syndrome associated endothelial dysfunctions? An assessment of the current evidence," *Antioxidants* 7, no. 2 (2018): 26. doi:10.3390/antiox7020026

26. Maciej Górecki and Ewelina Hallmann, "The antioxidant content of coffee and its in vitro activity as an effect of its production method and roasting and brewing time," *Antioxidants* 9, no. 4 (2020): 308. doi:10.3390/antiox9040308

27. M.L. Martins, H.M. Martins, and A. Gimeno, "Incidence of microflora and of ochratoxin A in green coffee beans (*Coffea Arabica*)," *Food Additives and Contaminants* 20, no. 12 (2003): 1127–31. doi:10.1080/02652030310001620405

28. Dave Asprey, *Head strong* (HarperCollins, 2017).

PART IV

1. Phillippa Lally, Cornelia H. van Jaarsveld, Henry W. Potts, and Jane Wardle, "How are habits formed: Modelling habit formation in the real world," *European Journal of Social Psychology* 40, no. 6 (2009): 998–1009. doi:10.1002/ejsp.674

CHAPTER 18: REVITALIZING YOUR BODY

1. Ananda L. Roy and Richard S. Conroy, "Toward mapping the human body at a cellular resolution," *Molecular Biology of the Cell* 29, no. 15 (2018): 1779–85. doi:10.1091/mbc.e18-04-0260

2. "What do cells need to survive?" *Reference.* IAC Publishing, April 17, 2020. https://www.reference.com/science-technology/cells-need-survive-8c862918c3e4a0b6

3. Simone Fulda, Adrienne M. Gorman, Osamu Hori, and Afshin Samali, "Cellular stress

responses: Cell survival and cell death," *International Journal of Cell Biology* (2010): 1-23. doi:10.1155/2010/214074

4. Lijing Jiang, "Alexis Carrel's immortal chick heart tissue cultures (1912-1946)," *The Embryo Project encyclopedia*, 2012. https://embryo.asu.edu/pages/alexis-carrels-immortal-chick-heart-tissue-cultures-1912-1946#:~:text=From%201912%20to%201946%2C%20this,the%20cells%20were%20deemed%20immortal

5. Leonard Hayflick, "Dr Alexis Carrel and tissue culture," *Journal of the American Medical Association* 252, no. 1 (1984): 44. doi:10.1001/jama.1984.03350010024012

6. Jerry W. Shay and Woodring E. Wright, "Hayflick, his limit, and cellular ageing," *Nature Reviews Molecular Cell Biology* 1, no. 1 (2000): 72-76. doi:10.1038/35036093

7. Piotr Zimniak, "Detoxification reactions: Relevance to aging," *Ageing Research Reviews* 7, no. 4 (2008): 281-300. doi:10.1016/j.arr.2008.04.001

8. Jonathan Myers, "Exercise and cardiovascular health," *Circulation* 107, no. 1 (2003). doi:10.1161/01.cir.0000048890.59383.8d

9. Jonathan Myers, Manish Prakash, Victor Froelicher, Dat Do, Sara Partington, and J. Edwin Atwood, "Exercise capacity and mortality among men referred for exercise yesting," *New England Journal of Medicine* 346, no. 11 (2002): 793-801. doi:10.1056/nejmoa011858

10. See note 9.

11. Tarja Porkka-Heiskanen, "Adenosine in sleep and wakefulness," *Annals of Medicine* 31, no. 2 (1999): 125-29. doi:10.3109/07853899908998788

12. Hans-Peter Landolt, "Sleep homeostasis: A role for adenosine in humans?" *Biochemical Pharmacology* 75, no. 11 (2008): 2070-79. doi:10.1016/j.bcp.2008.02.024

13. *Module 7. Napping, an important fatigue countermeasure, sleep inertia*, Centers for Disease Control and Prevention, March 31, 2020. https://www.cdc.gov/niosh/work-hour-training-for-nurses/longhours/mod7/03.html#:~:text=Sleep%20inertia%20is%20a%20temporary,reasoning%2C%20remembering%2C%20and%20learning

14. Rachel A. Newman, Gary H. Kamimori, Nancy J. Wesensten, Dante Picchioni, and Thomas J. Balkin, "Caffeine gum minimizes sleep inertia," *Perceptual and Motor Skills* 116, no. 1 (2013): 280-93. doi:10.2466/29.22.25.pms.116.1.280-293

15. Atsushi Ishida, Tatsushi Mutoh, Tomoko Ueyama, Hideki Bando, Satoru Masubuchi, Daiichiro Nakahara, Gozoh Tsujimoto, and Hitoshi Okamura, "Light activates the adrenal gland: Timing of gene expression and glucocorticoid release," *Cell Metabolism* 2, no. 5 (2005): 297-307. doi:10.1016/j.cmet.2005.09.009

16. Frank A. Scheer and Ruud M. Buijs, "Light affects morning salivary cortisol in humans," *Journal of Clinical Endocrinology and Metabolism* 84, no. 9 (1999): 3395-98. doi:10.1210/jcem.84.9.6102

17. "Cortisol (blood)," *Health encyclopedia*, University of Rochester Medical Center, 2023. https://www.urmc.rochester.edu/encyclopedia/content.aspx?contenttypeid=167&contentid=cortisol_serum#:~:text=In%20most%20people%2C%20cortisol%20levels,too%20high%20for%20too%20long

18. J. Thirthalli, G.H. Naveen, M.G. Rao, S. Varambally, R. Christopher, and B.N. Gangadhar, "Cortisol and antidepressant effects of yoga," *Indian Journal of Psychiatry* 55, no. 7 (2013): 405. doi:10.4103/0019-5545.116315

19. Dorothy Bruck, *The "sleep calculator" is just unscientific hype*, Sleep Health Foundation, September 12, 2021. https://www.sleephealthfoundation.org.au/news/latest-news/the-sleep-calculator-is-just-unscientific-hype.html#:~:text=Sleep%20cycles%20across%20the%20night%20are%20only%20approximately%2090%20minutes,individual%20from%20night%20to%20night

20. Timothy H. Monk, "The post-lunch dip in performance," *Clinics in Sports Medicine* 24, no. 2 (2005). doi:10.1016/j.csm.2004.12.002

21. Mikkel H. Vendelbo, Jens O. Jørgensen, Steen B. Pedersen, Lars C. Gormsen, Sten Lund, Ole Schmitz, Niels Jessen, and Niels Møller, "Exercise and fasting activate growth hormone-dependent myocellular signal transducer and activator of transcription-5b phosphorylation

and insulin-like growth factor-i messenger ribonucleic acid expression in humans," *Journal of Clinical Endocrinology and Metabolism* 95, no. 9 (2020). doi:10.1210/jc.2010-0689

22. Mark Sisson, "Post workout fasting," *Mark's Daily Apple*, December 8, 2022. https://www.marksdailyapple.com/post-workout-fasting/

23. Roberto Lanzi, Livio Luzi, Andrea Caumo, Anna Claudia Andreotti, Marco Federico Manzoni, Maria Elena Malighetti, Lucia Piceni Sereni, and Antonio Ettore Pontiroli, "Elevated insulin levels contribute to the reduced growth hormone (GH) response to GH-releasing hormone in obese subjects," *Metabolism* 48, no. 9 (1999): 1152–56. doi:10.1016/s0026-0495(99)90130-0

24. Dan Nemet, Yoav Meckel, Sheli Bar-Sela, Frank Zaldivar, Dan M. Cooper, and Alon Eliakim, "Effect of local cold-pack application on systemic anabolic and inflammatory response to sprint-interval training: A prospective comparative trial," *European Journal of Applied Physiology* 107, no. 4 (2009): 411–17. doi:10.1007/s00421-009-1138-y

25. Llion A. Roberts, Truls Raastad, James F. Markworth, Vandre C. Figueiredo, Ingrid M. Egner, Anthony Shield, David Cameron-Smith, Jeff S. Coombes, and Jonathan M. Peake, "Post-exercise cold water immersion attenuates acute anabolic signalling and long-term adaptations in muscle to strength training," *Journal of Physiology* 593, no. 18 (2015): 4285–301. doi:10.1113/jp270570

26. Vighnesh Vetrivel Venkatasamy, Sandeep Pericheria, Sachin Manthuruthil, and Shikha Mishra, "Effect of physical activity on insulin resistance, inflammation and oxidative stress in diabetes mellitus," *Journal of Clinical and Diagnostic Research* 7, no. 8 (2013): 1764–66. doi:10.7860/jcdr/2013/6518.3306

27. Marcelo Flores-Opazo, Sean L. McGee, and Mark Hargreaves, "Exercise and glut4," *Exercise and Sport Sciences Reviews* 48, no. 3 (2020): 110–18. doi:10.1249/jes.0000000000000224

28. Maria M. Mihaylova et al., "Fasting activates fatty acid oxidation to enhance intestinal stem cell function during homeostasis and aging," *Cell Stem Cell* 22, no. 5 (2018). doi:10.1016/j.stem.2018.04.001

29. Abu Shufian Ahmed, Matilda H.C. Sheng, Samiksha Wasnik, David J. Baylink, and Kin-Hing William Lau, "Effect of aging on stem cells," *World Journal of Experimental Medicine* 7, no. 1 (2017): 1. doi:10.5493/wjem.v7.i1.1

CHAPTER 19: MENTAL PARADIGM AND YOUR EMOTIONAL WELL-BEING

1. James Altucher, "The power of five," *James Altucher.com*, December 23, 2013. https://jamesaltucher.com/blog/the-5x5-trick-to-make-life-better/

2. Nicholas A. Christakis and James H. Fowler, "The collective dynamics of smoking in a large social network," *New England Journal of Medicine* 358, no. 21 (2008): 2249–58. doi:10.1056/nejmsa0706154

3. Nicholas A. Christakis and James H. Fowler, "The spread of obesity in a large social network over 32 years," *New England Journal of Medicine* 357, no. 4 (2007): 370–79. doi:10.1056/nejmsa066082

4. J.H. Fowler and N.A. Christakis, "Dynamic spread of happiness in a large social network: Longitudinal analysis over 20 years in the Framingham Heart Study," *British Medical Journal* 337, no. 2 (2008). doi:10.1136/bmj.a2338

5. John T. Cacioppo, James H. Fowler, and Nicholas A. Christakis, "Alone in the crowd: The structure and spread of loneliness in a large social network," *Journal of Personality and Social Psychology* 97, no. 6 (2009): 977–91. doi:10.1037/a0016076

6. Neil Pasricha, *The happiness equation – want nothing + do anything = have everything* (London: Ebury, 2017).

7. Rick Hanson, *Hardwiring happiness* (New York: Random House, 2015).

8. Ellen J. Langer, *Counterclockwise: Mindful health and the power of possibility* (New York: Ballantine, 2009).

9. *The power of positive thinking*, Johns Hopkins Medicine, November 1, 2021. https://www.hopkinsmedicine.org/health/wellness-and-prevention/the-power-of-positive-thinking

10. See note 9.
11. See note 9.
12. See note 9.

CHAPTER 20: DEFINING YOUR PURPOSE AND ENGAGING YOUR SPIRIT

1. Neil Pasricha, *The happiness equation – want nothing + do anything = have everything* (London: Ebury, 2017).
2. S. Miyagi, N. Iwama, T. Kawabata, and K. Hasegawa, "Longevity and diet in Okinawa, Japan: The past, present and future," *Asia Pacific Journal of Public Health* 15 (suppl 1) (2003). doi:10.1177/101053950301500s03
3. Aislinn Kotifani, "Bringing the 'blue zones' lifestyle to America: It takes a village," *Blue Zones*, February 12, 2021. https://www.bluezones.com/2018/08/future-of-health-care-is-creating-environmental-change/
4. Dan Buettner and Sam Skemp, "Blue zones," *American Journal of Lifestyle Medicine* 10, no. 5 (2016): 318–21. doi:10.1177/1559827616637066
5. Toshimasa Sone, Naoki Nakaya, Kaori Ohmori, Taichi Shimazu, Mizuka Higashiguchi, Masako Kakizaki, Nobutaka Kikuchi, Shinichi Kuriyama, and Ichiro Tsuji, "Sense of life worth living (ikigai) and mortality in Japan: Ohsaki Study," *Psychosomatic Medicine* 70, no. 6 (2008): 709–15. doi:10.1097/psy.0b013e31817e7e64
6. James E. Loehr and Tony Schwartz, *The power of full engagement: Managing energy, not time, is the key to high performance and personal renewal* (New York: Free Press, 2005).

Index

Berk, Lee S., 175–76
Bethesda, Dean, 109
bile, 125, 131
binaural beats, 61–62, 208
biohackers, 38
Biohacker's Handbook, 37–38,
  61–62, 229–30
bisphenol-A (BPA), 95, 96, 97, 98, 102,
  117–18
bisphenol-F, 118
bisphenol-S, 118
bladder cancer, 116
bloating, 122, 123, 127, 255
blood-brain barrier, 228, 243
blood cells: red, 109, 218, 231;
  white, 109, 215, 218, 225, 228
blood pressure, 106, 199, 210, 214,
  220, 265
blueberries, 125
body: body language, 178; breakdowns,
  12, 13–19, 25–26, 45; core
  temperature, 206, 228; harmonious
  flow-state, 108, 251; life cycles
  within, 108–9; listening to, 32, 45,
  119, 135
bone broth, 125, 257
books, baby, 97
BPA (bisphenol-A), 95, 96, 97, 98,
  102, 117–18
brain: brain fog, 25, 49, 102, 104,
  237, 255; gut-brain axis, 126–27;
  hypothalamus, 202; intermittent
  fasting and, 237, 240; mindfulness
  and, 189; suprachiasmatic nucleus
  (SCN), 202, 208; zinc deficiency and,
  222. *See also* subconscious mind
Branson, Richard, 320
bravery (courage), 52–53, 132, 144
breakdowns, 12, 13–19, 25–26, 45.
  See also burnout
breakfast, 27, 32, 235
breast cancer, 117
breathing: deep (diaphragmatic), 62,
  190, 191–93, 264, 273; heart rate
  variability (HRV) and, 193–94
Bretherton, Beatrice, 186
Breus, Michael, 203–4
Bristol Stool Scale, 130, 131
Brothers, Joyce, 302
Brown, Brené, 17, 32, 271
Brown, Les, 87
brown adipose tissue, 228, 243
Buddha, 78, 84, 94

bug sprays, 97–98
burnout, 36–37, 50.
  See also breakdowns

Cabelly, Harriet, 143, 176–77
Cafasso, Jacquelyn, 109
caffeine, 2, 5, 123, 205, 206, 240, 260
cancer: bladder, 116; breast, 117;
  emotional strength and, 58–60;
  intermittent fasting and, 239–40;
  leukemia, 97; lung, 25, 98; skin, 98;
  testicular, 96, 117
candida albicans (yeast), 103–4, 107–8
capacity, building, 34–36, 45, 140–41
cardiovascular health, 5, 115, 176, 224,
  239, 242
career. *See* work
carpe diem, 160
Carrey, Jim, 165
celiac disease, 122, 131
cells and cellular health, 109, 189, 225,
  238, 251–52
chewing, 125, 257
children: emotions and, 172; energy and,
  3; gastrointestinal health and, 121;
  playing with, 287, 295; subconscious
  mind and, 71–72
chlorine, 98, 116
choices: happiness and, 171, 241;
  healthy behaviors and, 1, 22–23, 45
circadian rhythm (chronobiology), 200,
  202–4, 208, 215, 267
circulation, 62, 220, 234
cirrhosis of the liver, 25
cleansing. *See* detoxification
clocks, 210
Clond, Morgan, 188
clothing, 161–62, 222, 254
coffee, 5, 240. *See also* caffeine
cold-water therapy: acclimating to,
  229–30; in author's optimal day,
  266; benefits, 227–28, 242–43;
  chest freezer conversion for, 229;
  comfort zone expansion and, 232–33;
  emotions and, 273; energy generation
  and, 263; exercise and, 231–32;
  face-washing with cold water, 190;
  laughter and, 295; mammalian dive
  reflex and, 230–31; Nordic Cycle and,
  214, 233–34; waking up and, 263
Coleman, Mark, 196
collagen, 125
colon (large intestine), 106

IF YOU'VE READ the book, done the exercises, and still desire to learn and adopt more, don't worry, I'm here for you! Scan the QR code and head over to discoveringoptimal.com to access more insight and information that will help you on your journey. From detailed information on breathing methods to tips on how to set up your own cold-water plunge, I promise you'll find something that will help you discover your optimal.

ABOUT THE AUTHOR

JOSEPH GIBBONS IS a professor at Humber College in Ontario, Canada, where he holds exemplary faculty status. He has 20 years of experience as a professor, exercise physiologist, health and lifestyle coach, and mental health first aid instructor.

Joseph's mission is to help people overcome the life obstacles that impede their journey toward optimal physical, mental, and spiritual health. *Discovering Optimal* is the result of more than a decade of study on the optimization of health and wellness.

In addition to his professional endeavors, Joseph is a small-town-living, sports-loving father to miracle twin boys, Jakoby and Elijah. His days are spent helping people improve their health and wellness; his nights are spent chasing his kids and listening to his wonderful wife, Lauren, sing.

REVIVE REINVIGORATE REJUVENATE
RETHINK REBUILD REVAMP RECLAIM
RECHARGE RECONNECT REFORM R
REIGNITE REINVEST REPLENISH RE\
RENEW REVITALIZE RESTORE REDISC
REALIGN REASSESS RECREATE REAFFIF
REGAIN REGENERATE REINVENT REIG
REINVIGORATE REJUVENATE RENEW
REBUILD REVAMP RECLAIM REALIGN
RECONNECT REFORM REFRESH REGAIN
REPLENISH REVAMP REVIVE REINVIGOR/
REDISCOVER RETHINK REBUILD REVA
REAFFIRM RECHARGE RECONNECT REFC
REIGNITE REINVEST REPLENISH RE\
RENEW REVITALIZE RESTORE REDISC
REALIGN REASSESS RECREATE REAFFIF
REGAIN REGENERATE REINVENT REIG
REINVIGORATE REJUVENATE RENEW
REBUILD REVAMP RECLAIM REALIGN
RECONNECT REFORM REFRESH REGAIN
REPLENISH REVAMP REVIVE REINVIGOR/
REDISCOVER RETHINK REBUILD REVA
REAFFIRM RECHARGE RECONNECT REFC
REIGNITE REINVEST REPLENISH REVAMI
REVITALIZE RESTORE REDISCOVER RE
REASSESS RECREATE REAFFIRM RECH/